Couples on the Fault Line

Couples on the Fault Line

New Directions for Therapists

Edited by
Peggy Papp

THE GUILFORD PRESS
New York   London

© 2000 The Guilford Press
A Division of Guilford Publications, Inc.
72 Spring Street, New York, NY 10012
www.guilford.com

Printed in the United States of America

This book is printed on acid-free paper.

Last digit is print number: 9 8 7 6 5 4 3

Library of Congress Cataloging-in-Publication Data

Couples on the fault line : new directions for therapists /
    edited by Peggy Papp
    p. cm.
    Includes bibliographical references and index.
    ISBN 1-57230-536-3 (cloth) — ISBN 1-57230-705-6 (pbk.)
    1. Marital psychotherapy. I. Papp, Peggy.
RC488.5.C6435 2000
616.89 156—dc21   99-086313

*To my parents, Vera Weiler Bennion
and Heber Bennion, Jr., who were married
for 52 years; and to couples everywhere who are
struggling to meet the challenges of our new age.*

—P.P.

About the Editor

Peggy Papp, MSW, is a senior training supervisor and director of the Depression Project at the Ackerman Institute for the Family. She served on the board of *Family Process* and was a cofounder of the Women's Project in Family Therapy, which won the 1986 American Family Therapy Academy award for distinguished contribution to the field of family therapy.

She was an associate director of the Center for Family Learning and has served on the faculty of the Philadelphia Child Guidance Clinic and the Family Studies Center of the Albert Einstein College of Medicine.

In 1991 she received a lifetime achievement award from the American Family Therapy Academy and in the same year was cited for her distinguished contribution to marital and family therapy by the American Association for Marital and Family Therapy. She is the editor of *Family Therapy: Full Length Case Studies;* author of *The Process of Change,* considered a classic in the field; and coauthor of the landmark book *The Invisible Web: Gender Patterns in Family Relationships;* as well as a video program, *Gender Differences in Depression* (with the Ackerman Institute's Depression Project). She has written numerous articles and has lectured in many countries around the world. She maintains a private practice in New York City.

Contributors

Anne C. Bernstein, PhD, The Wright Institute, Berkeley, California; Department of Psychology, University of California at Berkeley, Berkeley, California

Lascelles W. Black, MSW, Private practice, Mt. Vernon, New York

Peter Fraenkel, PhD, Doctoral Program in Clinical Psychology, Department of Psychology, City University of New York; Ackerman Institute for the Family, New York, New York

Wendy Greenspun, PhD, Columbia University Counseling and Psychological Services, New York, New York

Evan Imber-Black, PhD, Director of the Center for Families and Health, Ackerman Institute for the Family, New York, New York

Lawrence Levner, MSW, Family Therapy Practice Center, Washington, DC

Caroline Marvin, PhD, Family Institute of Cambridge, Watertown, Massachusetts

Dusty Miller, EdD, Director of Consultation, HRA/The Consortium, Holyoke, Massachusetts

Ruth Mohr, MSW, Director, Aging Family Project, Ackerman Institute for the Family, New York, New York

Peggy Papp, MSW, Depression Project, Ackerman Institute for the Family, New York, New York

Esther Perel, MA, Interfaith Couples Program, 92nd St. Y, New York, New York; Family Studies Unit, Department of Psychiatry, New York University Medical Center, New York, New York

Gary L. Sanders, MD, FRCP(C), Human Sexuality and Family Therapy Programs, Department of Psychiatry, Faculty of Medicine, University of Calgary, Alberta, Canada

Constance N. Scharf, MSW, Infertility Project, Ackerman Institute for the Family, New York, New York

Margot Weinshel, MSW, Infertility Project, Ackerman Institute for the Family, New York, New York

Skye Wilson, MPhil, Doctoral Program in Clinical Psychology, Department of Psychology, City University of New York, New York, New York; Ackerman Institute for the Family, New York, New York

Acknowledgments

The contributors to this book were asked to write about what they considered to be the most important changes taking place in their particular areas of expertise, how these changes were affecting couples' relationships, and what therapists and couples needed to know in order to deal with these changes. I wish to express my appreciation to each and every one of the authors for the special insights, wisdom, and imagination they brought to bear in exploring these questions. Combining historical and current perspectives, they examined both the possibilities and the problems of our contemporary age and came up with a rich variety of approaches for dealing with them. This book would not have been possible without the spirit of collaboration and commitment that fueled their creative thinking.

The impetus for this book came from listening to the couples in weekend workshops that Peter Fraenkel and I conducted at the Ackerman Institute for the Family. As the couples described the many different ways in which the outside pressures of daily life had had impact on their relationships, we realized the importance of designing a program that dealt with the interface between their inner and outer worlds. Peter's original ideas on the structure and use of time contributed a valuable dimension to our program. His open-mindedness and spirit of adventure lent a special kind of verve to our endeavor.

My deepest appreciation goes to the Ackerman Institute for the Family for having provided me with a professional home in which to develop my work. I consider myself most fortunate to be part of an institution that encourages experimentation, tolerates differences of opinion, and promotes innovation and creativity. I especially appreciate the support of the Institute's director, Peter Steinglass, and Marcia Scheinberg, director of training, who have provided an atmosphere in which new work and ideas can flourish.

A very special thanks goes to the team of the Depression Project— Gloria Klein, Paul Feinberg, Jeffrey Seibel, and Sania Rolovic. Without their continued devotion, commitment, and creative energy the project would not have been possible. The ideas expressed in my chapter "Gender Differences in Depression: His or Her Depression" are based on our collaborative thinking.

My years as part of the Women's Project in Family Therapy, with Marianne Walters, Olga Silverstein, and Betty Carter, helped raise my awareness of the many ways in which gender beliefs and cultural mandates shape couples' relationships. The concepts that emerged from our animated discussions laid the foundation for many of the ideas expressed in this book.

Collaborating with Evan Imber-Black in exploring the effect of themes, beliefs, secrets, and outside systems on the lives of couples has further expanded and enriched my thinking. Evan continues to be a source of inspiration and support both personally and professionally.

My loving daughter, Miranda, is a constant reminder that the future belongs to her generation; they will be called upon to deal with the marvels and perplexities of the new century. I am grateful for her everlasting optimism and enthusiasm in facing this challenge.

A good relationship with one's editor is paramount in shaping a book. For me, Kitty Moore possesses all the qualities of an ideal editor. Her critiques, suggestions, and comments were always direct and probing but balanced with warmth and encouragement. The combination of her generous availability and involvement, strong beliefs, and underlying patience were invaluable to me.

I wish it were possible to personally thank all the couples from whom we therapists learned so many valuable lessons about endurance and hope. By sharing their lives with us, they informed us about those issues most meaningful to them and pointed a direction for addressing them.

Contents

Couples on the Fault Line

CHAPTER 1

New Directions for Therapists

Peggy Papp

"I used to know what it was to be a man, but I don't know any more. At work I'm expected to be aggressive, take charge, have all the answers, and always be in control of my feelings. At home, I'm supposed to be nurturing, loving, sensitive, express all my feelings, and cry a lot. I don't know who I'm supposed to be anymore."

"Love? I don't have time for love! Between being a mother at home, a supervisor at work, a nurse to my sick mother, managing our social life—holidays, vacations, wedding, funerals—I don't have time for myself, let alone my husband."

These words were spoken, respectively, by a confused husband and a harassed wife in answer to the question "What do you find most difficult about being a man or a woman in today's world?" The question was raised in a weekend couples group lead by Peter Fraenkel and myself at the Ackerman Family Institute. Over and over we heard the couples expressing feelings of being overwhelmed, exhausted, and confused by the onerous demands, changing roles, and unprecedented pressure of our times.

For many years therapists have been primarily concerned with the interpersonal world of couples and helping them "improve their relationship," "learn to communicate," or "change dysfunctional patterns" through the use of a particular set of techniques or models of therapy.

But today therapists are facing a whole new set of complex and disquieting issues that render many of our previous models and techniques obsolete. Couples are having to hew their way through an uncharted landscape in which all the old roles, traditions, values, and practices no longer apply, and they are having to invent new ones as they go along. Developments such as commuter marriages, "Internet affairs," computer addictions, gay couples adopting children, gay spouses in heterosexual marriages "coming out," and genetically designed children are challenging us to reevaluate some of our most cherished concepts. Even such old and familiar situations as the challenges of dual careers, divorce, remarriage, stepparenting, infidelity, and retirement are taking place in a rapidly changing social context that requires a whole new set of assumptions regarding coupling, reproducing, love, marriage, commitment, and intimacy. We are having to reconsider what is normal or abnormal, natural or unnatural, healthy or unhealthy. The cutting edge of couple therapy is no longer methodological but ideological.

Currently popular books are conveying the message that couples have problems because they come from different planets, are aliens to one another, and speak a different language. By ignoring the cultural explosion that is taking place on Planet Earth, which is their natural habitat, these books make the differences between the genders seem innate and immutable. The only form of therapy that can follow from these assumptions is one of adaptation to each other's genetic predispositions. If therapists are to remain relevant to the experience of contemporary couples, they must help them look beyond their private worlds to the outside social forces that are currently shaping those worlds.

The revolutions taking place today in biology, technology, and genetics are changing the premises of therapists and the nature of therapy. Therapy is no longer a matter of helping couples adjust to the different stages of the life cycle because the life cycle itself has changed. Reproductive technology, life-extension regimes, mood-altering drugs, and electronic communication are changing the meaning of birth, marriage, parenting, aging, and death. They are raising questions of a third kind:

"How much is a baby worth?"
"Can a pill replace human will?"
"What is the optimum love–work ratio?"
"Are the boundaries between genders fluid?"
"Does commitment have a time limit?"

The answers to these questions require value judgments and a reordering and reconsideration of life priorities.

On the one hand, these changes give couples more freedom, options, and possibilities for developing better ways of being together. On the other hand, they can easily disorient individuals, exhaust them, and promote a new kind of alienation.

It is the goal of this book to present work that demonstrates the many different ways in which the ideology of social awareness can be translated into clinical practice to meet the new challenges of our times. In the following chapters the contributors, although coming from different theoretical orientations, demonstrate therapeutic perspectives that connect couples' lives to the world and times in which they live.

WHO WILL RAISE THE CHILDREN, THEN?

The inherent problems for two-career couples have grown rather than diminished over the past decade. Now that it is accepted that in most households both spouses have full- or part-time jobs, juggling work with domestic responsibilities and parenting has become more complicated. The myth that men and women have achieved equality in the domestic arena has been debunked by studies that find that women still come home from stressful jobs and do the larger percentage of child care and housework. The inequities and contradictory expectations of our society do not support equality in marriage. Arlie Hochschild recently shattered the myth that women want more time with their families in her book *The Time Bind: When Work Becomes Home and Home Becomes Work* (1997). Her study showed that many mothers would rather be at work than at home; indeed, some leave for work early just to get away from the house. They describe work as a place where they feel welcomed, appreciated, liked, and supported, as a place where they and have a rapport with peers. We have known for many years that fathers have been using work to get away from the home, but *mothers?* Who will raise the children then? This is one of the central issues of our time.

The greatest number of marriages break up after the first child is born. Clearly, coparenting and the division of domestic labor is a pivotal issue for couples today. Yet therapists continue to think in terms of "closeness," "intimacy," "trust," and "commitment" without taking into account the social conditions that interfere with their attainment. How can a wife feel close to her husband when she comes home every night from a stressful job and does most of the housework and child care? What happens to intimacy when she is too tired and resentful to have sex? How can a husband climb the fiercely competitive ladder of success and still find time to be a loving husband and father?

Books on how to keep passion alive in a relationship are flooding the market with techniques and advice of every kind. In the meantime, noted researcher John Gottman offers us statistics that link sexual satisfaction with equitably shared housework. In his book *The Seven Principles for Making Marriage Work* (Gittman & Silver, 1999) he discusses the connection between marital happiness and a husband's willingness to participate in the domestic chores: *"Women find a man's willingness to do housework extremely erotic.* When the husband does his share to maintain the home, both he and his wife report a more satisfying sex life than in marriages where the wife believes her husband is not doing his share" (pp. 205–206; italics in original).

This brings to mind a couple I saw in which the presenting problem was the wife's lack of sexual desire. Years of individual therapy had failed to arouse her sleeping libido. The husband, a writer, wrote at home while the wife went to work and supported the two of them. She was happy to do this, as she saw her husband as a talented man who was in the process of writing a Pulitzer Prize-winning novel. Her only complaint was that she hated to come home every night to dirty dishes in the sink, an unswept floor, and clothes scattered all over. The husband dismissed his wife's complaints as trivial and irrelevant to the real issue of her "sexual dysfunction."

Then one day, after a session in which the wife had vociferously expressed her anger, the couple came to a session surrounded by a radiant glow, blushing and holding hands. I asked them what had happened and the wife said shyly, "Well, this may sound ridiculous to you and I'm embarrassed to talk about it, but last night I came home and found Jim down on his hands and knees scrubbing the kitchen floor and I really got turned on! Just knowing that he cared enough to do that made me feel passionate toward him." So much for Viagra! What many husbands fail to realize is that for women whose sexual desire is dependent on emotional connection, the husband's willingness to share domestic burdens can act as a powerful aphrodisiac. It is not inconceivable that in the not-too-distant future someone may develop a kitchen floor sex therapy!

In Chapter 2, Lawrence Levner renames the "two-career couple" the "three-career couple," arguing that domestic responsibility be given the same priority as the couples' professional careers. This requires confronting each partner's hidden assumptions and beliefs regarding child rearing, the division of labor, nurturing, and responsibility. Therapists are prone to skip over conflicts regarding domestic issues as being "boring" and "superficial" and would prefer to get to the "deeper," more "meaningful" issues. They fail to see the sharing of domestic responsibility as a microcosm of the couples' deeply ingrained gender beliefs that touches on responsibility, freedom, entitlement, power, control, and independence. Women need the support of therapists in validating the importance of this issue and men need to become aware of the disparity between the lip service they pay to equality and what they actually do.

Many husbands today see themselves as modern liberated men who believe in equal rights for women, support their wives' career ambitions, and extol their wives' virtues in public. They also have the illusion that they have worked out an equal relationship at home. It is this illusion that confuses both men and women. On the one hand, men are doing more, for example, by changing diapers, taking the children to school, and doing the laundry. And women are feeling more entitled to ask for parity, not as afraid to speak out as in the past. On the other hand, the gendered role divisions still exist and are a common source of problems.

The techniques by which stereotypical gender assumptions are challenged are secondary to the therapist's conviction that they need to be challenged in order for an egalitarian relationship to become a reality instead of a myth. When Levner asks a husband who refers to his wife as the "primary parent," "Do you believe a child can have two primary parents?" he is challenging the husband's underlying assumption that his job is to "assist" his wife.

Levner examines the gendered construction of heterosexual relationships, particularly in relationship to work, and its impact on the couple, in terms of power, self-esteem, role definition, intimacy, and the experience of competency and capacity. He demonstrates the way in which therapy can move beyond merely helping couples to understand differences, communicate effectively, and make compromises to examining the way in which men and women internalize and play out socially defined roles.

He then both challenges traditional power arrangements and works toward fostering a relationship in which power and responsibility are shared.

THE TIME WARP

The management of time is often overlooked as an important issue in couples therapy. And yet how couples spend their time is indicative of their most basic values and priorities. Our information age has placed couples on "the fast track." They are pressured to do more, be more, have more, know more, think more, talk more, relate more—and do it all this as quickly as possible. The complaint, "There's never enough time to ____" (fill in the blank: have sex, talk to each other, go on vacations, take a walk, workout in the gym, see a movie, visit relatives or friends) is heard so often in therapists' offices it might well be the theme song of the 21st century. Our "time famine" is depriving couples of the leisure to love one another. How can they find time to sustain an intimate relationship when they are caught between frenetic work schedules, commuting time, business travel, raising families, solving problems, job burnout, and taking care of aging parents? Intimacy cannot be forced or manufactured on demand. It requires the nurturance of time, the space for unpredictable experiences, and quiet unscheduled moments that define the uniqueness of a relationship.

If one were to choose a quintessential cartoon for our time it might well be the one of the middle-aged woman sitting at her desk who suddenly looks up from her work and exclaims, "Oh, my God! I forgot to have children!" Another sign of our times is the increasing scenario of a couple sitting together in a fashionable restaurant, but turned away from each other and talking to someone else on separate cell phones. Dining out in a fancy restaurant, once the symbol of intimacy, is now just another occasion to conduct business.

In our weekend workshops, Peter Fraenkel and I ask the couples to draw a time pie and divide it into sections representing the time spent on various daily activities. The couples are often shocked to see in black and white how they spend their time. The diagram serves as a motivation for rearranging the temporal aspect of their lives to allow time for connecting to one another.

Besides daily routines and schedules, certain life events require adjustments in time. These life transitions include parenthood and adjusting to the routines of a new baby, the death of a parent, changing jobs, children getting married or leaving home, one partner going back to school or retiring, or the couple relocating. All of these life-cycle events require time to adjust to them emotionally, physically, and psychologically. If a couple tries to rush this process they may pay a heavy price later on.

I recall a couple who came in with the presenting problem of the wife's depression. The depression had come on gradually for no apparent reason. Both she and her husband were perplexed because up until then the wife had always seemed happy and energetic. Each considered their marriage to be a happy one. They enjoyed a full active life together, working, raising children, participating in community activities. In tracing back to find the beginning of the change in her mood, the wife remembered feeling somewhat disoriented a year earlier after she returned from her mother's funeral in a different part of the country. She had cut short her stay because she felt she could not allow herself to be away from home for more than 2 days. She had deadlines at work and her daughter's high school graduation was approaching. When I asked her how she had handled her grief, she burst into tears and admitted that there really hadn't been enough time for that. She then spoke of the deep longing she felt to stay on after the funeral, to comfort her father, to share her grief with her brothers and sisters, to look at family pictures, visit old friends, recall memories. She was quite embarrassed by her tears, confessing that she knew she shouldn't be crying after all this time because she had read somewhere that the grieving process should not last more than a year. I told her I was surprised to hear someone had established a time limit on grieving.

Clearly her depression was linked to her having suppressed all her natural feelings of sorrow. After this session, she agreed to go back to her hometown to see her father and her extended family, with no time limits on her stay. Her husband reassured her he would hold down the fort in her absence. When she returned from this trip her depression had disappeared.

The key premise of Peter Fraenkel and Skye Wilson's chapter, "Clocks, Calendars, and Couples" (Chapter 4), is that the manner in which couples experience and organize the temporal dimensions of their lives has a profound effect on their relationship. They refer to underlying conflicts around time as "couple arrhythmias," disjunctions in their daily rhythms that throw their time patterns out of joint. These arrhythmias often go unattended by therapists who focus on other issues such as "communication problems," "fear of intimacy," or "personality defects" rather than the conflicting time constraints that bind the couples' lives.

One of the most difficult arrythmias to resolve are those that arise from differences in personal life chronologies. Fraenkel and Wilson use the terms "projected timelines" and "personal life chronology" to describe life-cycle plans such as when to have children, reach a certain level of financial security, change jobs, move, or retire. Certain social changes have accentuated the differences in these projected timelines. Now that women have become more financially independent they no longer need to conform to their partner's time line as they once did. The increased trend toward multicultural marriages has also increased these differences as different cultures may hold different norms regarding the passage of life and the milestones along the way.

Fraenkel and Wilson offer a theoretical framework to assist couples to resolve these difficulties around time and rhythm so that they can have "time for love." They view time as a resource for healing and offer many clinical vignettes illustrating therapeutic interventions so couples can "take back time" from insidious work schedules.

CYBERSPACE ROMANCES

The awesome possibilities of the Internet have brought with them new symptoms and new problems into therapists' offices, ranging from "computer addictions" to "Internet affairs." Now that computers are in so many homes, a variety of electronic escapes are readily available to many people. You can conjure up a vicarious world at any hour of the day or night where you can meet new people, play games, express your opinions without censure, and be whomever you want to be. Safe behind the screen of anonymity, you are free to terminate the contact at your own discretion. How can a real home with real people compete with these virtual possibilities?

The human propensity for taking flights of fancy in order to periodically escape reality has, until the advent of the Internet, been fueled by movies, television, theater, and literature. A vital difference between these forms of escape and the Internet is that you can become an actual player in the drama of cyberspace rather than just a member of the audience. In fact, you can write your own drama, cast yourself in the leading role, and choose your own costar for an idealized electronic romance. In many cases, the computer becomes more than a communication device and technological marvel, it becomes a substitute for real life and plays havoc with relationships. Therapists are used to dealing with reality—but what about *virtual reality?* What are we to make of the seductive powers of this new technological siren? Do we have something to learn about the power of fantasy in intimate relationships, the meaning and nature of communication, the need for anonymity, the fear of vulnerability, and the conditions for closeness? Is it possible or even desirable to attempt to bring into on ongoing relationship the sense of adventure, discovery, excitement, and intoxication that some find on the computer?

On-line trysts, although generally described as "meaningless" by the person indulging in them, can disrupt a couple's relationship in strange and elusive ways. How do you compete with a fantasy? Unlike in a conventional affair, in which the two lovers meet in secret outside the home, in a computer affair the lover is always available in the next room, where the computer sits. Recently a "computer-cuckolded" husband moaned, "Every time I look at that damned computer it reminds me of him, whoever he is. I'd like to smash it to bits!"

These liaisons are often an indication of one partner's ongoing dissatisfactions in a relationship and can serve as a wake-up call for the other partner. One of the most seductive aspects of the Internet is the freedom to express oneself without critical feedback. In describing her fixation with a computer companion, a wife said, "I can share my secret fantasies with him—tell him anything—be myself with him. My husband would criticize me." This admission raised cogent questions relevant to the couple's relationship that were then open for exploration, such as What does it mean to be oneself in a relationship? When does being oneself infringe on the self of the other person? How can two people be themselves at the same time?

In discussing these questions, the wife was surprised to learn that her husband also found their relationship dreary and boring and was thinking of looking elsewhere for excitement and adventure. Until now she was unaware of his rakish side, which he had hidden under a serious and conservative demeanor. The husband had been afraid to reveal his more passionate self because he feared his wife's censure. As they shared more and more of their secret selves, they began to discover different aspects of each other for the first time. They ended up concluding that perhaps it was a good idea to get better acquainted with each other before leaving the relationship for someone else. The interactive processes that take place in the theater of real life are usually more difficult and prosaic than those that take place on-line, but hopefully they can lead to some new adventures in the real world that are more enduring.

Since cyberspace attachments are a recent development, little of value to therapists has been written on the subject. Unfortunately, too much of what has been written simplistically labels such attachments as a form of "addiction" comparable to "alcoholism," "drug addiction" and "compulsive gambling." Words such as "netaholics," "codependent," and "enabler" have appeared with prescribed individual treatment strategies for "recovery" and "cure." Clinical guides are offered in recognizing and treating computer dependency. On-line addiction support groups are being formed, hospitals and clinics are setting up counseling centers, and universities are holding seminars. On the Web we find the Center for On-Line Addiction designed to alert Internet users to the problems. Can a medication for computer addiction be far behind? Fortunately, computer addiction has not been slotted into a diagnostic category on the next revision of the *Diagnostic and Statistical Manual of Mental Disorders*. We can only hope that this complex phenomenon, with all its wide variety of meanings and rich relational and social implications, will never be reduced to a genetic defect or a single pathology category.

As with every technological advance, dazzling possibilities are accompanied by worrisome consequences and unfamiliar problems. Just as our interstate highway system brought new problems and casualties that called for new solutions, so the information highway has brought unprecedented problems that call for unprecedented solutions. Let us hope that the field of family therapy will bring to this new problem that which it has brought to so many other new problems, a unique systemic approach based on viewing and treating the situation within the interpersonal and social context in which it is developed and is maintained.

Evan Imber-Black takes a first step in this direction in Chapter 3, "The New Triangle: Couples and Technology." She sees technology in terms of the new family triangle and offers cogent and useful ways of dealing with it. Instead of offering a list of "warning signs," she looks at the meaning it holds in terms of peoples' lives and relationships, and she gives others many helpful suggestions about how a therapist might use technology to help couples communicate better, schedule their lives, improve communication and enhance relationships. She explores the hazards as well as the potential of the new technology so that couples may incorporate it into their interactions as a useful device rather then allowing it to dominate their lives.

TAILOR-MADE BABIES

Infertility is one of the most neglected areas in our field. Most therapists are lacking in the expert knowledge needed to guide couples through the complex and confusing labyrinth of infertility issues. The age-old miracle of giving birth has been transformed by advances in technology that have drastically altered the options for those who wish to have a baby. Infertility clinics are now advertising their products in newspapers and magazines. You can choose an egg donor from a catalog that includes photographs and vital statistics on the donors. Doctors can now mix human eggs and sperm in the lab to make a variety of embryos with different pedigrees. Do you want your baby to be short, tall, blue-eyed, brown-eyed, a lawyer, an artist, or a scientist? This is all part of the fast-emerging new world of assisted reproduction. Women can freeze their eggs and have babies at 63. Dead men can father children through postmortem sperm extraction. And it is possible to become your own grandmother through the use of a surrogate parent.

These and many other possibilities bring with them complex moral, ethical, and psychological decisions. And yet many childless couples are seeking aggressive fertility therapies with very little understanding of the complicated risks involved. The reckless use of infertility drugs has resulted in an alarming increase in the incidence of multiple births. The world was recently stunned by the birth of *eight* siblings who were born as a result of the use of these drugs. This was a wakeup call for the medical profession, which had largely ignored this issue until then. It prompted Dr. Alan Copperman, director of reproductive endocrinology at Mt. Sinai–New York University. Medical Center and Health System in New York to state, "the fact is that the vast majority of these cases end in disaster, sometimes for the mom, most often for the babies" (*New York Times,* December 22, 1998). We hope that it will also result in a wakeup call for our profession to acquire the knowledge necessary to counsel couples on the risks and dangers involved in the various infertility procedures and to become more sensitive to the multitude of meanings that surround this traumatic experience.

One wife, who had suffered through the ordeal and disappointment of eight failed *in vitro* fertilizations said emphatically this would be the last one because she could not tolerate another disappointment. Her husband wanted her to keep trying. Since the wife was 40 years old, both realized that this was her last chance to have a child, but not his. The issue that hung heavy in the air was whether he would leave her for a younger, more fertile woman. He assured her that he had no such thoughts and the ninth *in vitro* fertilization produced healthy twin boys. Unfortunately, such a happy ending is an exception. The inability to produce one's own progeny suddenly brings to the surface a multitude of questions and doubts—about one's sexual potency, what it means to be a man or a woman, failing to fulfill a natural life function, failing to carry on a family name and legacy, inability to pass on one's genes to future generations—that otherwise might lie dormant in a couple's relationship. Couples and therapists are suddenly confronted with meaning-of-life questions such as: How much is a baby worth? Do you set a limit on the price you are willing to pay in terms of finances, time, physical pain, humiliation, guilt, pride, disappointment?

In my work with couples I have been amazed at how often I have discovered the presenting problem to be connected with the aftermath of an infertility problem thought to have been buried and forgotten. The whole complex of feelings around this nightmarish experience had gone unacknowledged and unexpressed but remained festering underneath the couple's relationship and manifested itself in disguised forms in everyday conflicts.

Recently I treated a couple in their mid-40s who presented their problem as "constant tension and fighting—over everything, you name it. Half the time we can't even remember what we're fighting about." In an attempt to trace the triggers that set off the fighting, we went down many different paths that always seemed to end in more confusion and frustration. It wasn't until we were discussing a fight that took place at a family gathering that included many young children that the wife revealed her anger and bitterness over not being able to have children. The couple had been through 4 years of what she referred to as "the infertility nightmare." They had made the rounds of all the infertility clinics, had received conflicting opinions from doctors, and still didn't know if the problem was her eggs or his sperm. They both had endured invasive treatment procedures and had tried the most advanced approaches and the latest techniques only to have all of them fail. The wife ended this account by stating that she guessed she had never forgiven her husband for not pursuing a cure longer and more aggressively. She claimed to have sensed his reluctance to continue their search, and since she herself was ambivalent and felt guilty about exhausting their finances, she had agreed to stop. They had never discussed the termination as it was too painful a subject to broach.

The husband was astounded to learn of the feelings his wife had been harboring. He claimed he would have continued regardless of the expense if he had known how strongly she felt. In the course of their discussion his own disappointment over his wife's failure to recognize his feelings of loss emerged. He had refrained from expressing them at the time for fear of making her feel worse. Although it was too late to retrace their steps, this sharing of their joint disappointment and grief was important for the continuation of their relationship.

In Chapter 5, "Infertility and Late-Life Pregnancies," Constance Scharf and Margot Weinshel describe all the ramifications of the new reproductive technologies and the specific issues of infertility that need to be explored. Without specific knowledge of infertility, many therapists are unable to separate infertility issues from the couple's own unique problems and consequently tend to view the couples' functioning as pathological. Scharf and Weinshel describe what therapists need to know about sperm banks, *in vitro* fertilization, donor eggs, surrogate mothers, frozen eggs, and custom-designed embryos. They elaborate on the role that society, family, and friends play in the drama of trying to become a parent. They discuss the couple's feelings of being marginalized and out of step with other couples who are starting their families. Couples are better prepared to handle their difficulties and build on their strengths when their experiences are put in the context of the total impact of infertility.

BRIDGING TWO WORLDS

As our world shrinks and emigration from country to country increases, cultural taboos are falling away and more and more people are daring to cross the boundaries of race, religion, ethnicity, and class to enter into mixed marriages. These marriages are a microcosm of our postmodern world, which dissolves national boundaries and expands global connections.

This has resulted in a sharp upswing of couples whose daily interactional patterns are governed by clashing cultural beliefs. It is not uncommon for therapists to get stuck trying to resolve the couple's interactional patterns while ignoring the cultural differences in which the patterns are embedded. It is essential for therapists to distinguish between the content of the cultural material that is presented and the emotional dynamics surrounding it. Often, the process of therapy necessitates dealing with the latter before addressing the content itself.

Dealing with differences is central to all couple therapy, but with the mixed couple the differences in gender beliefs, commitment, intimacy, child rearing, family values, and family loyalties are rooted in different tribal affinities. Each partner has different interpretations, symbols, and rituals for managing shared life events. Since the core of one's identity originates in one's culture, underlying the manifest differences is an intense web of emotions and invisible loyalties. Esther Perel, in Chapter 8,

"A Tourist's View of Marriage: Cross-Cultural Couples—Challenges, Choices, and Implications for Therapy," describes how she helps couples to think of themselves as "tourists" exploring each other's traditional territory. This metaphor endows the process of acculturation with a sense of mutual adventure and discovery: "In the other, we discover ourselves." She also suggests that therapists develop a "tourist's sense" of learning the landmarks in an unfamiliar territory.

I remember feeling like a tourist driving on the wrong side of the road while working with a couple who were referred to the Depression Project at the Ackerman Institute. The English wife, married to a Middle-Eastern husband, was pregnant with their first child and was worried that she might experience postpartum depression. She had been susceptible to bouts of depression all her life and feared the recurrence of one that would interfere with her caring for the baby. The couple described many sources of tension between them, including the husband's language difficulty that limited his job possibilities, concerns about money, and quarrels over household responsibilities. But the most explosive issue arose when the husband's mother wanted to come and stay with them during the birth of the baby. The wife objected because she wanted the initial experience of the infant to be between the two of them. We helped them to compromise on an agreement by which the mother would come to this country but live separately until they had had time to adjust to the baby. Shortly after this session, the husband dropped out of therapy, saying it wasn't helping. The staff of the Depression Project spent a great deal of time reviewing the sessions and pondering why all our concerted efforts had not been helpful.

Several months later, the couple sent us an announcement of the birth of their baby girl. We responded with a congratulatory card saying how much we would enjoy seeing their baby. When they came as proud parents to show us their beautiful child, the husband reported that he had been to see an individual therapist who was helpful because she "understood him" and his feelings about his mother. We then realized we had been so focused on preventing the wife from falling into a postpartum depression that we had failed to fully understand the husband's deep commitment to his mother or to pay proper attention to his family traditions and beliefs about birth.

In their work with families of diverse cultures at the Family Center in New Zealand, Charles Waldegrave and Kiwi Tamasese make it a practice when treating families from a different culture to have a person from a similar cultural background present in the sessions. This person serves as a cultural interpreter of the family's beliefs, values, and traditions. Since this is not feasible for most practitioners, they themselves must serve as the interpreters.

One of the most common but unacknowledged experiences of displaced persons is that of homesickness. It is rarely expressed openly and often manifests itself in a low-grade depression. This leaves the partner mystified and gives rise to secret fantasies and conjectures.

(In *The Process of Change* (Papp, 1983) I describe a case in which a Norwegian wife's homesickness for her native land resulted in her husband harboring a secret fear she would one day return there to live with their children. Although they had never discussed this openly, it was an ever-present fear.)When it was brought out into the open, the wife was able to reassure her husband that she had no intentions of returning, but she did admit that she had been homesick ever since coming to this country. She missed her family, the music, food, landscape, and customs of her birthplace. Over the years she had continually compared them unfavorably with those of this country. Her husband was threatened by her attachment to her homeland and had tried to keep her from talking about it. He attempted to counteract her pessimistic attitude by extolling the virtues of everything American and all the advantages of living here. This only made her feel even more isolated and cut off from her roots, which she deeply resented.

I suggested to the husband that the cure for homesickness was not less connection with the missed home but more. If his wife were able to bring more of Norway into her life, she would probably be less homesick, Since her birthday was just 3 weeks away, I suggested it be declared "Norway Day" and that he and the children collaborate in planning a celebration of everything Norwegian. They followed through on the suggestion: they decorated the house with Norwegian flags, prepared Norwegian food, played Norwegian music, brought out old records and photo albums, invited friends from "the old country," and arranged a long-distance telephone call to her family. Feeling her heritage was honored rather than belittled and dismissed helped to banish the ghost of her homesickness.

Perel sees therapists as ambassadors who can resolve global conflicts by acquiring the cultural knowledge necessary to understand the deeply held passions of their clients. In order to do this, therapists need to be able to distill specific interpersonal dynamics from the broader sociocultural context; to understand each partner's basic assumptions regarding marriage, gender roles, intimacy, power, sex, and money management; and to anticipate the conflicts that may arise at key junctures in the life cycle such as weddings, birth, deaths, the observance of religious traditions, and the celebration of specific holidays.

Perel categorizes global cultural differences into "high context" and "low context" societies and lists the prominent characteristics of each. It is impossible to read the different descriptions without instantly recognize one's own values, traits, and tendencies. And if therapists' want a quick litmus test of where they themselves stand on issues of money, religion, sex, food, communication, achievement, responsibility, suffering, entitlement, and parenting, they should answer the questions on the "Exercise to Identify and Clarify Family Values." While they may not fall consistently into one category or another, they are sure to recognize many of their own traits that they take for granted. The therapist's recognition and acknowledgment his or her own attitudes toward these fundamental issues is crucial in helping couples understand their own.

DOMESTIC VIOLENCE: THE ABUSE OF POWER

Violence no longer lies in the hidden underbelly of society. Its prevalence is recognized and acknowledged by the mass media, the public, the police force, the mental health profession, and our legal system. In our profession, the idea that violence was the result of a reciprocal interaction in which the woman was equally to blame was abolished years ago, thanks to the feminist critique of the power differential existing between men and women.

I recall with a combination of shame and disbelief my first violence case 20 years ago when I turned to the wife and asked, "What do you do to provoke your husband's violence?" This was not a shocking question at that time; the common theoretical stance of the field was based on the systems concept of reciprocity, which held that everyone involved in an interaction plays an equal part in the maintenance of that interaction by reinforcing the behavior of the other. We have since come to recognize that this concept ignored the inequities of power and authority. Obviously a rape victim, abused wife, or abused child does not play an equal part in rape or abuse. The distinction between a person being *involved* in an interaction and being *responsible* for that interaction represents a seismic shift in our field. This led to the challenging of another cherished system's concept: neutrality. Physical abuse of any kind, whether it be spouse abuse, child abuse, rape, or incest, calls for moral and ethical positions. This gave rise to a new dilemma: How does a therapist take a strong ethical, moral, and legal position while still respecting the couple's strong bonds of caring and attachment? When does therapy cross the line into social control, which historically has been considered antithetical to therapy? If we relinquish our neutrality toward violence, how, then, do we establish a therapeutic relationship with an abusive man while still protecting the safety of the abused woman? Do we terminate the therapy if the violence continues? If so, are we not leaving the woman in a dangerous situation? At what point is it our obligation to persuade an abused woman to leave the relationship? And how does the therapist cope with his or her own feelings of anxiety and abhorrence that physical abuse is likely to evoke?

These are but a few of the perplexing issues facing therapists when entering this high-risk situation. The consequences of therapeutic failure are awesome. The stakes involved are not just the emotional well-being of our clients (as in most cases), but physical safety and possibly even life-and-death issues—as evidenced by weekly headlines. Therapists are bound to feel anxious. In this area, perhaps more than any other, they need concrete guidelines, ground rules, and a clear ethical stance. These are provided by Wendy Greenspun who describes the step-by-step process she follows in her "metasystemic approach" in Chapter 7, "Embracing the Controversy." She also addresses the current controversy in our field as to the best way to intervene. On the one hand, there are those who believe it is unethical to do couple therapy in cases of domestic violence since by definition domestic violence includes the battered woman in the problem definition. On the other hand, there are those who believe that such a refusal ignores the intense bond between the partners and fails to address some of the underlying dynamics that keep them locked in a dangerous relationship. Greenspun offers a comprehensive approach that takes both sides of this controversy into account, emphasizing the batterer's responsibility for violence, the woman's need for safety, and ways to address the complex web of underlying relational factors. She takes the basic ethical stance that a psychological and relational understanding can be used to deter violence, but it can never be used as the excuse for it. She weaves together a feminist, systemic, narrative, and neurobiological approach that addresses the variety of forces that lead to violence.

HIS OR HER DEPRESSION

During the past decade both the mental health field and the media have shined a spotlight on depression. Once stigmatized and hidden under the cloak of other problems such as alcoholism, domestic violence, gambling, and child abuse, where it went unacknowledged and untreated, depression is now being recognized in all its disguised forms. Therapists are being called upon more frequently to deal with depression as a distinct condition requiring a distinct approach, but are understandably confused by the conflicting viewpoints in our field regarding its cause and appropriate treatment.

Most of the popular and professional literature on depression published over the last decade has been biologically oriented. Vast amounts of money have been spent on researching medical solutions. The public has been inundated with information on the biochemistry of depression, with the latest data on genes and serotonin levels. Prozac has become a household word synonymous with achieving nirvana. Our age may well be remembered as the "Age of Prozac."

What is missing in this lopsided biochemical view of depression is the undiagnosable, unpredictable dimensions of personality and character that make up the human profile. Depression is more often than not an idiosyncratic response to the disappointments, failures, frustrations, and losses of life. More than brain chemistry is involved in this response. Individual beliefs, expectations, habitual behavior patterns, interpersonal relationships, and interpretations of life events are also involved. We know that the mind–body connection is circular and that we can change our brain chemistry by changing our thoughts and behavior. But this very circularity is often neglected in biological research.

A depressed wife who had managed to pull herself out of her depression by changing a debilitating interaction with her husband asked, "If I have a diseased brain, how come I, of my own free will, could overcome my depression?" This question goes to the heart of the controversy between the biological and the psychological camps. It is not an easy question to answer. We still know very little about the complex interaction between the mind and body that results in depression.

When confronted with a mysterious and devastating condition such as depression, it is easier to think in terms of a single cause and a single solution. There is a current trend in our society to describe every unwanted behavior in clinical terms and then to prescribe a pill. This trend has recently been extended to characters in literature. In a *New York Times* article, Peter Kramer (1997) reviewed Chekhov's play *Ivanov* and diagnosed Ivanov as suffering from depression and in need of an antidepressant. Thus, all the richness, complexities, and contradictions of Ivanov's character and his idiosyncratic response to the claustrophobic conditions in Russia were reduced to a psychiatric diagnosis. One shudders to think what will happen to great literature if all human behavior is categorized and labeled in clinical terms. Will someone suggest that Hamlet could have been cured with Zoloft or Romeo with Ritalin?

Most human problems are complex and mulitdetermined, and therefore require a multidimensional perspective. This is especially true of depression, which most clinicians and researchers now agree is a complex combination of biological, psychological, social, and cultural factors.

I became interested in depression because of a number of research studies that linked depression with gender and marriage. Ever since Jessie Bernard published her research in *The Future of Marriage: The His and Her Marriage* (1972) we have known that married women suffer more emotional, physical, and psychological disabilities than married men. These same results have since been replicated in many other research studies. Although some researchers acknowledge gender as a risk factor in depression, little work has been done to determine how this occurs and the implications for treatment.

In 1990 the American Psychological Association published a comprehensive report on women in depression sponsored by the National Institute of Mental Health with the following recommendation: "Understanding how to ameliorate the negative effects of gender roles and stereotypes is essential if optimal treatment outcomes are to be attained" (p. 71). I believe these statistics have profound implications for the diagnosis and treatment of depression, but they have been largely ignored by the mental health field.

In order to address this serious omission, I organized the Depression Project at the Ackerman Institute with the goal of developing a multidimensional treatment approach to depression highlighting gender differences as well as biological and interpersonal factors. My chapter, "Gender Differences in Depression: His or Her Depression" (Chapter 6), describes the results of this work. We are still in our infancy in understanding all the individual, familial, social, and cultural factors that contribute to this mysterious condition, but we believe it is important to address these complex issues as best we can right now.

REMARRIAGE: "THE TRIUMPH OF HOPE OVER EXPERIENCE"

The increasing prevalence of remarriage reflects our postmodern attitudes toward love and commitment: marriage is not forever or even until "death do us part," personal fulfillment takes precedence over duty, emotional fulfillment overrules obligation, happiness is a divine right, boundaries are fluid, roles and rules are negotiable, arrangements transitional, commitment circumstantial, accountability contextual, purpose and meaning improvisational. But despite these dramatic changes in the meaning, structure, and form of marriage, remarriage testifies to the human desire for intimate connection, which seems to remain constant throughout history.

And so couples come to this land of renewed hope seeking solace from all the heartache, disappointment, anger, guilt, and rejection they may have experienced in past unions, hopeful of finding that vital connection that eluded them previously. Having been tempered in the crucible of experience, they are determined not to make the same mistakes, to do it differently this time around. They soon discover that many surprises await them, some wondrous and others disappointing. It is difficult to think of a journey more fraught with unpredictable pitfalls. Despite the knowledge, understanding, and experience they may have gained from previous unions, they are bound to have their ingenuity and resources taxed to the limit as they suddenly have thrust upon them a whole new set of kinships, with many not necessarily of their own liking or choosing, that they must incorporate into their lives: stepchildren, in-laws, ex-spouses, stepgrandparents, and all of their extended families and friends. While attempting to form the appropriate connections with this complex new network, they must find the time and energy to nurture their relationship with their new partner, and at the same time deal with all the emotional hobgoblins from the past that may arise at the most unexpected and inconvenient moments: uninvited memories, past comparisons, echoes of unfulfilled dreams.

Since 40% of all marriages are remarriages, a high percentage of clinical practice now consists of helping couples deal with this new mixture of dreams and nightmares. Which relationship comes first? Who should one be accountable to, responsible for, protective of, loyal to? Where do one's personal as opposed to the couples collective rights begin and end? Which issues are worth fighting over? Which are best ignored? Where should the lines be drawn?

Each couple must find their own answers to these questions and fashion their own custom-made arrangements. Finding the answers to such questions requires the therapist and the couple to be flexible and resilient. As Anne Bernstein points out in Chapter 12, "Remarriage:

Redesigning Couplehood," successful remarriage is not so much a matter of developing new techniques as it is a matter of gaining new knowledge and transforming basic assumptions based on that knowledge. This means the therapist must also reevaluate some of his or her assumptions concerning family loyalties, priorities, boundaries, and responsibilities.

In working with remarried couples, more than working with other couples, I have found myself questioning my own values regarding privacy, entitlement, loyalty, and obligations. Like most of us, I was unaware of how many preconceived notions I had regarding these issues until they were called into question in certain situations. In one of these situations Julia, a divorced single-parent mother, was torn between spending time with her young son, David, and time with her fiancé, Glen. A year earlier, when the couple had been about to marry, both for the second time, Glen had backed out because of what he considered to be Julia's intense "overinvolvement" with her son. Since I too had a young son at the time and knew how much attention he needed, I was prone to be sympathetic toward Julia and believed that Glen was not paying due heed to a mother's obligation to her child.

My evaluation of the situation shifted somewhat after a session with the three of them. David turned out to be an extremely precocious and appealing 10-year-old who had learned that he had tremendous power over his mother. Taking on the role of a little authoritarian husband, he handed down dictums, ordered her about, and issued ultimatums. Julia, blinded by her guilt over having "robbed David of a father" and not wanting to "crush his masculinity," was allowing him to run their lives. Whenever his mother refused to allow him to do something, David with a lawyerlike demeanor would cry "unfair" and "children have rights too you know." This was Julia's achilles' heel and she would back down.

In the therapy that followed Julia was able to let go of her belief that she would "crush David's masculinity" if she set limits and established disciplinary rules. We worked together to connect David with his peer group and to use available relatives to relieve Julia of the burden of being David's sole caretaker. The couple married several months later. David's closing statement was that he didn't like it but thought he could get used to it.

The many social changes taking place have compelled our field to reevaluate some of our traditional concepts regarding divorce and remarriage. The common concept of complimentarity led us to the assumption that people inevitably choose the same kind of person when they remarry, and therefore are bound to repeat the same kind of relationship all over again.

Anne Bernstein takes a different, more contemporary, point of view based on the idea that every person has within him or her a wide repertoire of thoughts, feelings, and behaviors that emerge in different patterns in different relationships. Having a different partner and learning from experience can elicit different aspects of a person and result in a different kind of relationship.

In her chapter, she elucidates the different meanings of first and second marriages. She discusses the need to understand the misunderstandings that can arise in marriages composed of one partner who has never been married and one who has. She invites clinicians to view remarried couples as a collective rather than as a single unit and provides an in-depth description of the many different levels of this new collective that therapists should become aware of in order to help guide their couples through it. She provides insightful guidelines for stepparenting issues, emotional triangles, ex-spouses, gender arrangements, the needs of children, and respecting old relationships, while accommodating to new ones.

A THIRD SPACE: GAY AND LESBIAN COUPLES

More gay and lesbians couples are seeking therapy now that the mental health field has stopped viewing homosexuality as an "illness" or a "perversion" and has come to accept it as a normal human experience. The American Psychiatric Association removed homosexuality from its list of mental disorders in 1973 and no longer stigmatizes it as a "serious character disorder" that can be "cured." Even the more conservative Psychoanalytic Society recently acknowledged its past homophobia by presenting an open forum at its 1998 national meeting in Manhattan to which it invited the openly gay congressman Barney Frank to be a speaker.

However, even with the changing climate concerning homosexuality and advances in scientific knowledge about human sexuality, prejudice and bigotry still exist in our society. Many opportunities that same-gendered couples would wish to have, such as easy access to civil rights, social benefits, and adoptive children, are denied to homosexual couples. All these factors can raise significant concerns for same-gendered couples and cause them to seek therapeutic resources. Therapists need a different cultural lens to see the complexities of these couples' challenges, overlaid as they are with the shadow of homophobia and the fog of heterosexism.

Homosexual couples enjoy the opportunity to explore new definitions of coupling, for in a homosexual couple the usual hierarchical relationship of male and female, leader and follower, one role and another role, is much less strenuously dictated. As there are relatively few social role models for same-gendered couples to follow, this can allow for much greater flexibility and freedom in the construction of a same-gendered relationship. Additionally, the fact of a relationship existing solely from choice can be highlighted as an ongoing value as opposed to what too often becomes simply a marital state.

Gary Sanders, in Chapter 10, "Men Together," gives a historical overview of society's changing attitudes toward homosexuality and the meaning of these changes in the lives of gay men. He contends that the major impediments for gay men in developing, maintaining, and promoting intimate relationships is the "triad of tyranny": patriarchy, heterosexism, and homophobia. Sanders elucidates the belief systems of heterosexism and homophobia that operate in institutions, the community, and individuals. He emphasizes the importance of therapists understanding and acknowledging their own belief systems in relation to homophobia. Using a narrative approach, he presents therapeutic conversations that deal with the unique experiences of gay men, including pervasive loneliness, invisibility, unclear boundaries, lack of role models and "genitalization of the heart."

Caroline Marvin and Dusty Miller in Chapter 11, "Lesbian Couples Entering the 21st Century," look at some of the issues facing lesbian couples in the new century. Now that gays and lesbians are living less closeted lives, they are moving beyond issues of "coming out" and focusing more on concerns common to heterosexual couples, such as having children, coparenting, separation agreements, custody, and financial contracts. The resolution of these concerns is, however, not necessarily the same for gay and lesbian couples as it is for ordinary heterosexual couples because the legal sanctions are not the same. Lesbian couples face complicated questions such as: What are the rules, obligations and responsibilities of coparenting? Who is entitled to custody should the couple separate? Does a nonbiological partner have the right to be treated as a coparent by the school? Financial arrangements also become more complicated. Should partners name each other as the beneficiary of life insurance policies? Who owns the apartment or house? In case of death is the surviving partner entitled to continue to live there? If a couple breaks up, how will assets be divided with no formal divorce process to structure the decisions? Therapists are advised to encourage lesbian couples to take legal measures to ensure that their rights are fully protected, including creation of wills and the designation of health care proxies.

Miller and Marvin use the developmental stages of the life cycle to provide a unifying frame to consider lesbian couples as a group in need of special consideration. They contextualize lesbian relationships by looking at the tasks and accomplishments of five life-cycle stages: couple formation, ongoing couplehood, the middle years, generativity, and couples over 65. This alternative life cycle goes beyond the traditional family life-cycle paradigm of weddings, births, divorce, and midlife angst. The authors describe the special problems that can arise in each stage and offer innovative ways of resolving them.

THE INVISIBLE WALL OF RACISM

Demographic shifts taking place in our nation are changing our nation's racial and ethnic identity. People of color (this includes Native Americans, African Americans, Hispanic/Latino Americans, and Asian Americans) constitute the fastest growing population in the United States. It is estimated that by the year 2056 whites will be a minority in our country.

These demographic changes have brought about an increasing awareness in our field of the need to expand our current clinical theories and modalities to meet this new challenge. Most of our theoretical concepts have been constructed within our dominant cultural context and are inadequate to encompass the needs of minorities.

This is especially true of African Americans, who, although living side by side with White Americans for hundreds of years, still live in a different experiential world set off by an invisible wall of racism and prejudice. In order to prevent this wall from becoming an obstacle in therapy, the therapist's first step is to recognize its existence. While it is important to understand every couple's social and cultural context, it is doubly important to understand that of African Americans. Their experiences of prejudice and discrimination are part of their identity and are woven into their interpersonal reality.

Most white therapists condemn racism and see themselves as free of prejudice, but their unfamiliarity with African American culture and traditions makes them prone to many misconceptions and misunderstandings. Afraid they are going to say or do the wrong thing, they tend to walk on egg shells in therapy sessions, either bending over backward in an effort not to appear prejudiced or distancing themselves to avoid making a mistake. Their obvious discomfort interferes with their forming a strong therapeutic connection.

One of the best antidote to this discomfort is for therapists to arm themselves with knowledge about the African American experience. The more they know about this world, its traditions, beliefs, fears, and frustrations, the better prepared they will be to engage in meaningful therapeutic discussions regarding African Americans and their problems.

A prerequisite for understanding the cultural background of others is to first understand one's own. Toward this end, the minority social work program at the Ackerman Institute developed an exercise based on one created by Elaine Pinderhughes that engages our staff members in examining our own racial and ethnic beliefs and prejudices and understanding how these shape our lives and impact our therapy. The staff breaks up into small groups and discusses the following questions with one another:

1. Describe your cultural/racial/ethnic/class background and how you would identify yourself.
   - What aspects of your background are you most proud of? How have those aspects affected your life?
   - What aspects are you most ashamed of? How have they affected your life?
2. How did your family fit into the community?
   - What did you learn about people who were different from you?
   - Describe an experience that made you feel "different" because of your background. What was good or bad about the experience?
3. How do you think your background affects your way of being with the families you treat?
   - How is it a help? A hindrance?

Examining these issues in one's own life and discussing them with others is surprisingly revealing and deepens one's sensitivity to differences on many different levels.

In Chapter 9, "Therapy with African American Couples," Lascelles Black takes us into the experiential world of African Americans. He describes the impact of racism, the meaning of skin color, the importance of spirituality, the effect of social class, the need for community identity, and the different definition of family. This information should prove invaluable to therapists in helping them to be respectful of but not immobilized by differences.

A NEW VIEW FROM OVER THE HILL

The 1985 movie *Cocoon* worked to change the public image of the elderly from helpless, fragile invalids who needed to be helped across the street, to that of feisty romantic figures who could not only take care of themselves but could take off in a spaceship—a precursor to the real-life adventure of John Glenn at 78. The movie presented elderly couples cavorting on the edge of the grave with the same absurd mixture of jealousy, lust, competition, and romantic yearnings as their younger counterparts. They dealt with their bodily aches and pains by falling in love, having affairs, flexing their muscles, dancing, fighting, and competing with each other. Yes, it was a romantic fantasy, but one that more and more AARP (American Association of Retired Persons) members are attempting to realize.

This shift in our view of the elderly has also been reflected in popular literature and in our own professional literature. Elderly love, once thought to be slightly disgusting, was the subject of Gabriel García Márquez's book *Love in the Time of Cholera* (1988), which won the Nobel Prize for literature. In *Love's Executioner*, Irvin Yalom (1996) presents a fascinating case of a 70-year-old woman who falls in love with a younger man. Yalom describes how he overcame his own ageism during the process of doing therapy with her.

One sure sign that older people are no longer on the fringe of mainstream culture is that they are appearing more frequently in therapist's offices—a mark of normalcy in our psychologically oriented age. Gone are the days when we therapists quietly shunted those over 60 onto beginning students for "supportive" work because we believe that they were too old to change. We now know that elderly couples sometimes have more motivation for changing than younger couples because they have more invested in staying together at this point in their lives and fewer options if they separate. In their declining years they need each other more than ever. As their resources dwindle, they are more dependent on one another for physical as well as emotional support. The main limitation to treatment is in the minds of those therapists who continue to believe there is an age limit to change.

One of the first couples we treated in the Depression Project at the Ackerman Institute was a couple in their 70s who had been married 47 years and were having a sexual problem. At the end of the first session the wife looked beseechingly at us and said, "When we were coming here today, I thought maybe it would not be worth your time to spend with us because we're older and—." Her voice choked with tears. Characterizing our new clinical attitude, the therapist (Mark Finn) replied, "We were thinking about it from the exact opposite point of view. We were thinking how much time you've invested in your lives and how important it would be to try and help you at this point."

Ruth Mohr's chapter, "Reflections on Golden Pond" (Chapter 13) deals with the many different stages and exigencies of elderly love. Mohr sees the major challenge to growing old together as being able to "stay connected" while "letting go." This is the guiding principle she uses in helping couples adjust to retirement, deal with adult children and mental health workers, readjust their gender roles, and confront illness and death. She provides specific guidelines for renegotiating the marriage contract in order to accommodate to life changes and create a different story elderly couples can live by.

LOOKING AHEAD

Over the years, the field of family therapy has reflected the changing ideas and values of the historical times to which it belonged, expanding its concepts to accommodate to the social, cultural, and political upheavals of each era. Our field has a unique contribution to make in this new century, based as it is on the systems theory that no phenomenon in the universe can be understood outside its context. Each new scientific, technological, biological, political, and social development changes our context and requires an accompanying shift in our ideology. It is important to understand the impact of these changing contexts that shape our lives and relationships in order to avoid the pitfalls and take advantage of the promises they offer.

The couple relationship in the past was prefabricated according to a specific structure and style and built on a foundation of stability, dependability, and familiarity. The air inside the house may have been stale, but it was safe and certain. There are those in our field who are trying desperately to rebuild the old foundation on sunken ground rather than finding new, more suitable terrain.

In the following chapters, each author explores a different social terrain with his or her clients, encouraging them to examine some of their old myths, beliefs, and expectations that keep them stuck in old territory and urging them to turn their attention toward designing a new home on fresh earth.

REFERENCES

Bernard, J. (1972). *The future of marriage: The his and her marriage.* New York: Bantam.

Gottman, J. M., & Silver, N. (1999). *The seven principles for making marriage work.* New York: Metropolitan Books.

Grinfeld, M. J. (1996). Mental illnesses to be among most prevalent by 2020, WHO study says. *Psychiatric Times, 13*(11), 1, 79.

Hochschild, A. R. (1997). *The time bind: When work becomes home and home becomes work.* New York: Metropolitan Books.

Kramer, P. D. (1997, December 21). What Ivanov needs in the 90's is an antidepressant. *New York Times,* Section C, p. 5.

García Márquez, G. (1988). *Love in the time of cholera.* New York: Knopf.

Papp, P. (1983). *The process of change.* New York: Guilford Press.

Papp, P. (1996). Finding a third space. *In the Family, 2,* 4–26.

Yalom, I. D. (1996). *Love's executioner.* New York: Harper Collins.

CHAPTER 2

The Three-Career Family

Lawrence Levner

Reconceptualizing the "two-career family" as a family with "three careers" (the third being family life) involves a major change in values that places domestic life on a par with work and offers an expanded frame of reference inclusive of all areas of the couple's relationship. The inclusion of three equal spheres of activity, "her career," "his career," and the "career of the family," opens the door to a therapeutic discussion requiring women and men to "own" both the instrumental and the relational domains of work and family. It raises therapy to a level of importance beyond the negotiation of tasks—"who drives the children" or "who does the laundry"—to a dialogue in which equal significance is assigned to work and family in the lives of both women and men.

The popular term "two-career family" implies that work is more important than domestic life. If there are only "two careers," women's careers are seen as secondary even if these women earn higher incomes, while men are not seen as primary at home no matter how much they are involved. In U.S. society, mothers are still thought to be primary in child rearing. Men are identified with work in terms of social and self-esteem, while women's work outside the home is considered secondary (see Coontz, 1992, p. 3).

Despite a dramatic shift in the content and structure of family life over the last 30 years, the actual dynamics of heterosexual relationships have seemingly changed very little. "The exodus of women into the economy has not been accompanied by a cultural understanding of marriage and worth that would make this transition smooth" (Hochschild, 1989, p. 12). Couples continue to experience relationships in terms of traditional role divisions: he is from "Mars" and she is from "Venus"; he is instrumental, she is relational; he is the "caveman" and the hunter, she tends to the home; he feels constrained by commitment, while she craves it (see Rubin, 1994, p. 76).

This process of dividing things up according to gender limits both women and men (even if they both have careers) to traditional roles: women nurture, while men are task-oriented; women are supportive, while men are competitive; women share feelings, while men control their emotions (see Tavris, 1992, p. 263). Couples get stuck in this belief that "he" does not have sufficient emotional capacity to take responsibility for relationships and family life, that he is disengaged and fearful of intimacy, while "she" not only has the skill but the responsibility to pursue and manage the relationship and to foster emotional connection in the family. "This shared belief system makes men feel incompetent in relationships, and makes women feel crazy because they are constantly seeking to get what both of them believe is not there to be had. So, in their coupling, he feels inadequate and she feels disappointed" (Walters, Carter, Papp, & Silverstein, 1988, p. 242).

Therapeutic concepts, terminology, and metaphors should challenge belief systems that assign women and men these different roles, skills, and unequal status. This is not an easy task since couples are understandably more responsive to frameworks that are consistent with their existing social context. Moreover, therapists find it easier to organize treatment around ways in which men and women are different as opposed to encouraging them to transcend these differences. Clinical strategies that seem most comfortable to the couple and clinically expedient to the therapist often result in reinforcing existing roles and patterns of interaction, facilitating negotiation within traditional belief systems as opposed to challenging them.

Following are suggestions for recontextualizing work and family:

1. Refer to both partners as primary in both work and family, and point out when women are categorized as secondary in their careers and men are categorized as secondary in family relationships. Men do not "baby-sit" their own children, they *parent* them.

2. Think of women as trying to protect men from emotional vulnerability instead of referring to women's identification with nurturing and relationship as "overfunctioning" or as "intrusive" (terms that marginalize women's roles in families), thus validating women's emotionality and relationality while expecting and assuming the same capacity in men.

3. Discuss personal styles of connection and attachment, affirming relationality as a competence for women and reflecting belief in men's emotional capacity.

4. Point out instrumental, task-oriented skills and relational, interpersonal skills in both men and women, thus challenging the popular belief that each gender brings a different capacity to the relationship and that expectations for men and women are inherently different.

5. Ask couples to reflect on the common and shared as well as the differential experiences of balancing work and family. Encourage a discourse that signifies domestic roles of both partners along with the interrelatedness of work and career (see Galinsky, 1999, p. xvi).

6. Encourage couples to develop extrafamilial emotional and social support systems within which they can ask for help with the tasks of sharing work and family as well as benefit from identification with other couples with similar experiences.

GREAT EXPECTATIONS

I recently had the opportunity to work with Bob and Fran, before and after they had their first child. The couple's ideology clearly places work and family on equal footing, while their transactional pattern reveals very traditional values about their roles. What follows is a clinical study of two therapy sessions. In the first session, prior to the birth of their son, we discussed their expectations, beliefs, and conflicts regarding family life and parenting. The second session focused on their initial experiences as a couple with a child and the conflicts that arose from their attempts to strike a balance between work and family as they began to understand their internalization of traditional roles and values.

Bob and Fran are both in their early 30s and have been married for 8 years. They grew up together and knew each other and each other's families well. Fran recently completed her PhD and is the executive director of a small foundation. Bob is a college professor. They moved from their hometown for Fran's career, after which Bob looked for his job. Her income is greater than his. They describe their relationship as egalitarian and take pride in their "role reversal," a term that indicates a keen awareness of the roles they are supposed to play as a couple and as parents. Although they have doubts about their decision that Fran return to work full time after 6 weeks of maternity leave, Bob boasts, "She's the executive and I'm the schoolteacher." She frequently travels and is trying to reduce the number of her business trips, though she expects to continue being away from home. In planning for their baby, they found daycare convenient to Bob's job because he will be the parent doing most of the driving before and after work. They have had what they term "the usual conflicts" over household responsibilities but are generally pleased with their ability to negotiate and accommodate.

It is important, initially, to construct the belief system that both family and work are equally important endeavors. As Bob starts by identifying himself as responsible for getting the baby to child care, the therapist frames his choice of a teaching career as a decision to be an available parent. When Bob downplays the importance of his job (as women often do when they decide to prioritize the family), Fran supports him, speaking about the meaning of his role. The therapist frames this as the importance to her of his sense of personal competence. The therapist labels Bob as primary in a way that is inclusive of both Bob and Fran as parents and introduces the notion that two parents can both be primary.

BOB: I'll take the baby to the sitter and pick him up, all except the two nights that I teach.

FRAN: I'm trying to hire another person for my staff at work, someone who can take on some of the travel so I don't have to be away as much. I worry about working so much. I hate it more now that I'm going to have a baby.

BOB: Fran has the more traditional man's type of job while I have the woman's job since I teach school and she works in an office and directs a project. Other women we know stay in teaching because it gives them more flexibility to be with the children.

THERAPIST: (to Bob) So you've decided that a good reason to stay in your career is that it gives you the opportunity to be the kind of parent you want to be?

BOB: It gives one of us the chance to be more flexible. It's different because I'm the man. I'll take the baby, most days. It will change how I work, but it's an important sacrifice. No more hanging around, talking to students. No big deal.

THERAPIST: Are you saying that your work isn't as important as Fran's?

BOB: Au contraire! (*laughter*)

THERAPIST: It sounded that way—the way you said "hanging around" and "no big deal."

FRAN: (*sounding defensive*) He means that it's his schedule that will be different. He will have more time with the baby than if he had a traditional office job. It's going to be hard for him to work—to grade papers at home with the baby.

BOB: Yes, yes. I'm going to have to make my time mesh with the baby's. I'm going to have to be more organized. (*Fran seems relieved.*)

THERAPIST: (*to Fran*) You interrupted him when he was saying that there is nothing to it, to be responsible for the baby. It's important to you that he feel good about this?

FRAN: Yes, I feel guilty that he has to do this because I'm working.

THERAPIST: (*to Bob*) Are you looking forward to being a primary parent?

BOB: Well I don't know about primary. . . . Fran is the mother and she will be nursing.

THERAPIST: Do you believe that a baby can have two primary parents?

FRAN: I think so. Breast-feeding is just a small part of caring for a baby.

The following discussion about work "once the baby comes" points to an uncharacteristic shift from this couple's balanced perspective concerning family and work toward a more traditional ideology in which Bob identifies himself as the provider and takes on extra work in response to the need to maintain their income. Fran, on the other hand, begins to "distance" herself from her job in anticipation of being a mother. This shift highlights the couple's conflict and ambiguity about their arrangement and how each defines competency in the relationship. Fran earns more money, Bob has the more flexible job; she will continue to work full time and travel, he will be responsible for getting their child to and from daycare. Despite these nontraditional arrangements, their anticipations about the first weeks of parenting are reflective of a traditional, gendered construction of relationship. The economic power of the higher salary does not translate, for Fran, into a greater sense of power and role differentiation in her marriage. Bob, on the other hand, despite his availability and aptitude for parenting, identifies his contribution as wage earning "so that Fran can have more time with the baby." This reflects his sense that he will be a secondary parent. Fran begins to be responsible for his relationship with their child, feeling "guilty that he's taking on too much." This narrow identification of the male role as instrumental and the female role as relational speaks to the couple's internalization of social rules about competence and empowerment. A man's power tends to be independent, often extrafamilial, while a women believes her power and status is derived from maintaining her family.

The couple's identification as "role-reversed" conveys an underlying belief in dominant social stereotypes that if Fran identifies too strongly with work, she is playing the man's role, and conversely that if Bob identifies too much with parenting, he is acting like a mother. Their identification with these rigidly constructed social roles becomes the context for conflict and unhappiness. The therapist introduces the frame of a "third career" in response to this conflict. Bob jokes that two careers are already too much for him, while Fran identifies the need for figuring out how to manage "all three."

BOB: I am taking on more [work]. I have a noncredit class, an email class, a night class—two nights a week—and I have advising to do. If I do all these things, I'll be busy.

FRAN: My job drives me crazy but my attitude toward things has changed the last 6 months or so since I've known about the baby. I thought we had a role reversal—you know, my job and all—but I have begun to distance from work a little more. I just focus on the baby being most important and I don't want to be stressed out and bring work home. My attitude has definitely changed.

BOB: *Your* attitude is much different.

THERAPIST: (*to Bob*) You say that as if yours isn't, yet you're more focused on work now.

BOB: My attitude is different in the sense that usually in the summer, I work less—I look forward to not working so much. That's not my priority this summer so that Fran can have more time with the baby.

THERAPIST: What about your time with the baby?

BOB: I don't want Fran to feel that she has to go back because of the money . . .

FRAN: *(interjects)* I feel guilty that he's taking on too much—that he'll be gone at least two nights a week for 8 weeks right when the baby will be a newborn—that he won't get to bond with the baby right away.

THERAPIST: It sounds as if the baby . . . your family and all you have to do is kind of third career.

BOB: Don't say that! Two careers are enough *(laughter)*!

FRAN: Well, we are going to have to figure out a way to do all three.

Despite his plan to be involved in the family, Bob expresses fear of losing his relationship once Fran becomes too "busy" working and mothering. He does not identify himself as sharing her experience or being in a similar position of having to balance career, parenting, and relationship. The therapist challenges Bob's perspective, suggesting that his involvement is a way to create the intimacy that he fears will be lost.

BOB: If Fran is busy with the baby and has her job—to me, it creates a division between the two of us.

THERAPIST: Tell me how that would be.

BOB: Her attention will be taken up with work and with the baby. Her responsibility would increase and mine wouldn't.

FRAN: *(looking down, shaking her head negatively)* I don't want that.

THERAPIST: *(to Bob)* You plan to be very involved with the baby as well as with your job, yet you say that Fran's responsibility would increase and yours wouldn't. You don't identify yourself as involved even though you plan to be. You talked about Fran having less time, about her being busy with work and the baby. What about your involvement? You didn't say anything about that.

BOB: That's what I mean. I enjoy being around so much, I don't want less time with her.

THERAPIST: So don't you think that being involved will help you feel closer to Fran?

In the next sequence, Fran responds enthusiastically to the idea that their closeness will be enhanced through mutuality and role diversification, while Bob continues to identify the obstacles to sharing the responsibility for work and parenting. The therapist again uses the "third career" metaphor to encourage both Bob and Fran to identify themselves as parents.

FRAN: Yes, we would be closer. The baby should get attention and that wouldn't be something I would automatically think to do or have to do . . . that I would always be the one to get off the couch or stop what I am doing to take care of the baby. The assumption should be that *one of us* will do it, and it wouldn't have to be me. This would make me feel closer.

THERAPIST: (*to Bob*) Does that help you in any way?

BOB: I go along with that, but . . . and this will be what gets me hit on the head . . . if I am going to be working this summer, Fran will be the one who gets up most of the time at night. (*Looks at Fran, who raises her eyebrows.*) Well, (*jokingly*) we'll probably be doing that equally.

THERAPIST: When he talks that way, even though he's joking, you start to think, "This isn't going to be a shared endeavor."

FRAN: Yes, it worries me. The baby is going to need both of us and we are going to need each other. I don't want it to be all on either one of us. What is it going to do to our time together . . . to our relationship?

BOB: I've seen it happen to other people—to my sister. They have a baby and its like "circle the wagons." The mother and baby in the middle and the father is out there on the periphery.

THERAPIST: Why do you think that happens?

BOB: The husband can take care of himself, the baby can't.

FRAN: If the baby can't take care of itself, it doesn't mean it is the mother who always has to be the one to do it. We can both take care of the baby.

THERAPIST: (*to Fran*) The last thing you said is very important and also very different from the traditional view that a baby needs only mothering because it can't care for itself. It's that third career that you both will share.

FRAN: That's right. It needs parenting from both of us.

Bob is unsure, despite his best intentions, that he has the skill and the capacity to be a primary parent while continuing to work. Intellectually, he recognizes the importance and necessity of his involvement, but as he begins to struggle with the meaning and experience of balancing his work and relationship he expresses uncertainty and discomfort. His uncertainty leaves him open to traditional beliefs about gender roles. Fran speaks with more certainty about her expectations and her belief in Bob's capacity, but her protectiveness and feelings of guilt when he is stressed, point to her underlying doubts about his relational competence. The therapist asks Bob to identify the skills of being a parent. In different ways, Fran and Bob have begun to recognize how important being traditional has been to their success in balancing work and family. Bob responds to the therapist's question about relational skills by identifying the need to see things differently. Fran frames it in terms of giving up her storybook ideas about marriage.

BOB: Last night in the birthing class, we heard a doctor who was talking about having someone to help the mother, and he said that any girl 12 years or older has the mothering skills. . . . He said that men just don't have these, no matter who or how old . . . a man just doesn't have the skills of a 12-year-old girl.

THERAPIST: (*as Fran makes a face*) Do you object to that?

FRAN: Give me a break!

THERAPIST: (*to Bob*) Your response?

BOB: (*doubtfully*) I think a man can have the skills . . .

THERAPIST: When you think about the skills of the 12-year-old girl versus the grown man in taking care of a baby—the skills each of you will need to make this happen—to parent and to work and to be fulfilled by your careers, by your child, and by each other—what do you think those skills are?

BOB: We have to be willing to see things differently. Having the baby will help us to do that. I know a guy who was talking about his job that kept him away and he said, "That's what my dad did." It didn't bother him that he was going to do the same thing—not be focused on his family. He figured that that's just the way you do it. I can't let myself think this way. It's hard to see things differently. It seems almost natural just to do it the way everyone else does.

FRAN: I guess this means that it will be different from all the storybook stuff about marriage that I grew up with (*laughs*).

THERAPIST: It is not taking on traditional storybook roles that will keep you together.

Fran and Bob experience themselves as isolated both in the conceptualization of their dilemma and in finding physical and emotional support and encouragement. They see themselves as each other's sole mainstays, other than their parents and siblings, in responding to stress and in making difficult situations manageable. Having moved a few hundred miles from their extended families, they are isolated from support systems that might help them make the difficult adjustment to parenthood. In this final sequence of the first session, the therapist expands the discussion to include "support systems" in response to the couple's isolation. The couple does not understand their situation as universal or their experience as commonplace. Fran, in particular, is sensitive to the ways in which she may be different from other working mothers. She has difficulty thinking of her boss as a support since he and his wife have made a more traditional decision about parenting. Her reluctance to engage their willing neighbors in helping reflects the social value that she should not need extrafamilial assistance. Similarly, she does not look to Bob as someone to be responsible for networking and he does not involve himself in the discussion. The therapist challenges him directly about his role in "arranging for supports."

THERAPIST: Who will help you out? What about your support systems?

FRAN: *Official* child care is worked out for when I go back full time, and I feel pretty good about the person who we arranged for. We could ask neighbors—some have volunteered—to watch the baby to give us a break, but I wouldn't want to bother them on a regular basis—only in an emergency.

BOB: If it were family, they would have to help us (*laughter*).

THERAPIST: I know you can count on each other . . . there is no one else?

FRAN: I've talked to my boss, who has a 3-year-old daughter. He seems to understand but his wife and daughter have never been apart from each other overnight. We don't even have the baby yet (*shaky voice*) and I'm already upset thinking about this. I don't know if we're doing the right thing.

THERAPIST: So you are trying to find a support system at work?

FRAN: Yes . . . but I don't know . . . in my job . . . I may have to change my position.

THERAPIST: (*to Bob*) What is your role in this, in arranging for supports?

Five weeks and a baby boy later, an exhausted Bob and Fran bring their son for his first family therapy session. He is a good baby: sleeping as much as can be expected, nursing well, healthy, and content. Labor and delivery were difficult. Despite having gone to "baby school," Bob felt irrelevant during the birth process. Both Fran's and Bob's families came to help and have since returned home. Fran's emotions, both highs and lows, have been exaggerated and Bob does not quite know how to help her. He began his summer routine at work. She hated for him to leave the house and became tearful when he did.

Bob responds defensively and anxiously when asked about helping Fran when she is sad. Again, he feels helpless to make a difference. Fran senses Bob's discomfort and protects him by supporting his going to work and attributing her tears to "something chemical." The therapist validates Fran's worrying as helping and protecting Bob, and then encourages Bob to consider the ways in which he reciprocates.

FRAN: Life is *very* different.

THERAPIST: Is it what you expected?

FRAN: For me, it has been busier and much more emotional. Ever since he was born, everything, happy and sad, gets me to cry. I am not usually like this. I mean, I'll cry, but not every day like this. I know Bob feels guilty about going to work 'cause every time he leaves, I just ball like a baby. I know that he needs to go, that it's the best thing for him to do, and I tell him that, but at the same time I'm sobbing. (*Bob looks down.*) It's overwhelming. I know it's partially something chemical . . .

THERAPIST: It's not just chemical. You worry about yourself and about Bob—that he feels guilty and that your tears overwhelm him. You protect him and that's terrific. Bob, can you help her—take care of her when she is sad?

BOB: I stayed home the week the baby was born. . . . In comparison to those people who work 70–80 hours a week, I only have a couple of long days, it's not every day. I know it's not easy on Fran. Neither of us does well when we're home by ourselves. I asked some neighbors to come over. I can't stay home with the baby for very long because she's nursing.

FRAN: The baby's doing really well, gaining weight. He seems happy.

THERAPIST: You feel Bob's anxiety, don't you? It helps to change the focus to the baby.

BOB: We didn't anticipate the effect of being awake at night. I thought the 2:00 A.M. feeding would be baby wakes up, eats, goes back to sleep, but he stays up for hours.

THERAPIST: Do you stay up with Fran through all of this ?

FRAN: He stays up as much as possible, but the night before he has to get up to go to work he can't stay up with me.

BOB: Some nights I have to bail out, go to another room, turn on the air conditioning, and go to sleep.

FRAN: Which makes me sad.

BOB: And it makes me feel very guilty—going to work, going to sleep, doing anything that doesn't help Fran or the baby. I feel that there is this test of being the good modern dad, but you never know if you have what it takes to do enough and you can never do as much as the woman. Work is easier, I recognize that. I get a break, leave the house, see other people.

THERAPIST: Well, Bob, it's a good thing that you feel guilty for not making it better for Fran the way you would like to. It's the feeling guilty and responsible that let's you both know how much she matters to you. Sometimes, when it's impossible to help in other ways, feeling guilty creates an attachment.

BOB: (looking at Fran) I just have to figure out how to be there to make her feel supported.

THERAPIST: Do you see how much better that sounds than the way you were speaking earlier?

Framing Bob's guilt as a positive function to create attachment (in the last segment) sets the stage for the therapist to challenge Bob to connect to Fran in other ways, helping him to consider his relational competency even as he is feeling useless and irrelevant to Fran and the baby. Bob becomes less defensive and creates a more manageable frame for the problem that the therapist quickly validates. This frees

Fran to begin to speak about her experience of being home with the baby without feeling that she has to protect Bob from her ambivalence and her anger. It also opens up their conflict about housework—something Fran had previously been reluctant to discuss. Despite their disagreement over housework, Fran and Bob share a belief system about their roles in the family. As annoyed as she is with Bob, Fran feels guilty about not doing the preponderance of the housework, believing it to be her role. Bob prioritizes work, recreation, and relaxation, and doesn't feel the same need to wash and clean. Fran's compulsion is framed as maintaining Bob "right where he is." Their agreement on roles is another indication that they both see Fran as primarily responsible for the household even though Bob has the more flexible job.

FRAN: It really is a break to be able to get away, but I couldn't leave the baby—it bothers me to be in a different room, I feel so connected to him. It's a Catch-22 situation. I need to be near him, but, on the other hand, I can't get anything else done. When he naps, I end up scurrying around trying to do housework instead of resting or doing something peaceful. If I were to let go of it, the housework wouldn't get done (*begins to weep*). It's all too much.

BOB: Well, two afternoons, I go to work, and besides, I don't feel the same urgency about it that she does. Fran has always felt this urgency about floors—that floors have to be clean. To me, they're floors. People walk on them. They are never spotless. It's summer, the dogs are shedding, and every once in awhile you clean it up, but it bothers Fran all of the time.

THERAPIST: (*to Bob*) Do you know why she is so upset?

BOB: I don't know why this is coming up now. It has never been a problem before. I've always done things around the house. I clean the basement and take care of the outside. Fran has gotten so she keeps the house clean but her room was a mess when she did her dissertation. I don't see why this is coming up.

THERAPIST: You really don't see what is different now? (*Bob laughs.*) Now you are facing a situation where Fran is exhausted and still feels that while the baby is asleep she has to do all these things. What you have to ask yourself is "How do you see your role? How do you see yourself involved?"

BOB: I try to encourage her to relax, take time, and that kind of thing—thinking it makes things better because it does for me. If I stay up one night to watch a video—it makes it seem like I've had some time for myself. If I felt the same urgency about cleaning the house along with grading papers, going to work, and the baby—it would drive me crazy! I don't want to take all the anxiety about the house that Fran feels. I don't think it's necessary. To me, it's more important to have time for myself than to have dog hair off the floor.

FRAN: (*tearful*) He makes sense, but I feel no less compulsion to try to clean up.

THERAPIST: Do you think that if Bob did feel the need, would you still have the compulsion, or would you be able to relax? For instance, when the baby naps and you have a list of things to do, were Bob to say "Here, let me do those, you take a rest," would you still feel the compulsion?

FRAN: I think I would because it's my job. His attitude is that we have the baby to take care of, he has work to do, and in the meantime the diapers pile up, the trash piles up, the dishes pile up, laundry has to be done—because there are things we don't have enough of, and I hate to ask him to do any of that because I feel guilty because he is going to work.

THERAPIST: (*to Fran*) So you would do it anyway? Do you see how that contributes to keeping Bob right where he is? Even though you're angry with him, you behave as if the housework is entirely your responsibility.

As they look for resolution through negotiating housework, Bob continues to respond defensively ("It's not my role to beat her to things"), while Fran "wishes she hadn't brought it up," worrying that Bob will "back away." The therapist frames her "not wanting it to become an issue" as helpful in not upsetting him, validating her role as protective, and maintaining their attachment and connection despite the conflict. The therapist frames her "paying so much attention" to housework as maintaining Bob in the position of not having to focus on it.

BOB: If she's going to do laundry and housework and spend all her free time working on the floor, I'm not going to feel guilty about it and I don't think I should. It's not my role to beat her to things.

THERAPIST: What do you think your role is?

BOB: In the past, I've suggested that we work on things in 30-minute intervals but she never did it. It never got done.

FRAN: Is this payback time (*tearful*)?

BOB: Until a few minutes ago, I never thought there was a problem.

THERAPIST: There is a way to understand why you didn't think it was a problem. To the extent that you (*to Fran*) paid so much attention to it, it didn't have to occur to you (*to Bob*). You didn't have to be focused on it. You were so used to Fran taking it on, it didn't seem so important.

FRAN: I don't want there to be a problem. You are upset with me because it is too much [work] now and that's making you back away from me.

THERAPIST: (*to Fran*) What are you responding to that makes you think he is backing away?

FRAN: He sounds really angry. I don't want him to be upset, to back off. But I don't know what to do. I do as much as I can but I'm tired. I wish I hadn't brought it up.

BOB: I am angry about trying to do all the things I'm doing now and I am getting the sense that I'm not doing enough and that I should be doing more, but before it wasn't an issue. I'd like to feel that I don't have to take on all that Fran does in order to feel responsible. When you ask me to help, I feel as if you think I don't do anything at all. I've been helpful all these years . . .

THERAPIST: (*to Fran*) So you've helped this to not become an issue—because Bob didn't want to talk about it or you didn't want to upset him?

BOB: But I have wanted to talk about it. I didn't know what to do and she never brought it up, so I didn't think it was a big problem.

THERAPIST: Do you understand why she didn't bring it up?

BOB: She didn't want to upset me. She knew it would bother me.

FRAN: You're already so tired—you have so much work to do, you have long days, you have too much on you already, so I don't want to ask you to do anything more but I'd like to feel that it is OK to ask you (*cries*).

THERAPIST: Do you see what's happening? She's asking for help and you feel criticized. She asks "Can you do the laundry" and you say "Are you calling me a lazy so-and-so?" You are responding to something totally different to what she is asking.

When Bob responds with humor ("let a floor be a floor"), the therapist challenges him to think about why it is easier for him to have a lighter point of view than it is for Fran. Bob refers the question to Fran, who initially protects him by saying that she doesn't know why housework has become such a serious topic. It is not until the therapist encourages a shift in focus from the practical division of labor to the paradigm of "three careers" that Bob begins to accept their dilemma as more than just a difference of opinion.

BOB: You know my feeling: let a floor be a floor. (*Both laugh.*)

THERAPIST: Bob, do you see why it is so much easier for you to have that point of view than for Fran?

BOB: Why is it so important now when it wasn't before?

FRAN: Honey, I don't know.

THERAPIST: Oh, yes you do! This is another of those things you don't talk about so as not to upset him.

FRAN: Well, the stakes are higher—we have a baby!

BOB: Why are the stakes higher? I'm not making the connection to housework. (*Both exasperated, look at therapist.*)

THERAPIST: It is what the two of you have been saying since you walked in the door—the time, the focus your son requires, the additional housework, the exhaustion, all while you have your jobs. Now you have a third full-time career. How will you manage it?

BOB: I just thought we had a difference of opinion. Now it feels like so much more. I never paid much attention to who did the housework. It didn't bother me.

As often happens when therapy dislocates a system, the therapist gets caught responding to the disequilibrium by becoming inducted and re-creating the homeostasis in the relationship. In the next sequence, he responds to Bob's question about what to do by enjoining him to be less defensive so that Fran will be more comfortable "asking for help"—a frame that the therapist was expressly trying to avoid.

BOB: I guess we know who will nurse the baby (*laughter*). So, I am still not sure. Tell me what I have to do again? (*Fran hugs him.*)

THERAPIST: (*to Bob*) You have to figure out what your defensiveness is all about so that Fran who is nursing, feeling emotional, and over-burdened can come to you and say, "Can you help me" without having to feel that she's making your life miserable.

FRAN: I just need a little help, sometimes.

BOB: I can do that.

This intervention seems to result in accommodation and reduced tension, but in effect it reinforces the existing transactional pattern of the woman taking primary responsibility for the family while the man helps her. The therapist catches this and changes the frame of reference to one that encourages both Bob and Fran to experience themselves as primary.

THERAPIST: To go one step further, you (*to Bob*) might assess the situation independently and say to yourself "Hmmm, there is more laundry coming through here than there used to be—I guess I need to attend to it" without Fran having to ask at all.

BOB: (*laughing*) I don't like that as much.

THERAPIST: (*as baby sighs*) See! He agrees with me. He wants you to be primary.

As Bob struggles with what it means to be a primary parent, Fran, as much as she has pursued him to be more involved, protects him from the therapist's challenge, again framing the problem as just needing his help and expressing her guilt for needing it. She is also challenged by the therapist's notion that both parents are primary in that her sense of competence is vested in being a mother, even though she has a successful career.

FRAN: You area great husband and father. I just need a little help. Remember the other night when you wanted to go downstairs to exercise, I told you it was OK but in retrospect it probably wasn't. I was really tired and I needed a break. I felt guilty for not giving you that time to yourself. I know exercising is important to you and you had a long day and you are working and I haven't gone back to work yet.

At the end of the session, Bob, for the first time, equates work at home with the workplace. He feels the increased expectations of being a father, and, with only slight prompting from the therapist, he identifies them as his self-expectations, not Fran's. He no longer defines his role in the family as contingent on Fran. As he begins to refer to himself as primary, Fran, less cautious and protective, begins to talk to him about her fear of being held totally responsible for the family.

BOB: You are working too—I mean now, at home, not only when you go back. I know you are but I still feel that now that I am a father, the expectations on the husband are way up.

FRAN: And so are the expectations on me.

THERAPIST: Where do these expectations come from?

BOB: Well, I want to say "from Fran" but I think that's the wrong answer (*both laugh*).

THERAPIST: What's the right answer?

BOB: I think they are my own [expectations] about being a good father.

THERAPIST: Exactly!

FRAN: You know that I am going to be held much more accountable for what happens to him (*pointing to the baby*) than you—I mean by everyone's expectations (*tears*).

BOB: That's probably true and it's not fair (*comforting Fran*). Maybe if we do it together it will help.

FRAN: I guess what it means is that we will both have to do everything and that feels OK.

TRADITION

"It's hard to see things differently. It seems almost natural just to do it the way everyone else does" is Bob's sense of why it has been so difficult for him and for Fran to feel that they have the skills to parent, to work, to be fulfilled by career, by their child, and by each other (see pp. 39–40). This goes directly to the core of what brings couples into therapy, why they feel stuck, and what therapy should be about. He is referring to the power of traditional, gendered, social rules in defining the couple's relationship even as they have adopted egalitarian beliefs and values, ideas of inclusion, and equality.

Tradition guides people through difficult times, delineating rules and standards for behavior and relationship, facilitating the negotiation of new and uncertain life stages. But tradition is also grounded in socially dominant beliefs that prescribe very different roles for men and women; defining each gender as having different skills and capacities, limiting their sense of competence. Bob and Fran were proud, at first, of being a nontraditional couple who planned to share work and parenting responsibilities equally, but the dissonance between their perspective and their process increased along with their anxiety in anticipating the birth of their baby. They became more traditionally gender-defined in their transactional patterns, Fran with domestic life, Bob with career, experiencing increased disagreement and conflict as they tried to define their new roles.

In a parallel fashion, the therapist also has to "see things differently;" replacing traditional perspectives with ideas and metaphors that make it possible for Bob and Fran to struggle not so much with each other, their differences and conflicts, but with the dichotomy between their belief in the equal sharing of roles and the patterns of transaction that found them traditionally defined.

Bob and Fran are a three-career couple, the third career being the family, within a tradition of work being valued as domestic life is marginalized. Fran's conclusion at the end of the second session sums up the message of therapy: "I guess what it means is that we will both have to do everything and that feels OK."

REFERENCES

Coontz, S. (1992). *The way we never were*. New York: Basic Books.

Galinsky, E. (1999). *Ask the children*. New York: Morrow.

Hochschild, A. (1989) *The Second Shift*. New York: Avon Books.

Rubin, L. (1994). *Families on the fault line*. New York: Harper Perennial.

Tavris, C. (1992). *The mismeasure of woman*. New York: Simon and Schuster.

Walters, M., Carter, B., Papp, P., & Silverstein, O. (1988). *The Invisible Web: Gender Patterns In Family Relationships*. New York: Guilford Press.

◆ CHAPTER 3

The New Triangle

Couples and Technology

Evan Imber-Black

> Ms. Chang . . . placed a long, poetic ad in the personals section of Yahoo, the Internet service. . . .
>
> Within moments she began receiving E-mail responses, and over the next few weeks she heard from 107 people. "There were some complete sex maniacs," she said. "There were some nice, normal people. There was more than one business man who was in town for the weekend and logged in from his hotel room. None were quite right. It was like Goldilocks—too hot, too cold."
>
> Buried among the responses was one response so right it gave her goosebumps. It was Randall dean te Velde. . . . Like her, he plays the sax, places some faith in tarot cards, enjoys ballroom dancing and has a sly, intellectual writing style. . . .
>
> They began an on-line relationship that quickly became intense. "By the third E-mail, I was in love," Ms. Chang said. . . . "It was so great to have someone to share all your thoughts with, *someone you didn't even know.* We likened it to having someone to confide in behind a dark screen."
>
> —*New York Times* (Styles section, Weddings, June 28, 1998, p. 7; italics added); copyright © 1998 by the New York Times Co.; reprinted by permission.

Marital and family therapists have a reserved front-row seat in the theater of social change. Before a trend captures the media's attention, we begin to see its impact on the intimate lives of the couples with whom we work. In recent years, the influence of technology on couple's relationships has entered our consulting rooms. Personal computers, laptops, e-mail, the Internet, cell phones, call-waiting, call-forward-ing, caller ID, fax machines, 160-channel television—all these and more have begun to challenge and reshape couples' mutual communication, their search for meaning, experience of time, choices for leisure activi-ties, daily rituals, boundaries between work and family life, parent–child interaction, and critical definitions of secrecy and privacy. And all of this is being played out in a context in which intergenerational maps are of little use—our parents may have watched Ralph and Alice Kramden or Lucy and Ricky Ricardo, but the screen was 10 inches, not 40, and a test pattern forced them to turn the TV off at 10 P.M. Our grandparents wrote letters, not e-mail, and waited an hour for the oper-ator to connect their long-distance call.

VOICES FROM "TECHNO-LAND"

In the past 2 or 3 years I began to hear a new set of issues from the couples I was working with in therapy. Recent developments in technology were entering their lives with a speed faster than our capacity to think through their impact on relationships. For many of these couples, the therapy arena would be the first place to take a careful look at this new triangle, a triangle comprising each member of a couple and the technology in their lives. Here are some snapshots from recent therapy sessions:

> "I called Sheila 14 times in 40 minutes," Sam complained in our third marital therapy session. "We have 'call-waiting'—there's simply no excuse for her not to have picked up my call. I'm abso-lutely furious that she wouldn't respond to me when I wanted her to."
>
> "The call-waiting was his idea in the first place," Sheila re-torted. "We put it in when his mother was ill, and his family felt he needed to be instantly available. My mother-in-law's been well for over a year. I hate being interrupted by the call-waiting when I'm talking to someone. And I hate that I have to be instantly available. I want to get rid of it, but Sam refuses."

> "My husband, Kevin, drags in every night at 8 o'clock. He used to say hello to me," Sandra said sadly. "Now he heads straight to his study. First he listens to his answering machine, then he checks his e-mail and reads his faxes. He wolfs down his dinner and then disappears to his computer for the rest of the night. I'm a 'technology widow' and I'm tired of it."

✳ Kevin had sent me a fax just prior to this first session, stating that he was too busy to attend and would "catch up" the following week.

"I woke up at 3 A.M. to find that Carolyn was gone from our bed," Peter began in our first marital therapy session. "A small light was on in our den. I found my wife at the computer, writing intimate messages to a man she's never met."

"It's all just a fantasy," Carolyn responded. "I'm bored—the Internet eases my boredom. I wish he'd get over it."

"We've both been looking at pornography on the Internet," James remarked. "Sara liked it at first, but now she wants to stop. Quite frankly, I think it spices up our sex life, which goodness knows we need."

"I was so embarrassed," Ellen exclaimed. "Embarrassed and furious. It was our first night out together in months. I got tickets to one of the best shows in town. Twenty minutes into the first act, his damn cell phone started to ring. And James actually sat there and answered it! Everyone around us was telling him to be quiet. Just once I want to go out and have him leave that stupid phone at home."

"I know it was wrong to stay in my seat and talk," James responded. "I heard the phone ring, and I just forgot where I was. What she refuses to get is that I was in the middle of an important business deal—I can't just turn the phone off."

"I checked his caller ID one night after work," Steven began. "I saw that Andrew had four calls from his former lover. I'm sort of sorry I snooped. I think I would have rather not known, but the caller ID was there, and I couldn't resist."

"To me, it's like he read my mail," Andrew said. "He violated my privacy. It's my apartment. He had no right to check on who called me."

"My husband, Alan, and my 11-year-old son, Jake, spend all of their free time at the computer. They've even made their own webpage—whatever that is," Donna protested. "I don't understand how any of it works, and I really don't want to. I'm also tired of all of our money going for more and more computer equipment. Every time I turn around something new has come into the house. There's no room for me in their relationship with those damn machines."

"I've tried and tried to show Donna how to get involved with us, but she refuses," Alan replied. "Jake has learning disabilities, but he adores the computer. Why can't she see that and stop being so jealous?"

WHO'S IN CHARGE?—PEOPLE OR TECHNOLOGY?

Several key areas for inquiry in couple therapy emerge from these illustrations concerning couples' engagement with the technological revolution of our time. Many couples in therapy speak about the technology that has entered their lives and their homes in terms that sound as if the technology is in charge of them, rather than vice versa. One role for couple therapists as we approach the 21st century is to help couples to address their relationship to technology and to consider its impact on their lives.

Technology in Daily Life

During the assessment phase at the beginning of any couple's therapy, I always explore the couple's typical day, searching for repeating interactional patterns: areas of conflict, proximity, and distance; and meaningful rituals. In addition, I now routinely ask about the place of technology in their lives. Unless technology has become a central source of their arguments or interpersonal pain, most couples will not include in their description of their lives all of the ways that technology affects their relationship. How much time is spent, for instance, reading or composing e-mail at home? Does this take too much time away from face-to-face conversation by the couple?

Who uses the Internet and when? Is the Internet a useful source of information for a household, or has it become a place where one member of a couple retreats every evening until long past the time his or her partner has gone to bed? Has what began as a tool to monitor stocks, pay bills, and do on-line banking become, as with one couple who came to therapy, a nightly 3-hour activity for a husband while a wife seethes with a sense of neglect?

Questions and conversation in therapy about whether the presence of three televisions, two computers, and a home fax machine have eroded or enhanced a couple's relationship offer an opportunity to begin a reflective process about the place of technology in any couple's daily life.

Of course, while technology can be a source of stress for couples and families, it can also be an important daily source of support. It can offer new ways to solve old problems. For instance, for couples who live far away from their extended families, e-mail enables connection with the extended family in ways that enhance support for a couple. I have worked with couples who regularly e-mail their grown siblings whom they might see only once or twice a year. Grandparents and grandchildren are increasingly staying connected across computer networks. These electronic relationships can provide important affiliations for couples and their children.

Technology and the Boundary between Work and Family

The explosive growth of home computers linked to offices has radically shifted the boundary between work and family. A home office (or, often with two-career couples, *two* home offices) can either obliterate the boundary between work and family (Fraenkel, 1998), eating into couple and family time in ways that would have been unheard of a decade ago, or it can open new possibilities for reorganizing the relationship between office and home in positive ways. I have worked with couples for whom a home office has meant that work never stops. Here it is important to sort out what are the realistic—although almost always unreasonable—demands of a corporate structure that a decade ago might have required long hours at work and now requires these same long hours on site and more hours in the home setting, and what are the alternatives for a spouse when retreating to the home office is truly not necessary. Often, a couple will polarize: he insists that his career demands that he spend 4 hours a night at the computer, while she believes he's using the computer to put distance between them. By the time they come to therapy, some part of each of these positions are probably true. It's important to facilitate a thorough and frank conversation about the meaning of work and career advancement in their lives, while helping the couple to be allies in this examination. A therapist's questions regarding career and financial goals, intergenerational beliefs about the connection between work and marital relationships, and values in the wider culture will help couples sort out how much work time at home fits who they truly want to be as individuals, as a couple, and as a family.

On the other hand, home computers and fax machines can be put to good use to enhance family functioning, creating a flexible boundary between work and home. Because gender roles have changed, more and more fathers want to take a larger parenting role in the lives of their children. I have coached expectant parents to use the presence of a home office to negotiate with their employers so that a new father could telecommute 2 days a week during the first year of his baby's life, thus enabling a parenting involvement that would otherwise be impossible.

Technology and Daily Rituals

Daily rituals in many couples' lives have been impacted powerfully by technology. Participating in daily rituals tells couples over and over again who they are to each other in ways that are reliable. Such rituals help define a boundary between a couple and the outside world, between home and work. A couple's relationship may be continually evoked without words through the repetition of familiar daily rituals (Imber-Black & Roberts, 1998). The young wife in one couple who came to therapy sadly remarked during our first session that a meaningful evening ritual of tea and talking together had simply disappeared after her husband installed a new satellite dish that brought every possible sports event into their living room. In another couple, a husband complained bitterly that his wife, a successful stockbroker, insists on bringing her cell phone along when they go out for a Friday-night dinner—ironically, a ritual originally initiated by him to give them some time alone together in their hectic lives.

At least 65% of American families no longer sit down for an evening meal together (Imber-Black & Roberts, 1998). The disappearance of this daily ritual has been hastened by our overly busy lives, extended work days, and the intrusion of all manner of technology in the home.

Conversation in couple therapy about daily rituals allows couples to begin to think through whether they want to create a boundary around dinner time that excludes television or telephone. Putting technology to use rather than allowing it to rule relationships means, for instance, that phone calls can be picked up by an answering machine while a couple or family share some protected time.

Technology can also be used to create new and meaningful daily rituals. I worked with one two-career couple who had become estranged due to their hectic and overly busy lives. Earlier in their marriage, they had talked on the phone once a day at an agreed-upon time, but this ritual had become impossible in their current work settings. I asked them if they could imagine any ways to use the vast technology in each of their offices to connect once a day. Together, they created a new daily ritual of leaving one another an endearing afternoon e-mail message, thereby turning the available technology into a method of connection.

How Did the Technology Enter a Couple's Life?

Many couples talk about the technology in their lives as if it were a living, breathing entity that simply decided, unbidden, to take up residence in their home. When one couple sat and reflected with me about how a now troublesome call-waiting system made its way onto their telephone line, the wife said, "You know, the phone company offered it for free for 3 months when we moved into our new house. Until this moment, I never thought about how the marketing of all these gadgets just brings them into our home, and we forget that we have some choice about what we really want."

When I inquire about how decisions get made regarding what technology to bring into a couple's life, I am left with the sense that the available technology is driving them, rather than their being proactive about what to select. Whatever is newer, speedier, or trendier necessarily shows up in their household. In one therapy conversation on this topic, a couple decided to review all the technology in their lives on an annual basis in order to determine what they truly wanted and needed, what was no longer necessary, what perhaps had come into their lives due to marketing pressures or without careful thought, and what, if any, new items they might like to try.

In some couples, one partner seems to make all the decisions about what new piece of equipment the household must have. One young woman began our first couple session angrily telling me that her fiancé had bought her a tiny cell phone for Valentine's Day when what she really wanted was a romantic bottle of perfume. He, in turn, expressed bewilderment that she didn't want this newest, lightest, smallest phone that she could carry in her purse. As this anecdote suggests, communication about who decides to buy the new computer, install the second telephone line, or bring the fax machine into the bedroom can lead to significant conversation about other decisions, including money, allocation of resources, and time commitments.

Neo-Luddites versus Technocrats

Differing viewpoints regarding experiences with technology can lead to sharp polarizations in couples. Often one member of a couple becomes devoted to increasing the presence and use of all that technology has to offer, while the other partner is less involved. What might begin simply as a difference in interests can all too quickly become diametrically opposed positions. Characterizations of "neo-Luddites" versus "technocrats" take the place of meaningful conversation about the desired place of technology in individual and couple life.

Therapy needs to help couples get beyond the often stuck and escalating polarization about the place of technology in their lives to a level of deeper meanings.

In one family I worked with, a father, Jeff, and his 11-year-old son, Kyle, spent all their free time on the computer. In a somewhat typical systemic process, the more the mother, Sara, complained, the more Jeff and Kyle found new and exciting reasons to use the computer. As we talked, it became apparent that the technology, which Sara didn't understand, contributed to her feeling ignorant, a feeling she had, in fact, struggled with long before the computer joined their household. She was an artist who came from a family where her father was an engineer who denigrated her talents and showed interest only in her scientifically inclined brother. Sara experienced her husband and son's close relationship, facilitated by their passion for the computer, as a replication of her father's closer relationship with her brother. Unpacking these earlier experiences and their meanings in the present helped shift the family conversation from an escalating argument about computers to a far more important conversation about the kind of relationships they wanted with one another. As Jeff began to give Sara what she truly needed from him—validation for her talents and her creative contributions to their marriage and family—so Sara grew far less defensive about learning what the computer might, in fact, have to offer her. Gradually, she allowed Kyle to teach her how to use his computer. I coached her about the possibility of surprising both Jeff and Kyle by taking a computer graphic arts course. When we ended therapy, Sara was teaching Jeff and Kyle some of her newfound knowledge.

Speedier Is Not Necessarily Better

The new technology has impacted the ways that we experience time (see Chapter 4, "Clocks, Calendars, and Couples"). Demands for immediate interpersonal responses and constant availability arise from the presence of technology in our lives. One woman threatened to divorce her husband when he didn't respond to her beeper, until she discovered that the satellite that controls beepers went out for the day (*New*

York Times, May 20, 1998, p. A1). Since authentic couple interaction and reliable relationship building require a process of getting to know one another over time, the expectation of instantaneous replies bred by cell phones, e-mail, faxes, and the like, can prevent deeper and more reflective conversation. I often remind clients that while microwave ovens are great for quick meals and warming over leftovers, they seldom produce the creative, gourmet repasts that sustain us and build memories.

When I meet with individuals or couples who bring a sense of impatience to their every interaction, I no longer assume that they learned this impatience in their own family of origin. Rather, we look together at the many ways that technology has changed their expectations concerning the time that responses from partners and children should take. Couples therapy should be a place to challenge the cultural assumption that faster is necessarily better.

Technology and Parenting

Technology has a powerful and often unacknowledged impact on relationships between parents and children. Young children today are often computer wizards, and may know more than their parents about the Internet, modems, and complex computer programs. It is important that technology be employed as a resource, and not be allowed to drive a wedge between the generations. I have worked in therapy with parents who are so intimidated by their children's superior knowledge in the area of technology that I need to remind them that they still have the right to decide what is good for their children, whether it comes into their home via the television or by the Internet.

In a two-parent family, when one parent is far more interested than the other in all that cyberspace has to offer, then time, activities, and relationships with their children can begin to be shaped by this mutual enthusiasm, which may put the other parent at a distance. Therapy may be the place to examine both the benefits and the costs of the new technology to parent–child relationships, and, in turn, how these benefits and costs affect a couple.

While all of the foregoing suggested areas for exploration in couple therapy begin with a focus on the specific content of technology, they lead us, as with all content areas in systemic work, to an examination of interpersonal process, the elaboration of core themes across time, an increased tolerance for difference between members of a couple, and the development of shared meanings.

SEX AND THE INTERNET

The Internet is expected to reach 75–80% of the American population within the next few years. Perhaps it comes as no surprise that sex is the most searched-for topic on the Internet (Quinn, 1998). There are presently some 70,000 sex-related websites, accounting for a sizable amount of the $4 billion U.S. adult entertainment industry. In circular fashion, the demand for sex via the Internet has led to computer innovations such as the better delivery of high-quality images and secure credit card systems, leading in turn to more sex-related Internet sites (Swartz, 1998). Intriguing gender differences are evident in the fact that the majority of men who visit on-line sex sites prefer sites that include visual erotica rather than chat rooms, while the majority of women prefer chat rooms rather than visual erotica ("Numbers," 1998, p. 23).

The availability of cybersex has generated a new problem in couple therapy: "Internet infidelity." Ranging from brief, fleeting fantasies fueled by role-play in chat rooms, to ongoing and daily electronic conversations between two people who contact one another with urgency, to mutual masturbation with an on-line lover, to a decision to shift a virtual affair to an actual one, Internet infidelity is most often a *secret* activity that one spouse keeps from the other.

The Internet allows us to communicate with untold numbers of faceless others. In previous generations, children wrote a secret on paper, put the note in a bottle, and then cast it into the sea, never knowing if anyone would find or read it and never expecting an answer. In our computer culture, a marital partner can send a secret note out to a multitude of anonymous possible recipients, and some of them will probably write back. Communication with strangers via the Internet creates a context of secrecy. Indeed, on-line communication per se is a solitary activity. One can reveal shameful secrets to a stranger, make up sensational stories, explore pornography, create a fantasy life—all the while keeping such on-line explorations a secret from one's spouse. But when a net-surfing lover is discovered by his or her mate, a predictable marital crisis ensues that often brings the couple to therapy.

Making Sense of an Internet Affair

"I never thought we'd be coming to a marital therapist, and certainly not for something like this," Alan remarked with bewilderment. This was the first session of marital therapy with Alan, 47, and Elinor, 46, a therapy that would last 10 months and take us from a crisis over cybersex to the interior of a 16-year marriage whose intergenerational themes and current conflicts ultimately played out on a technological tightrope.

"When I first discovered last year that Elinor was using our computer for 'sexual encounters,' I was totally shocked," Alan declared. Elinor sat with her head in her hands, tears streaming down her face as Alan continued. "She said she was lonely because I was traveling so much. She promised never to do it again, and I believed her. We put it behind us and agreed never to speak of it again. Then last week I came home early from a trip, and there she was at the computer. She quickly turned it off when she saw me, and I knew she was doing it again. I just feel so betrayed. I don't know if I can get over it this time."

Slowly Elinor raised her head and began to speak. "I think I'm as confused as Alan over this. I don't know what any of it means. I just know I was so tired of being alone in the house with my 5-year-old twins while Alan jets all over the world for his work. I think it all began as a way to have some company in my life, and then it all just got a lot more complicated. What I feel the worst about is that I promised Alan last year that I wouldn't do it again, and I broke my word. I'm not that kind of person. I want my marriage and I want Alan to trust me again."

Alan and Elinor were a white, upper-middle-class couple who were at a point in their marriage when many issues needed to be renegotiated. Alan was a high-powered lawyer, a partner in a successful and demanding law firm. He traveled about 25% of the time. Elinor was also a lawyer, but she had put her career on hold when she became pregnant with twins through *in vitro* fertilization after several years of grueling fertility treatment. "We got the Internet when we were trying to get pregnant. It was a terrific source of information," Alan remarked. "What started out as our friend has ended up as my enemy," Alan continued, personifying the computer as if it were a member of their social network.

This couple had married just as both were beginning their careers. During the early part of their marriage, they had spent little time building their relationship. Many parts of their lives were separate, including bank accounts, friendships, and visits to their extended families, who lived in different parts of the country. They had worked well together on the pragmatics related to fertility treatments, but they had not shared the deep emotional distress of infertility with each other. Rather, Alan kept all his feelings to himself, and Elinor e-mailed her sister daily for support.Shortly after the twins were born, Alan received a job offer that required them to move across the country. In a mode that had become quite common in their marriage, they talked over all of the practical aspects of the move and none of the affective elements. Elinor's resentment at leaving her close friends went underground. Her enormous loneliness and lack of confidence as an isolated new mother of twins in a suburb where she knew no one went unmentioned by her and unnoticed by Alan. Her daily e-mails to her sister gradually evolved into visits to chat rooms. Over time, she found herself revealing her most intimate thoughts and feelings to total strangers. And one night while Alan was out of town, Elinor began an electronic relationship with a man that started with an exchange of kindness and led rapidly to an on-line "love affair."

"I had no intention of ever meeting this man," Elinor insisted. "It was exciting and fun. I only wrote to him when Alan was out of town. I could be anyone I wanted to be. I could pour out everything I felt about my life. I could imagine a different life and pretend it was happening. I never meant to harm Alan, and when he found out last year and was so upset I promised to stop. I stopped for a while, and then one day I just got curious again, and began writing to someone else. It's not like I was unfaithful. It wasn't even with a real person. At least that's how I see it."

In our third session, Alan remarked that he came close to throwing the computer out of the house. "If it's not there, I won't think about this so much, and she won't be tempted." I told Alan that thinking about what happened to them was not a bad thing, framing Elinor's on-line "affair" as a signal that many aspects of their marriage were no longer working for them. I also suggested that removing the computer would not rebuild trust, but rather would nail down the idea that Elinor couldn't be trusted.

My work with Alan and Elinor focused initially on this crisis and all that it meant in terms of the kind of marriage they had constructed. The beginning of our marital therapy was frightening for them, as this was the first time in their marriage that each spouse was able to be emotionally open and vulnerable. Elinor expressed surprise that her Internet infidelity had hurt Alan so deeply. In turn, Alan was stunned to find out that Elinor believed she didn't matter to him very much. Three months into the therapy, as we began a process centering primarily on how little time they had spent together for many years, how estranged they had become, and how they needed to build an intimate connection, our work took a surprising turn.

"Alan says he can't get over what I've done," Elinor tearfully began our tenth session. "I've felt so optimistic this last month. We've been talking in ways that we've never talked. Alan's been coming home for dinner with the twins and me. I thought we were putting this incident behind us. Then this weekend he said he doesn't know if he'll ever be able to trust me."

As I talked with Alan that day, he said he was haunted by the fact that Elinor had kept a secret from him. "I do believe her when she says it's over, and I don't really think it'll happen again because of all that's changing between us. But how do I know for sure?" Alan said with a sigh. "Why did she have to keep a secret from me?" I asked Alan what his experience with secrets had been before he ever met Elinor. Tears flooded Alan's eyes and he started to tremble. After several silent minutes, Alan told a story he had never spoken.

"When I was a kid, I was always being shuttled out of the house, told to go play outside. That would be just before my parents would have a roaring fight. By the time I came back, my father would have stormed off and my mother would be in tears. He often stayed gone overnight. I never knew what it was all about. I just knew there was never enough money, even though my dad had a good job. Two years ago, right after my dad's funeral, my older sister told me that he had been a compulsive gambler. I never knew, but it all makes sense now." Filled with shame, Alan had not confided in Elinor when he discovered the truth about his father. "He just grew more distant after his dad's death," Elinor remarked sadly. "He worked even longer hours, and I turned to the Internet."

I questioned Alan about the experience of being a child who knew something terrible was going on in his family, but could never find out what it was. Like many children who grow up knowing secrets are being kept from them, he was filled with pervasive and unattended to anxiety (Imber-Black, 1998). He learned to hunker down, not ask, not pay conscious attention to the emotional turmoil around him. When Alan married Elinor, their pragmatic marital contract seemed to work for him, until her secret computer affair unleashed all that he had hidden for so many years. The depth of Alan's feelings about a secret being kept from him now made a different kind of sense.

This session proved to be a turning point in our work. Alan became able to separate the impact of secrets in his childhood from Elinor's previously secret computer activities. At this juncture, I urged Elinor to spend less time talking about how guilty she felt and more time looking at what her computer affair might have been telling her about what she needed to do in her life. She had presented herself on-line as a woman with a thriving and creative career in the arts. It turned out she had never really wanted to be a lawyer, and had become one because her parents believed a fine arts degree would be worthless. As we ended therapy, Elinor applied to a master's program in museum arts administration. She also revealed a steamy, passionate side of herself to her on-line "lover," a side she had never unveiled to Alan until now. Their marriage changed profoundly from one marked by distance, silence, and practicalities to a relationship that included personal conversation, time together, and emotional and sexual intimacy.

Alan and Elinor are among several couples I have seen in the last few years whose entry into therapy is precipitated by Internet infidelity. Just as a given couple must struggle with the meanings of an on-line affair in a context without historical precedent, so today's couple therapists must begin to create effective ways to work with this new phenomenon. Presently, our own biases that any meaningful relationship development requires face-to-face contact may prevent us from hearing what an Internet relationship means to a participant. The immediate relevance of physical attraction is, in fact, removed in an electronic relationship. Physical appearance, eye contact, voice tone, and nonverbal behavior are all missing in on-line affairs (Lea & Spears, 1995). Our beliefs in the critical importance of these dimensions in relationship building are now put in question as we discover more about a form of communication that relies on disembodied words and mutual fantasies. Our challenge as couples therapists is to use what we already know about relationships, while remaining open to our clients' experiences in ways that do not force them into preexisting and potentially nonrelevant categories. For instance, the current primary approach to Internet affairs is to subsume them under the category of "addiction" (Young, 1998). Doing so can easily cause important complexities to be missed. Computer-mediated communication can allow exploration of both sexual and nonsexual fantasies. Elinor's wish to develop a different work life along with her need to have a closer and more emotionally connected relationship appeared in highly disguised form in her computer affair. Our work together in therapy examined what parts of these fantasies she truly wanted to make real.

CONCLUSIONS

Tiny computer chips have permanently altered our lives in ways that are obvious and will continue to change them in ways that we cannot yet imagine. Contemporary couple therapy can be a safe container to hold and transform the unanticipated pain of untamed technology. Couple therapists can create a venue to enable spouses to make conscious and informed decisions about the desired role of technology in their lives and their relationships.

REFERENCES

Fraenkel, P. (1998, February). The time crunch. *Parent Guide*, pp. 14–15.

Imber-Black, E. (1998). *The secret life of families: Truth-telling, privacy, and reconciliation in a tell-all society.* New York: Bantam.

Imber-Black, E., & Roberts, J. (1998). *Rituals for our time: Celebrating, healing, and changing our lives and our relationships.* New York: Aronson.

Lea, M., & Spears, R. (1995) Love at first byte? Building personal relationships over computer networks. In J. T. Wood & S. Duck (Eds.), *Under-studied relationships: Off the beaten track* (pp. 197–233). Thousand Oaks, CA: Sage.

"Numbers." (1998, June 22). *Time*, p. 23.

Quinn, A.(1998, March 19). U.S. web site poll to investigate cybersex. *Reuters News Service.*

Swartz, J. (1998, April 16). Surveyor of cybersex. *San Francisco Chronicle*, p. D3.

Young, K. (1998). *Caught in the net: How to recognize the signs of computer addiction and a winning strategy for recovery.* New York: Wiley.

CHAPTER 4

Clocks, Calendars, and Couples

Time and the Rhythms of Relationships

Peter Fraenkel
Skye Wilson

Time is one of the most powerful and yet largely unrecognized influences on the quality and organization of couples' lives) With an ever-increasing number of couples describing frantic, pressured lives, the contemporary couple therapist has many reasons to tune in to the temporal aspect of couples' lives and difficulties. For couples in distress, time-related problems—for example, differences in pace, mismatched daily schedules, different preferences for amount of time spent together versus apart, or one partner's annoyance at the other's chronic lateness—may be one of the explicit reasons they seek therapy. For others, problems in the temporal organization or patterning of their lives may underlie other problems, such as difficulty achieving intimacy, a lack of trust, or poor communication.

Consider the following brief vignettes of couples in therapy.[1] How is time involved in their problems?

Margaret, 39, and Fred, 38, both academics, had been friends before they became romantically involved. Two years later, Margaret, who wanted to have children, began suggesting that they move in together and think about getting married. At the time, Fred responded that he didn't feel ready; he was considering further graduate studies, and couldn't imagine beginning these studies, married life, and a family at the same time. It is now 4 years since they first became involved, and Margaret argues that it is time for Fred to "grow up," stop being a student, and assume adult responsibilities. She describes anxiety about her "biological clock" ticking, while Fred argues that if having children was so important to Margaret, she should have found someone else, angrily rejecting her implication that he is depriving her of children. The couple is deadlocked: the more Margaret insists on her vision of their future, the more Fred holds to his current plans.

Bill, a 40-year-old hospital administrator, and Mary Lou, a 38-year-old accountant, had been living together for 14 months and were considering marriage, the second for both. They were troubled by the frequency and intensity of their arguments over every aspect of maintaining the house. Bill took much longer to complete chores and "fix-it" tasks, although he always completed them and took pride in his results. In contrast, Mary Lou typically started her chores immediately and worked extremely rapidly. Each believed the other's pace reflected the other's lack of commitment to doing a good job: Bill saw Mary Lou's speediness as sloppiness; Mary Lou saw Bill as a "tinkerer" who dragged out tasks because he resented doing them.

Cecile, 26, and Tom, 27, both from wealthy families and each working for their own families' companies, describe themselves as having a passionate relationship and plan to marry. However, they describe frequent fights about when to go to bed. Cecile likes to take each evening as it comes, going to bed early if she feels like it, staying up late if the spirit moves her. Tom, on the other hand, believes strongly in adhering to a specific bedtime and waking time, and gets extremely tense and irritated when Cecile pushes him to change their bedtime. As the couple talks more, it appears this difference extends to other areas, such as plans for the weekend: Tom likes to schedule things in advance; Cecile likes a more spontaneous approach. Each attributes the other's preferences to negative personality characteristics: Cecile sees Tom as uptight and "anal," while Tom sees Cecile as irresponsible and "flighty." Cecile wants to "go with the flow"; Tom wants "to take charge of [his] destiny."

We contend that a core issue for all of these couples is how they handle time, and how the partners experience each other from the perspective of time. The first couple struggles with being "out-of-sync" in terms of what we call "projected life chronologies" or "personal timelines," what the partners would like to be doing now and how that relates to their imagined and planned futures. The second couple struggles with differences in each partner's pace or speed of doing things, which leads each partner to attribute negative intentions to the other's behavior. In the third couple, each partner feels quite differently about the need for regularity in schedules, for future planning versus living in the moment—a difference in what we call "time perspective"—and for monitoring how they use time: "going with the flow" versus being accountable to every minute.

The purpose of this chapter is to provide therapists with a way of thinking about time as a key issue for couples. We do not believe that therapists need entirely new sets of practices or techniques to work with time issues. Rather, in work with couples and time, our most common tools have been tried-and-true ones: detailed identification of here-and-now patterns and themes; exploration of the links between current patterns and sensitivities, experiences, and beliefs based in family of origin and culture of origin; and collaborative problem solving that allows couples to construct and experience new realities (Fraenkel, 1994, 1996, 1997; see also Papp & Imber-Black, 1996, for an approach to couple therapy that exemplifies our ways of working). A major purpose of our current research—in which we interview couples and families about the types of issues they have with time and the approaches they have found successful in solving them—is to develop new approaches to intervention that are based not on theory or therapist expertise but on what has actually worked for couples.

As well as being a source of problems, the dimension of time can be a powerful resource for change. In many cases, by helping couples identify and address the "time side" of their difficulties and the temporal demands impinging on them from the larger system, therapists can help partners move from "head-to-head" conflict—in which problems are attributed to each other's negative characteristics—to a "side-by-side" position in which partners work as a team to overcome a shared challenge. For some couples, this involves recognizing the power of contextual factors that limit or structure time in ways that negatively affect the relationship, and then joining together to change these factors.

As a simple example, one distressed couple in which the partners felt extremely disconnected from and critical of each other was surprised to find how much these feelings decreased once they each committed to spending 2 evenings a week together, during which time they agreed not to return phone calls or worry about the next day's schedule. It turned out that behind the irritation each felt toward the other lay intense loneliness. Having taken the first step toward reconnecting in time, they now realized they could talk about how much they missed each other.

For other couples, relief comes from recognizing how the same temporal differences that sometimes cause conflict also serve positive, complementary functions in the relationship. For instance, although Bill and Mary Lou's pace difference around household chores led to conflict, in other areas of their lives their pace difference enhanced their relationship and their appreciation of each other. For instance, on vacations Mary Lou benefited from Bill's predilection to take it "slow and easy," so that they always began and ended their trips with some "down time" by a lake or beach. Concomitantly, Bill took pleasure from Mary Lou's tendency to seek faster paced activities, which led them to do things like take a high-speed boat trip, go on rides at an amusement park, and visit three museums in a day (a practice they called "speed-viewing"). Once I (as the therapist) pointed out the fundamental difference in their paces, noted how this difference had resulted in mutual misapprehension about chores, and helped them see how this pace difference worked for them in many ways, the partners had a wider frame within which to understand their relationship and to anticipate, explain, and resolve problems.

We begin by identifying aspects of contemporary life that affect couples' time. We will discuss the impact of work, technology, the demands of larger systems agencies, multiple caretaking responsibilities, biological and health factors, divorce and remarriage, and culture and family of origin. Two of these factors—work and technology—are currently drawing increasing attention to time as a critical but seemingly ever-shrinking resource for maintaining the quality of intimate relations. We move next to a general theory of time in couples that is useful in clinical work as a guide to assessment and treatment. Clinical vignettes will be used to illustrate key theoretical points. We end with further clinical vignettes that illustrate creative use of time as a resource for change.

THE GROWING AWARENESS OF TIME
AND ITS CHALLENGES

Despite, or maybe because of, the "ever-presentness" of time as an element of relationships, social scientists and therapists have paid relatively little attention to how time affects the lives of couples. Certain events in the life of many couples have long been known to require major adjustments in how time is managed and experienced—for instance, the transition to parenthood (Belsky, Spanier, & Rovine,1983), children entering school, the retirement of one or both partners. Yet as we head into the new millennium, changing social and economic realities have increased the awareness of both professionals and laypersons about the powerful impact of time on relationships. As has been the case with other resources, such as space, money, energy, or a clean environment, awareness of how essential a resource is increases when there is (or at least seems to be) less of it, and this concern now appears to be the case with time. In fact, some have called time "the most precious resource" (Lagerfeld, 1998, p. 60) and the commodity of the 1990s (Markman, Stanley, & Blumberg, 1994). Because of certain trends in our culture, time is likely to become seemingly even more sparse and therefore more valuable, in the 21st century. Even now there is a growing sense that we have less and less time in which to conduct our complex lives. The notions of "time scarcity" (Pronovost, 1989) or "time famine" (Daly, 1996; Hochschild, 1997) have permeated professional and public discourse (Daly, 1996; Galinsky, 1996; McGuire, 1999), prompting numerous theories to explain this sense of diminished time, the sense of increased time pressures and of a frenetic pace of life, of fragmented, complicated schedules, and other signs of a subjective sense that there is a shortage of time (Daly, 1996; Fraenkel, 1994; Hochschild, 1997).

The Impact of Work on Relationship Time

The harried pace of work life, complex and often mismatched work schedules of partners, increased commuting times, prolonged periods of physical separation due to long work hours, and the rise of business travel—all these and more affect partners' amount and quality of time together, creating new challenges for couples in how they get "in sync" so as to sustain intimacy and shared enjoyment, raise families, solve problems, and build a life together. In addition, the continued imbalance between men and women in the division of labor around child care and the household can be exacerbated by the temporal pressures of work. Thus, when couples describe feeling distant, having heated arguments and poor communication, sexual difficulties, or other common couple concerns, it is important for therapists to inquire about the partners' temporal patterns of work, as these constitute one of the most powerful contextual forces giving form to their relationship. By the time couples come to therapy, they may have lost sight of the degree to which larger systems issues of work pressures and schedules—over which they may experience little control—may play a part in their distress. By inquiring about the interface between work time and relationship time, the therapist can help warring partners become allies by viewing their problems in terms of the larger context. The therapist may also need to help partners recognize their right to stand up to the often insidious, unreasonable demands of work, and to assist them to develop joint plans and strategies to "take back the time" for their relationship and their families.

Impact of Hours Worked

An overall trend toward spending more hours at work has been the single most powerful factor leading to the sense of diminished time for couple and family relationships. Over the past 20 years, across socioeconomic classes, there has been an increase in time devoted to work (Schor, 1991) and a decline in leisure time, resulting in a "time squeeze" (Leete & Schor, 1994). One national study found that about half of workers report working more than a 40-hour week; almost one-fifth report working 50 hours a week or more; and 18% report working more than 5 days per week (Galinsky, Bond, & Friedman, 1993). A "part-time" job now often involves working 35 to 40 hours per week (Abelson, 1998). Compared with those working 40 hours or less, those working longer hours generally report more job autonomy and control over their schedules, but have more demanding and hectic jobs (Galinsky et al., 1993). And the demandingness/hecticness of one's job—essentially, the *pace* at which one must get things done, another temporal aspect of life—is significantly associated with job burnout, negative spillover from job to home, stress, and a sense of one's inability to cope effectively (Lagerfeld, 1998). What is the impact of all this work time on relationships? Simply stated, "The majority of workers do not feel they have enough time with their spouse/partner and/or their children" (Galinsky, 1996, p. 7). And this sense of not enough time with family directly relates to the number of hours worked.[2]

In another study (Families and Work Institute, 1995), a nationally representative sample of women indicated that their "greatest family concern" was the family not having enough time together—this despite both men and women defining "success at home" as having time together with the family. Galinsky (1996) writes, "These findings provide further evidence that individuals in the U.S. experience a time famine" (p. 10).

Of course, the impact of long work hours affects couples gay or straight, with or without children. A gay couple, Roger, 32, a corporate lawyer, and Tim, 30, an actor and waiter, came to therapy because of what they described as "trust issues." Tim had engaged in a number of casual sexual affairs, all while Roger was working late. Roger was devastated. Tim states that he loves Roger and is quite committed to the relationship, but complains that he gets frustrated "waiting around" for Roger to come home from work every night. Roger bitterly counters that he provides the bulk of the couple's financial support, and that if Tim worked a regular job Tim would be more understanding of the pressures under which he lives. In this couple, Tim felt less powerful than Roger, and distanced by him, largely because Roger's work schedule affected the regularity and amount of their time together; Tim attempted to redress this power difference and his loneliness by going outside the relationship for intimacy.

Impact of Different Schedules Due to Work

The challenges posed to couples by the sheer number of work hours of one or both partners, and by the need to "downshift" from the fast pace of work life to the slower pace of relationships, are increased by the reality that the *daily schedules* of both partners often may not coincide (Daly, 1996; Hochschild, 1989; Rowe & Bentley, 1992). Schedule disjunctions may occur in both single-earner and dual-earner households. The most dramatic version of this occurs when one partner works a day shift (including partners whose work is child care and/or housework, typically daytime activities), and the other works a night shift. Shift workers have long been identified as being at greater risk for relationship and family difficulties (Hoffman, 1987; Voydanoff, 1988; Voydanoff & Kelly, 1984). However, sometimes it is relatively small disjunctions in schedules that separate partners enough so that they share virtually no daily activities together.

For example, in one couple seen in therapy, the husband rose at 5:30 A.M. each day so as to catch a 6:20 A.M. train to the city. His wife, who worked until 9:00 P.M. each night and often did not get home until 10:30 P.M., rose at 7:00 A.M. By the time she returned—"wired and ready to talk"—her husband, having returned home by 8:00 P.M., would typically be winding down and getting ready for bed, or even already be asleep. Although they spoke over the phone daily, they shared no meals together and essentially no time together during the week. In this case, the temporal dyssynchrony between partners was not huge—1½ hours different in the morning and 2½ hours in the evening—but it was large enough to place them in two temporally separate lives. Before implementing any other changes in their presenting problem—which they described as a lack of "sexual and emotional intimacy"—this couple needed to renegotiate and recalibrate the boundary between work and home life that preempted time together and even the *possibility* of intimacy.

These issues of schedule disjunction are likely to affect many couples, as recent statistics show that both partners work in more than half of all married couples, and the numbers are steadily increasing (Bureau of Labor Statistics, 1997a). More than 800,000 couples were added to this group in the period 1995–1997 alone. As the above clinical example demonstrates, when two persons work outside the home, and each is "entrained," or scheduled by the requirements of their workplace (as well as by the commuting times and schedules to and fro), it often becomes extraordinarily complex to arrange simple acts like conversation and meals together.[3] Even more than many single-earner couples, dual-earner families are likely to be "time poor" (Crouter & Crowley, 1990, p. 297).

One potentially positive result of this time disjunction between partners' work schedules is that it leads some fathers, either by default or by choice, to do more child care.[4] However, from the perspective of family time and couple time together, the increasing disjunction of work schedules between partners remains highly problematic.

In addition, studies of dual-earner couples have found partners struggling even harder than single-earner couples to keep a boundary between work and home life (Lewis & Cooper, 1989). Not surprisingly, dual-earner parents report that one of their most challenging issues is time management (Lewis & Cooper, 1989).

Impact of Commuting

Obviously, commuting adds to the already long work hours away from partner and family. But even worse, commuting time has increased for many people (Federal Highway Administration, 1997). In addition, the need to fit at least some chores and other family responsibilities into the workday has led commute times to be filled with increasingly complex sequences of activity—a phenomenon known as "trip chaining." A typical "trip chain" might involve bringing the children to daycare or school and dropping off dry cleaning on the way to work; and on the way back from work, picking the kids up and bringing them to play dates or lessons, shopping, and picking the kids up again to go home. Not surprisingly, because women still handle most of the home and child care responsibilities, women workers—especially mothers with small children—are "substantially more likely to link trips and to link multiple trips when they do" than are men (Rosenbloom, 1998, p. 77). The complex sequencing necessary to carry out trip chaining can add to the frantic quality of the day, resulting in exhaustion and stress that may affect the quality of the couple's interaction once they reunite in the evening. It may further contribute to resentments of wives toward husbands in couples where the burdens of trip chaining are unequally distributed.

For an increasing number of long-distance couples, the commute to and from work requires living apart some or much of the time. Work may require partners to live in separate cities, states, or countries for months or years, seeing each other only on weekends or even less frequently. These couples often "live in different temporal worlds with relatively low levels of intersection" (Daly, 1996, p. 34), creating great challenges to sustaining a sense of closeness and a shared life. Recent census reports indicate a growth of these commuter relationships, from 1.45 million in 1990 to 2.1 million in 1996.[5]

Impact of Business Travel

Numerous relationship problems can result when one or both partners regularly travel for business. Most obviously, such travel drastically reduces the amount of time partners have for each other. This issue is increasing due to the globalization of the world's economy, which in turn has led to the growing cohort of so-called frequent business travelers. These FBTs spend a significant proportion of their time far away from home—often working in several countries in as many days. As with commuter relationships, frequent business travel also may limit or entirely eliminate a sense of temporal regularity or rhythmicity in couples' lives together: rhythms of time apart versus time together, rhythms of sharing household chores, and so on. Although the work may be exciting and the potential for national or international travel may initially seem a glamorous job perk, many business travelers soon tire of the grind and accompanying separation from partners and children (Rayner, 1998).

In addition, the transitions of the traveling partner's departures and returns can be extremely stressful (Rayner, 1998): emotionally, through the repeated separations and reunifications; and logistically, in terms of the need to center the couple's life (meals, sleep schedules, sex, socializing, family time) around these transitions, as well as due to shifting back and forth from a two-partner or two-parent to a one-partner/one-parent household. For instance, struggles may occur when the traveling partner/parent expects on return to instantly reassume a position of power, decision making, or nurturance in the family—or conversely, when he or she is slow to resume this position and leaves these responsibilities to the other partner. Trust may also be difficult to maintain with frequent and long separations.

Gender Differences in Work–Family Pressures

Although the challenge of balancing work, relationship, and family is experienced by both men and women, data show that women continue to shoulder more of the burden of temporal complexity than do men (Hochschild, 1989). For instance, although men in dual-earner couples provide more child care than men who are the sole providers, women remain by far the primary caregivers, whether they also work or not (Galinsky et al., 1993). Given this role, working women may face far more tension than do men around the decision to raise children. In addition to the challenges of managing their time to include both work and child care (Hochschild, 1989), women more than men may experience a daily, jarring psychological conflict between two "senses" of time: the time frame of work and career, in which projects, goals, and promotions are laid out in a linear, stepwise, and fast-paced fashion, and the slower, cyclical time frame of child rearing, especially during the preschool years (Daly, 1996).

Regarding the division of household responsibilities, in couples in which women contribute at least 50% of the family income, men were found to do more cooking but fewer household repairs than in couples in which women contribute less than 50% of the income (Galinsky et al., 1993). As noted above, women also do much more home- and child care–related trip chaining on their commutes to and from work than do men. The gender inequity in handling child care and household responsibilities has not changed for couples in the younger, post–feminist revolution generation (Galinsky et al., 1993). Also, it is interesting to note that when women work nonday shifts, the reason most frequently cited is the need to balance child care or care for other family members (e.g., elderly parents, to be discussed shortly). Thirteen percent of women cited this as the reason for working nonday shifts, as opposed to 3% of men (Galinsky et al., 1993).

With the current increase in home-based work for both men and women (Rowe & Bentley, 1992), it is interesting to ask whether the typical gender split around work versus child care and household responsibilities is more equitable for home-based workers. Data suggest that, once again, home-based working women in single-parent and two-parent families carry out more of these family responsibilities than do home-based working men. Additionally, home-based working women make less money, are less likely to have a separate work space than are men, and do more restructuring of their time than do men (Rowe & Bentley, 1992).

Men directly face certain work-related time problems more than do women. Most notably, they are more likely to be FBTs and have generally longer commutes (Galinsky et al., 1993). However, it could be argued that these commuting problems create equal problems for women, as men's work-related absence is likely to result in even more of a gender split regarding child and home care. Clearly, although both men and women struggle and suffer with juggling work and couple/family life, working women, especially women with children, have more to juggle than do men.

The Impact of Technology on Couple Time

Over the past 20 years, the rapid development and availability of communication and information technology has had powerful effects on couples, families, and their time (Silverstone, 1993). Computers, and especially the Internet, provide a powerful, stimulating source of activities that more often separate partners than bring them together (Kraut et al., 1998). In addition, the advent of home-based personal computers and laptops, e-mail, and facsimile machines has essentially erased the physical boundary between the home and the workplace. As a result, the only boundary left between work and home (and the couple's relationship) is the *temporal boundary* set by one or both partners. The challenge of establishing and maintaining this temporal boundary is that—unlike the physical distance between the office and the home—it is essentially arbitrary, and based on a choice. When faced with a pressing deadline or a crisis at work, or when things are getting difficult in the relationship for other reasons, one partner may find it relatively easy to suspend the temporal boundary, to go online, and to get back to work. In addition, even the age-old couple's strategy of "getting away from it all" by spending a night on the town or vacationing in a geographically remote spot no longer guarantees a break from work—not as long as cell phones, long-range pagers, and laptops come along on the trip.

One couple's problems well illustrate the impact of technology on time together. Judy and Bert, both in their early 30s, came to therapy because Judy had concerns about the relationship that prevented her from agreeing to get married. She stated that they rarely had an uninterrupted evening together, and she attributed this to Bert's "boundary issues." Asked to elaborate, she noted that Bert wore his beeper at all times. He even brought it into bed—until she refused to sleep with him. Bert argued that his job required him to be on call for emergencies, especially now, during a critical period in the company's growth. Judy countered that she had spoken to the partners of some of Bert's work colleagues, and they said they had simply insisted that their partners not respond to the phone, beeper, or e-mail after a certain hour in the evening. Bert responded that his role in the company was different (he was in technical support) and required him to be more accessible. He also feared that if he set any boundaries between himself and work, he might not be considered for the next promotion. Bert also argued that Judy's schedule of writing from 11:00 P.M. until 3:00 A.M., and waking up at 10:00 A.M.—long after he'd gone off to work—was as much to blame for their lack of evenings and "quality time" as was his off-site availability to work.

In addition to decreasing the boundary between the couple and other parts of its world, the speed at which information/communication technologies operate provides both a sense of acceleration and a compression of time, as well as a powerful metaphor of speed being good and progressive and slowness being old and retrograde (Gleick, 1999). Technological acceleration has fed "an intolerance for waiting and a desire for immediate results and gratification" (Daly, 1996, p. 34). Solving complex relationship problems, getting to know one another's most intimate feelings, changing an old habit at the request of one's partner—all these tasks become more difficult in relationships guided by a speed metaphor. Electronic communication and data processing greatly outpace the speed of human emotion.

The sense of acceleration in the society at large also presents new challenges to couples as they attempt to "downshift" from the fast-paced life of work, commuting, and technology-based communication to the slower pace of human relationships. Probably at no time does this shift seem as dramatic as when a couple has their first child. Infants operate largely on biologically determined sleep–wake cycles, and require more sustained and slower paced attention as they develop their attachments to the primary caregivers. As children grow older, they are socialized to pick up the pace. Often, the plethora of afterschool activities, intertwined with parents' complex work schedules, results in an even more frenetic daily schedule. The current generation of children is the first to be raised "wired"—surrounded by advanced technology that equates speed with power and possibility. Electronic organizers, in wide use, create the impression that a limitless number of activities can be included and coordinated in a family's life. Yet "family calendars that are filled with work, lessons, and appointments create angst about 'fitting it all in.' The dominant discourse of current social time patterns is a discourse of 'crisis' that rests on the notion of an ever-increasing acceleration of time" (Pasero, 1994, quoted in Daly, 1996, p. 14). The struggle of partners to slow the pace enough to connect with each other, and for parents to connect with their children, may be one of the major challenges of our era.

The Impact of Larger Systems on Couple Time

Although the time issues posed by work and technology may affect mostly working-class to upper-class couples, working-poor or unemployed, welfare-dependent couples may experience some of these issues as well as other time problems more unique to them. For many poor couples, heightened involvement with and dependency on social service agencies and other public institutions dictates their daily and weekly schedules, the pace of life, even their ability to realistically plan for the future. In our current study of time issues for unemployed homeless families living in shelters in the South Bronx, we have heard repeatedly of the frustrations couples experience in having to dedicate hours per week to appointments with welfare workers, parole officers, and housing officials. Couples often wait weeks or months for decisions on such matters as permanent housing or changes in benefits, experiencing the pace of life as slowed to a standstill, and then may be given short notice about the need to quickly complete critical further appointments or paperwork. Failure to respond promptly to these demands or to be punctual for appointments may be followed by severe sanctions, including returning to the bottom of the list to start the application process anew. In addition, in some shelters, the strict and relatively early nightly curfew (9:00 P.M.) imposed on residents forces them inside their small units. If a couple is experiencing distress, this enforced closeness can at times escalate tensions, as partners cannot avail themselves of the adaptive option of getting some time away from each other during an argument.

The Impact of Multiple Caretaking Responsibilities on Couple Time

With an increasing number of persons living well into their 70s, 80s, and 90s, the children of these older adults are often placed in a position of caring for their parents as they raise families of their own (Miller, 1981; Neal, Chapman, Ingersoll-Dayton, & Emlen, 1993).[6] According to Daly (1996), "An analysis of the current research indicates approximately one-quarter to one-third of employees provide care to an elderly person, that most (72%) adult children caring for parents are women, and that almost half of these caregivers were parents to children under the age of eighteen living in their household" (p. 196). As members of the older generation age, they may develop chronic illnesses, need supportive housing, and have financial constraints. Along with the need to allocate financial and sometimes space resources to meet these needs, adult children typically experience an increased time crunch in tending to their parents. Daly (1996) writes, "The greatest impact of trying to manage caregiving responsibilities, paid work, family, and personal roles is with respect to time: Caregivers report that they have less time and energy available for meeting the demands of any of their roles—for work, caregiving, or themselves" (p. 196).

Because women shoulder the bulk of caregiving both for their children and the elder parents—irrespective of whether they work or not—women in particular may feel that they have little or no free time for themselves since they are constantly responding to the needs of others (Henderson & Allen, 1991). This gender difference in "caretaking time" and its greater impact on women's careers than on men's careers may breed resentment and conflict between partners (Scharlach, 1994).

The Impact of Biological and Health Factors on Couple Time

A wide range of biological and health factors can influence couple time. For instance, when one partner develops a medical condition such as a chronic illness or suffers a debilitating injury, the demands of the condition can radically reshape the pace of life (usually by slowing things down), as well as the daily schedules and time allocation of the couple. Gonzalez, Steinglass, and Reiss (1989) have noted that the lives of couples and families with a chronically ill member often become centered on that member's medical care. The rhythm of couple or family life may be structured largely by the need to attend to the ill member. Serious psychiatric disorders—for instance, major depression or bipolar disorder—may temporally pattern the life of a couple or family in ways similar to physical conditions.

The Impact of Divorce and Remarriage on Couple Time

Couples in which one or more partners have been previously married and/or had children find themselves juggling time with their children from the previous marriage, children from the current relationship, and sometimes their partner's children from a previous marriage, along with the usual struggles of balancing work and home time, and time together as a couple versus time alone (Visher & Visher, 1993). Partners may disagree around how much time to spend with whom, revealing hidden loyalty conflicts, for instance, when one partner shows greater enthusiasm for spending longer amounts of time with his or her children by a previous marriage than with the partner's children or with the partner alone.

The Impact of Beliefs from Family and Culture of Origin on Couple Time

In addition to factors that may fairly directly affect the temporal patterns of couples' lives, other factors, such as family and culture of origin, may contribute belief systems that affect the preferences and the range of options partners consider when they create the temporal patterns of their lives. As the world becomes a global community, a growing number of couple relationships are formed of partners from different cultural, racial, and ethnic backgrounds. Given that different cultures often embody quite different beliefs about time and patterns of pace, scheduling, punctuality, time perspective, and time allocation (Hall, 1983; Levine, 1997), partners coming together from different cultures may bring with them certain temporal expectations that clash with one another. In some cases, the conflicts that emerge reflect stereotyped differences between cultures; in others, the differences between partners contradict stereotypes. As in all work with culture and couples, therapists working with temporal problems in bicultural couples need to use general assumptions as no more than a starting point from which to explore the nature of each partner's understanding of and identification with his or her culture(s) of origin (Falicov, 1995). Below are three vignettes that illustrate how partners' differing family- and culture-of-origin experiences can lend widely discrepant meanings to acts such as being punctual or late, planning for the future, and structuring the use of time.

In one couple I worked with in Kenya, a temporal issue led partners who shared many other beliefs and personal attributes to recognize the vast cultural differences between them. The female partner, Grace, was Black African and the male partner, Richard, was African American. He described feeling continually frustrated with his partner's seeming indifference regarding the future: she never seemed to worry about maintaining health insurance or putting money away for the future. She explained that in her culture, the focus was on the present, and that fate and "God's will" would take care of things in the future. For her part, she was continually irritated with Richard's attempts to plan everything out in advance. Interestingly, they were Christians and had met in church, yet they interpreted their faith differently when it came to beliefs about time. As noted, Grace put her trust in God to determine the future, whereas Richard believed "God only helps those who help themselves." For Richard, who had come to Kenya in part to connect with his African roots, the stark difference in their orientation to time was one of the key experiences that led him frequently to remark, "I've realized now that I'm more Western and American than I am African."

While some partners' beliefs about time reflect the stereotypes of their cultures of origin, others' beliefs and temporal difficulties violate these stereotypes. Joseph was Italian American, the third generation of his family in the United States, whereas Alexandra was a first-generation German. Their conflicts centered around her chronic lateness to appointments and airline flights. Joseph noted with frustration that he could not understand how his wife was always so late, because he thought Germans valued punctuality. He noted further that her parents and siblings appeared to share her tendency toward lateness, which further puzzled him. He noted that, if anything, Italians were supposed to be the "laid-back" ones about time, but that he himself was typically on time.

As they explored the family-of-origin roots of each of their beliefs and practices regarding punctuality, both realized that their families had developed their respective practices regarding punctuality as part of *distinguishing* themselves from the stereotypes about their cultural groups. Alexandra's parents, who were children during the Nazi era, were deeply ashamed of much that was German, especially the "uptightness," orderliness, and efficiency that they saw linked to the attempted extermination of the Jews. One salient manifestation of this orderliness was the German emphasis on punctuality, so the parents, and then their children, made it a practice always to be a bit late and to reject worrying about being on time. Joseph's immigrant grandparents, who had their beginnings in working-class professions, had started businesses that built considerable family fortunes. One family tradition, especially drawn from the paternal grandparents, was to be on time for everything, and to view those who were late as "peasants." Understanding the family-of-origin roots of their beliefs and habits regarding punctuality brought each partner greater empathy for the other, and allowed the couple the freedom to begin to build their own family traditions that blended the best from each of their backgrounds.

As was true for this couple, partners' beliefs about time typically represent a blend derived from their culture(s) of origin and their particular family-of-origin experiences. Cecile and Tom, the white upper-middle-class couple mentioned at the beginning of this chapter, came to understand their differing beliefs about the need to monitor the use of time as being rooted partly in their ethnic cultures and partly in their particular families of origin. Remember that Cecile liked to let time flow and to invite spontaneity, whereas Tom believed in making every minute count. Both had come from wealthy families, but with a difference: Cecile's father was a "self-made man" from a humble Italian American background (his parents had immigrated to the United States), and so money was "new" for the family. In contrast, Tom came from a WASP family with many generations in the United States, and the family money had been made by a great-grandfather. Cecile's parents, having suffered hardships and constraints while the father built his business, wanted to see Cecile enjoy life ("Goditi la vita!" her father would say in Italian) in a way that they couldn't have at her age and encouraged her to spend money—and time—freely. On the other hand, because of the long history of wealth in Tom's family, value was placed on not taking this wealth for granted—and one key way to do this was not to take advantage of the money by "frittering away" time. Tom's family believed in industriousness, and Tom was under great pressure from his family to prove that he could be a responsible, serious person, not a "trust-fund kid" or a "spoiled brat," as he often called Cecile.

The result of these differing belief systems on the couple's day-to-day orientation to time was great tension—not only around the degree of flexibility versus regularity each wanted for their bedtimes but in all of the couple's activities. Predictably, Tom took the role of anxiously checking his watch to make sure they were on time when they were going to social engagements: whether on trips, vacations, or just spending a Sunday together, he would periodically express his frustration that they were "wasting time." In contrast, Cecile took the role of telling Tom to relax and of looking for serendipitous moments or opportunities to extend their trips in unplanned ways. Therapy was effective in reducing the extreme, tension-provoking level of this polarized pattern, largely through exploring the roots of their different beliefs, substituting empathy for disdain about each other's point of view, and recognizing that they had probably chosen each other to supplement and balance their own perspectives. Eventually, they each were able to find useful and acceptable compromises, in which Cecile came to appreciate more the value of structured time and Tom could loosen up and let time flow more.

A THEORY OF TIME IN COUPLE RELATIONSHIPS

A decade ago, Fraenkel (1990, 1994) introduced a theory of time in couple relationships. This theory forms the basis of our ongoing research in the Ackerman Institute Study of Time, Work, Technology, and the Family (Fraenkel & Wilson, 1998). For the clinician, this theory offers a set of premises to understand how time problems begin and are maintained, as well as concepts to guide assessment of the types of time problems experienced by couples. In turn, these concepts provide a map of possible entry points for intervention. Table 4.1 summarizes the key premises and concepts of the theory.

Key Premises

The first key premise is that *the manner in which couples evolve, organize, and experience the temporal dimension of their lives can greatly affect their overall satisfaction with the relationship*. In another words, time matters to couples. The second premise is that *the relationship between time patterns and couple satisfaction is bidirectional and often recursive*. For some couples, problems in coordinating schedules, synchronizing paces, or allocating time—among other time struggles—may lead to distress. For other couples, distress due to other reasons may lead partners to change their schedules so that they have little time together, may encourage partners to allow work or other time-consuming activities to intrude at home, or may lead to frequent arguments about how to spend time, all of which only furthers their distress.

TABLE 4.1. Time and Rhythm for Couples: Key Premises and Concepts

Key premises

How couples evolve/organize/experience temporal patterns affects relationship
   satisfaction
Recursive relationship between time patterns and couple satisfaction
No single or simple temporal pattern associated with couple satisfaction
How couple evolves and maintains rhythms reveals themes of power and
   closeness
Temporal patterns have multiple determinants
• Work
• Technology
• Larger systems
• Multiple caretaking responsibilities
• Biological/health factors
• Divorce and remarriage
• Beliefs from culture and family of origin

Key temporal concepts

Single instance versus repeated/recursive events
• Recursive events either irregularly (arrhythmic) or regularly occurring
   (rhythmic)

Temporal attributes of activities
• Position of occurrence: when in clock or calendar time
• Duration: length of time
• Pace or tempo: speed
• Frequency: how often
• Sequence: in what order

Three temporal levels or lengths of activities
• Micro (microseconds to seconds)
• Molar (seconds to 24 hours)
• Macro (days to years)

Temporal ideation
• Time perspective
• Time valuation
• Projected life chronologies

The third premise is that *there is not one single, or simple, temporal
pattern that correlates best with couple harmony or disharmony.* More important than the objective, quantifiable pattern of time allocation, a pace
difference between partners, schedules, and so on are the *meanings*
partners attribute to these patterns (Daly, 1996; Fraenkel, 1994). For instance, from a distance, a couple in which partners have highly synchro-

nized schedules and spend a lot of time together might be assumed to be close, until one learns that this schedule is enforced against the will of one partner by the threats and demands of the other.

This example leads well into a fourth premise of the theory: *how couples evolve their daily, weekly, and yearly rhythms, and handles time issues more generally, reflects much about their issues and preferences regarding the core relationship dimensions of closeness/connectedness and power.* Therefore, hearing accounts from couples of how their rhythms and time patterns evolved, who had the most to say about the form of these patterns, and each partner's degree of satisfaction with these patterns is an efficient way for the therapist to obtain a sense of how each partner feels about the degree of closeness and degree of power sharing between them.

A fifth premise of the theory is that *temporal patterns have multiple determinants.* Although we have emphasized the importance of eliciting from the couple the history of the evolution of their temporal patterns and difficulties, we do not thereby mean to imply that couples (or individual partners) have total choice and control over how their time is arranged. One couple's temporal patterns may be the result of deliberate decisions or actions, whereas other couples may experience themselves as having simply "fallen into" their particular patterns. In instances where one partner believes the other has total control over his or her schedule and can change it at will (e.g., in the forthcoming example of Mike and Laura), it is often therapeutic to identify the ways in which that person's schedule is tied to other temporal forces partially or entirely beyond his or her control. As we described earlier, common temporal determinants include work, technology, the demands of larger systems agencies, multiple caretaking responsibilities, biological and health factors, the complex relational demands that may accompany divorce and remarriage, and beliefs from family and culture of origin.

Thus, couples' temporal patterns acquire their meaning from:

- The process through which partners create and sustain them.
- The narrative recounted about this process.
- The degree to which the pattern is under the influence of the couple or controlled by outside forces.
- The degree to which the pattern represents broader themes around power and closeness/connectedness, and the degree to which the pattern reflects each partner's core values and goals.
- The links to each partner's family and culture(s) of origin.

The following two vignettes illustrate, in turn, how the meaning attributed to time patterns is more important than the actual pattern itself, and how temporal patterns represent and reveal issues of power and connection.

The Importance of Meaning in Temporal Patterns: A Vignette

Rick and Elaine, a couple in their early 30s, both have demanding jobs in finance. One of the only areas of conflict between them—but one that threatens to end their relationship—is Rick's aggravation when Elaine is late. She frequently comes home late from the office—on average, 1 hour later than the time she indicates when she calls him, when she is already running 1 to 2 hours late. Elaine states that she is frequently overwhelmed with work, finds it better to stay and complete a task rather than leave it half done for tomorrow, and agrees that it is hard for her to set limits at work. Her attempts to respond to Rick's upset by getting home earlier have not been consistent.

In tracing the theme of time in both of their families, it became clear that for Rick, punctuality was one of the only ways in which he experienced a sense of "normalcy" and "regularity" (his words) in his family. His mother had a severe bipolar disorder, which made her mood (and therefore the mood of the family) quite unpredictable. Rick's access to his mother for caretaking was likewise unpredictable. His father's attempts to control his wife's behavior during these episodes often involved high levels of verbal intimidation, which was extremely upsetting to Rick. However, the one "rule" that the whole family adhered to readily—including his mother, whether in or out of a manic or depressive episode—was the need to be on time for family meals, for getting out the door for family trips, and so on. Likewise, being on time was the one area of family life that Rick's father monitored and guided without intimidation. Thus, punctuality represented an aspect of family life that Rick could count on amid the turmoil; it was an oasis in the high levels of negative affect that otherwise characterized the family.

For Elaine, being late was the one way she felt she could exercise some degree of control and independence from her family. She described herself as the "good child" in her family, studious and responsible, while her brother had school and drug problems. She went into business ambivalently, largely at the urging of her father. Now she frequently found herself overwhelmed by and unhappy at her work, yet she felt that she had to show her family and herself that she could master the profession. As we explored the meaning of "lateness" for her, two facets emerged: First, being late coming home from work demonstrated to "everyone" (mostly to herself and to her internalized parents) that she was working as hard as she could, that she was beyond reproach. It was her nonverbal way of saying, "Don't ask one more thing from me." Second, being late was her nonverbal way of saying, "You can't control me."

The session with Rick in which we discussed the meaning of time in his family occurred one evening when Elaine was running so late that she missed the entire appointment. In fact, it was her lateness to the session that led him to return to this topic, which the couple had spoken about in the first session. In the following week, Rick arrived on time, and Elaine again was late, not arriving until a half-hour later. Asked how he felt about Elaine's lateness this week and this evening, Rick seemed genuinely relaxed about it. He noted that throughout the week, he found himself accepting Elaine's lateness without upset—with just a longing that she would come home so that they could spend more time together. Asked what he thought led to the dramatic shift, he said that understanding the family-of-origin basis of his own intense reaction to her lateness, and hearing what lateness meant to Elaine, had completely changed his perspective. Two weeks later (in the first session that Elaine came to on time—she was never late to sessions after this), both partners noted that they were no longer struggling about time. Both reported that Elaine continued to come home late, but not as often or as late. Asked to explain the change, Elaine commented, "I've got to confess, I think for me it was a power thing—the more he asked me to be on time, the more I was late. Now that Rick isn't bugging me about being late, I'm on time."

Thus, for this couple, understanding the meaning of the time pattern for each partner initially had more impact on relieving their tensions about it than actually changing the pattern; and the change in meaning led to a shift in the day-to-day interactions around time that actually led to a shift in Elaine's temporal behavior.

The Themes of Power and Closeness in Time: A Vignette

In addition to illustrating the centrality of meaning in defining and changing time problems, the example of Rick and Elaine illustrates how struggles around closeness and power emerge in the dimension of time. The problems of another couple, Mike and Laura, exemplify how the typical gender dynamic in heterosexual couples of men having more power than women is often constructed and largely maintained by the temporal demands of the workplace.

Mike, an international lawyer, travels for business at least twice a month. When in town, his daily schedule is erratic, dependent on the demands of clients for meetings, dinners, emergency phone calls, and so on. In contrast, Laura, a graphic designer, has a regular schedule: at work by 8:00 A.M., home by 6:00 P.M. As a result of their differing schedules, each day Laura asks Mike, "When will you be home?" Mike becomes anxious at this question, knowing that the answer he gives in the morning may need to be changed by the afternoon. Laura has become increasingly frustrated with Mike and his unpredictable schedule, as it keeps them from being able to make definite plans about dinner and social engagements. In addition, at times when she speaks to him (often by cell phone) when he is out of town or in town with clients, he sounds happy, and Laura finds herself feeling angry and resentful, as she believes that if they are going to be apart because of his business, he should at least be unhappy about it. In turn, Mike finds Laura's attitude selfish and unreasonable, and feels he can be unhappy that they're apart while at the same time being happy that business is going well—especially, he notes, because he provides the bulk of their income. The conflict around the temporal irregularity of Mike's schedule has become one of the major issues preventing Mike from proposing marriage.

As we explored this issue in therapy, it emerged that Laura felt Mike held all the control in this relationship. For her, his erratic schedule and her need to wait on him if they were to have time together represented both a symbol of his greater control and the most salient actual example of his greater power. Laura also perceived Mike to have greater control because of his significantly higher salary and more prestigious career. For his part, Mike acknowledged how his higher salary seemed to give him more power in the relationship, and he could see how Laura felt he had more control of their time together and daily rhythms. However, he emphasized that he often felt out of control of his schedule. He explained how his clients and their often last-minute demands forced him to bend his preferred schedule to their needs. He noted that he felt Laura often confused his happiness that things were going well at work with her belief that he completely enjoyed his work life. He spoke with much emotion of feeling torn on a daily basis between his work demands (which also felt tied to their financial well-being and future) and his wish to have a more relaxed and temporally regular life, with plenty of time for Laura and the family they hoped to have one day.

Before launching into attempts to solve their temporal problem, I asked each to reflect back on what had attracted each to the other when they first met. In addition to the physical and intellectual attraction each held for the other, Mike noted that he had dated other "high-powered lawyer and business types" with schedules similar to his and found these relationships unappealing in the end because "between the two of us, we could never seem to see each other long enough to develop the relationship." Mike found Laura's "normal" work day and her balance between career and other aspects of life extremely appealing—she had the balance to which he aspired but never seemed to achieve. For her part, Laura found Mike's career intensity and travel initially exciting, and it helped her focus on building her own career, which had stagnated. She also acknowledged that she liked the financial security and lifestyle that came with his career. However, she came to realize that his work life was better viewed "from a distance" now that the quality of her life was directly tied to it.

I suggested that we attempt to find ways to make small but significant changes in the balance between work and couple time so that they could preserve the appealing aspects of each other's approach to work, but in a way that their daily rhythms might become less of a power issue and provide a more satisfactory amount of time together. As a first step, Mike acknowledged that although he felt torn about work versus couple time, work always won out, as it had in his previous relationships. He recognized the message this sent to Laura about what he seemed to value most. At the same time, Laura acknowledged that Mike was more beholden to the whims of his clients than she had realized, and said she better saw how difficult it is for him to set limits.

Nevertheless, Mike believed that only he, and not Laura, could take the first steps to rectify this problem. As a start, he committed to one planned evening together a week, an evening that he would preserve no matter what. As it turned out, in the first week of this experiment, a client flew into town and wanted a dinner meeting that very night. Mike held his ground, explaining that he had social commitments for that evening, and was surprised to find that the client suggested lunch the next day instead. Laura felt extremely gratified by Mike's taking a stand against his work demands. Within a few weeks, Mike had added a second "work off-limits" evening for time with Laura. For those weeks when Mike was traveling, the couple arranged to have regular morning and nightly phone calls. Over the weeks of adapting these ideas, the night calls—initially designed just as times to talk—became intense sexual encounters as well. Several weeks after initiating these strategies, both partners reported feeling much closer and more at ease, and viewed time no longer as a power struggle.

It is important to note that, as in any systematic approach to identifying the nature of couples' problems, a focus on time does not exclude or substitute for other, complementary explanations. In other words, we are not suggesting that all couple problems should now be understood as only centering around time issues. Rather, we suggest that time is an underappreciated dimension of problems, and that by adding a focus on the temporal challenges and patterns of couples' lives, we can amplify the usefulness of existing systemic clinical approaches that understand couple problems as due to circular sequences, structural issues of closeness and hierarchy, intergenerational patterns and loyalty binds, constraining narratives, and so on (Fraenkel, 1996).

A Guide to Identifying Time Problems in Couples

Sometimes when couples complain about aspects of their lives, it initially appears that the solutions will need to involve finding new activities (e.g., changing their sexual repertoire, finding new ways to communicate, developing new recreational activities or ways of expressing tenderness) to substitute for the old, unsatisfying ones. However, when one listens with time in mind, a whole other set of options for change reveals itself, options that are often less difficult for couples to enact— for instance, changing the *degree of rhythmicity* of the acts rather than changing the acts themselves. In other words, often couples agree on what they want to do, but may disagree on how often or regularly, in what sequence, at what pace, and so on.

To assist therapists to identify and describe the temporal side of couple problems, we present briefly a taxonomy or organizational framework of time problems (described in detail in Fraenkel, 1994).

First, a specific temporal problem may occur only once or may occur repeatedly in the life of the couple ("recursive events"; Breunlin & Schwartz, 1986). As examples of one-time problems, consider a couple in which once, and only once, one partner kept the other waiting for hours after promising to be home in time for dinner, or in which one partner rushed the other through what was supposed to be a leisurely weekend day trip. Recursive events can be further subdivided into those that occur repeatedly at *regular* times versus those that repeat at *irregular* times. Recursive events that occur at regular, predictable intervals and at regular clock or calendar times are referred to as "rhythms" (Chapple, 1980; McGrath & Kelley, 1986; Moore-Ede, Sulzman, & Fuller, 1982).

Recursive events are the most common in the problems that couples bring to therapy. At the broadest level, one partner may not like the degree of responsibility that she or he must shoulder to ensure that the mutual rhythm occurs at all (e.g., the morning routine, weekly nights out, monthly visits to in-laws). Or one partner may be frustrated with the lack of a predictable daily rhythm of time apart versus time together (think of Mike and Laura), of bedtimes (think of Cecile and Tom), of daily meals, or of time to talk about kids and household management. In such cases, the solution may center around partners negotiating a rhythm that suits both of their needs and takes into account other constraints on their time.

Conversely, one or both partners may complain that certain repeated events occur *all too predictably*—that is, the rhythmicity of the act makes it feel routine, mechanical, boring. A good example of this for many couples is how their sexual life becomes restricted to the same time each week, and how the act itself moves predictably from familiar forms (and durations) of foreplay to coitus. In such instances, the solution may center around "shaking up" the rhythm by introducing temporal novelty.

Second, any act or event has five temporal aspects or attributes, and couple problems can occur around one or more of these attributes:

- *Position of occurrence*: *when* something happens in clock or calendar time.
- *Duration*: the length of time the activity/event happens.
- *Pace or tempo*: the speed at which the activity/event occurs.
- *Frequency*: how often something occurs in a specified period (day, week, month, year, lifetime).
- *Sequence*: the placement of the activity/event in terms of what comes before and what comes after, as well as the order of the component parts of the activity/event.

Take sex for example: One or both partners may be unhappy with the time of day that they typically have sex (clock time) or the day of the week (calendar time); with the length of time of their sexual encounters or with the relative length of time of foreplay versus coitus; with the pace or tempo of movements during sex ("Ow! You move too fast! Slow down!" or "Why are you taking soooo long to come?"); with the frequency of sex (just think of the classic scene from Woody Allen's *Annie Hall*: she's complaining to her psychiatrist how often they have sex—"constantly, I'd say, three times a week!"—while at the same time he's complaining to his psychiatrist how infrequently they have sex: "hardly ever, maybe three times a week!"); and with the sequence of sex in the context of their other activities (e.g., one likes to get the household chores done before relaxing and having sex, while the other wants to have sex and then take on the chores).

Third, time problems can occur in extremely short activities, lasting microseconds to seconds (*micro* level), in medium-length activities lasting from a few minutes up to a full day (*molar* level), and in activities whose durations are from days to weeks to months to years (*macro* level). Once again, couples can have temporal difficulties at one or more level of activity; sometimes, problems at one level reflect literally or metaphorically problems at another level. For example, in the case of Mike and Laura, Mike's arrhythmic daily schedule meant that Laura was always waiting for him to tell her when he'd be available for couple time (molar level). On the macro level, Laura was the one pressing for marriage, whereas Mike still felt unsure and wanted to wait to see if they could "work things out" better before he made this commitment. Thus, on both the day-to-day (molar) and life-as-a-whole (macro) levels, Laura waited for Mike, which infuriated her and often led her to explode angrily (which made him more reluctant to marry). A major insight for this couple came when the therapist noted this parallel, and how Mike's daily unpredictability constantly reminded Laura of the power difference between them and of how she was waiting for him to make the "big decision" about their future together. Change on one level (more predictability in terms of the daily schedule of when they came back together at the end of the day) lessened the tension each experienced about the larger, macro-level decision of when to get married. They married 1 year later.

Temporal Ideation

Throughout this chapter, we have emphasized the therapeutic value of exploring the range of partners' beliefs and preferences about aspects of time that contribute to conflict. However, there are three particular types of ideas about time worth emphasizing, as they come up frequently as areas of difficulty for couples: time perspective, time valuation, and personal life chronologies.

Partners, like cultures (Kluckhohn & Strodbeck, 1961; Levine, 1997) may differ in their *time perspective*, their orientation to past, present, or future. *Past-oriented people* may enjoy reminiscing, keeping in touch with old friends (and sometimes past partners), and going back to familiar vacation spots, and they may also be good at cataloguing in memory both the highlights and the unpleasant moments in the couple's life. *Present-oriented people* focus more on the here-and-now, enjoy trying new things and keeping up with the latest trends, like to spend money now rather than saving, and like to "let the past go." *Future-oriented people* use the present to plan for and work toward future goals, and present-moment pleasures may be put off in the service of achieving those goals. These people may have little patience for those who focus on the past, and may disdain those who "fritter away" the present on experiences that do not serve a larger end. Conflict can erupt for couples in which partners have different time perspectives.

For example, one couple requested marital therapy to discuss "lifestyle issues." Despite sensing that they communicated and solved problems well, the partners reported that they had never been able to agree on certain issues—foremost among them, how much money to put aside for retirement. The wife wanted to put aside a much larger proportion of the husband's earnings, whereas he argued that they should enjoy the money now and worry about retirement later. Their differences around this and other lifestyle issues (e.g., whether to spontaneously invite friends over for dinner or plan such meals well in advance) appeared to be rooted in a difference in time perspective: the husband was more present-oriented, the wife more future-oriented.

Time valuation is another key category of temporal ideas around which couples may struggle. Partners may differ in their beliefs and feelings about how important monitoring time is—that is, how important it is to be aware of (and attempt to control) the flow of time, to structure time, and to coordinate couple activities in time. One partner may be more concerned than the other about the use of time or about adherence to temporal agreements—for instance, about being punctual—and may play a monitoring function for the couple (Kantor & Lehr, 1975). Rick and Elaine struggled over differences in the meaning of punctuality, and Tom and Cecile had different beliefs about the importance of enjoying the flow of time versus making every minute count.

Differences in partners' *projected life chronologies*, or personal timelines, was the problem that caused great difficulty for Marcia and Fred, the couple described in the first vignette at the beginning of this chapter. Again, the term *projected life chronologies* refers to the individual's plans for the future: when she or he hopes to achieve certain life goals, in what sequence, how quickly, and the degree to which she or he sees current activities as promoting or blocking these goals. The issue of matching or synchronizing each partner's personal life chronologies has increasingly become a challenge for couples in the 1990s, with both men and women educated and in the work force, attempting to juggle careers, relationship, and family time, and with the feminist legacy that men's careers are not automatically assumed to be more important than women's. Another reason more couples seem to be facing this temporal challenge is that the average age of people getting married for the first time has increased (Bumpass & Sweet, 1989). As a result, partners may be more set in their individual lives and goals, and further along their chosen trajectories when they meet and marry, making it more difficult for them to compromise.

TIME-CENTERED INTERVENTIONS

Over the years, we have developed and experimented with some time-centered interventions. Our interventions include both ideas meant to shift how the couple views time and themselves in time, and practices that directly transform the couple's relationship to time. These ideas and activities build awareness of temporal patterns and constraints, help couples affirm acceptable patterns and alter unsatisfactory ones, and encourage them toward taking a position of activism regarding unreasonable demands by larger forces that control their time.

Three Myths about Time

One idea we suggest to couples, both in individual therapy sessions and in workshops, is the notion of "three myths" that interfere with coping successfully with time pressures: the myth of spontaneity, the myth of infinite perfectibility, and the myth of total control.

The Myth of Spontaneity

This is the notion that no matter how mismatched partners' schedules are—or how hectic and overstuffed their lives are with work and other extrarelationship involvements—fun, pleasure, sex, and other couple activities should somehow just "happen" spontaneously. We suggest instead that couple time needs to be scheduled. One idea many couples have found useful is the seemingly paradoxical notion of "scheduling unscheduled time" or "scheduling spontaneity." In this way, time is clearly partitioned for couple activities, but the nature of those activities can be created on the spot, or one partner can surprise the other with an activity, rather than having everything planned out.

The Myth of Infinite Perfectibility

Another maladaptive myth is the notion that the couple—and each partner in it—can "have it all": do all of their customary activities, work just as hard as ever, and still find more time for each other. Couples who think this way typically try to solve their time problems mathematically or organizationally—approaching the problem of "no time" as a time-management puzzle that can be solved through increasingly complex sequencing of activities. Sometimes, one or both partners will attempt to use a time-management computer program to solve the problem; of course, the time required to learn the program takes away even more time from the couple and generally does not solve the problem.

Instead, we suggest that couples need to make choices and set priorities. This involves partners thinking individually and talking together about what their core values are, what they want in their lives, and what they can do with less of or without. This is simple to say, and not so simple to do—yet this kind of "soul-searching" and prioritizing is critical when partners experience themselves as too busy for one another.

For many people in contemporary Western society, particularly those in the middle to upper classes, the last few decades of relative economic prosperity, the broader culture's emphasis on "self-actualization," exposure to a wide range of possible careers and leisure opportunities, and the relentless marketing of these possibilities through a wide variety of media, have led to a phenomenon we think of as "experience greed." Experience greed, a preoccupation with all the alternative paths one could take in one's life and the experiences one could seek, makes it difficult to select and develop just one (or a few!). Rather, many people seem to try to fit as much as possible into the time available, and end up frazzled as they run from one activity to the other.

Experience greed may lead people not only to overstuff their time away from work but (for some) drives decisions about how much work to take on. Although for many, job insecurity, competition, employer expectations, and financial concerns may motivate overwork, for others, work may be viewed as the best route to self-actualization, preferable to and more predictable than time spent with one's partner or children (Hochschild, 1997; Lagerfeld, 1998). For such persons, it may be difficult after a while to distinguish between opportunity and obligation (what they want to do vs. what they have to do).

In sum, while we believe much of the time pressure couples face today results from work and other factors over which they have less immediate control, some of the time pressures are self-imposed, and therefore require choices between a variety of excellent opportunities. Couples may need to give up the fantasy of somehow having a life in which limitless careers, all desired leisure activities, raising children, romance and a great sex life, and plenty of "down time" are delicately yet perfectly balanced, if they are to reduce the sense of time pressure and experience the creative, serendipitous, social pleasures of idleness, about which philosopher Bertrand Russell wrote over half a century ago.

The Myth of Total Control

In a sense, this belief underlies the notion of infinite perfectibility. It is the belief that couples (and their constituent partners) are completely in charge of their destinies, and that if their lives are frustrating it is all their fault. This belief is based on not recognizing the power of the various systemic forces that shape their lives, and so, their time. We suggest that couples laboring under this belief need to engage in a variety of exercises designed to increase their awareness of the forces that control their actual time, as well as their beliefs about and experiences of time. Once aware of these systemic factors, couples are better positioned to change them or to choose to "go with the flow."

For instance, partners can keep track of the number of daily occasions in which their lives are structured by the clock or calendar. They can count the number of times they use their calendars or organizers, check the time, confront a deadline or other requirement to do something by a certain time, and so on.

Exercises That Reveal Temporal Preferences

Here are exercises that increase awareness of partners' points of difference and agreement about time.

Time Pies

This exercise helps partners begin a conversation about how they view the allocation of time to various activities in their lives, and how they would most like to divide their time. Have each partner draw two identical large circles on 8½" × 11" paper. Label the first circles "Actual Time" and the second "Ideal Time." Now, ask the couple to decide on a category of activity—for instance, the time spent in work versus nonwork activities (leisure, couple/family time) or the different aspects of social time (including time spent alone as a couple vs. as a couple with children vs. with extended family vs. with friends vs. each partner alone). Usually, the relevant category has emerged in previous discussions about the couple's time problems. Now, with each working independently on their own pies, have each partner divide the first pie in terms of the amount or percentage of time actually devoted to each type of activity within the category (in a day, week, month—whatever unit of time makes sense). Next, have the partners use the second pie to indicate their *ideal* preferences for how to divide time among these activities. Have the partners compare their first pies, and encourage them to discuss ways in which their estimates of how time is actually divided concurred or differed, and if different, to explore reasons why this might be so. Then, in similar fashion, have them compare and discuss their ideal time allocations. Discussion of ideals and preferences about how to spend time can often be usefully informed by locating the family or culture-of-origin roots of these preferences. Finally, have the partners discuss ways they might combine their preferences and compromise as needed.

Time Lines: Projected Life Chronologies

As we noted above, partners often agree on major goals for their lives but disagree about *when* they want to achieve them. To assist couples in identifying possible differences in their projected life chronologies, have each partner draw a timeline on a piece of 8½" × 11" paper (turned on its side—or if more space is needed, connect two or even three pieces). Have the partners standardize the correspondence between inches and years (e.g., a half-inch equals 1 year). Have them label the left-hand side of the time line "Now" (and write the current date), and label the right-hand side "Death." (Alternatively, the partners might choose to use their timelines to chart their entire lives, from birth to death—the advantage of this approach is that it allows partners to visualize what they have already achieved up to this point, including meeting their partner.) Now have them write on the timeline all the goals they have for their lives, and when they hope to achieve them. Then have them compare timelines and encourage a discussion about how their temporal expectations converge and differ, and, if they wish to, what they can do to bring them more into alignment. However, be forewarned that in our clinical experience, differences in personal life chronologies are one of the most challenging time-related problems; in some cases, as couple partners more clearly identify discrepancies in their projected futures, they may decide to end the relationship.

The Life Pace Questionnaire

The Life Pace Questionnaire (LPQ; Fraenkel, 1989) is a 43-item inventory that asks partners to rate how quickly or slowly they conduct a wide range of daily activities, such as walking, talking, eating, showering, responding to phone messages, and so on. It also asks partners to rate the degree of match they experience with their partner on pace, and their level of comfort with the degree of match. Preliminary data suggest that the degree to which partners are matched on the dimension of satisfaction or dissatisfaction with the pace of life is highly correlated with overall relationship satisfaction. Having partners compare their responses to the LPQ item by item can serve as a structured exercise to locate problematic pace difference, which is the first step in understanding, adjusting to, or accommodating to this difference.

Affirming Existing Patterns

As is common in couple and family therapy today, we always attempt to assist couples to locate not only their problems but also their strengths—in this case, those temporal patterns and rhythms that work for them. Often, we find time-pressed couples have hidden resources of time that only need to be drawn forth and put to work more effectively.

Sacred Time

One of the ideas we suggest is to consider existing but overlooked and underutilized time together as "sacred." For instance, Judy and Bert—he went to bed and rose early, she wrote late into the night—actually had 2 hours each evening together (8:00 P.M.–10:00 P.M.) that they rarely used as couple time. By highlighting this time as their "sacred time" together, they were able to increase their sense of connection markedly in 1 week. Once they had set aside this time for themselves, each was better able to accommodate the other's different bedtimes and wake times.

One key to "sacred time" is to set a clear boundary between couple-related activities and other activities. For Judy and Bert, this meant a commitment on Bert's part to turn off his pager and not answer work-related phone calls during their time together.

Establishing Rhythms

Like creating "sacred time," establishing rhythms involves taking what couples already do and reorganizing it so that it becomes more built into their lives. We have observed that many of even the most time-starved couples have fun time together, but because these events occur sporadically and haphazardly the partners mistakenly believe that they never have couple time. By creating daily, weekly, or monthly rhythms of couple time, this time is woven more clearly into the fabric of their lives: it becomes something they can count on in their futures and look back to in their memories. By regularizing or rhythmicizing couple time, its occurrence becomes more automatic, and so, less likely that one or the other partner will forget to preserve the time. In fact, having rhythms of small amounts of time together (e.g., a rhythm of coming together at the end of each day or the once-a-week date) may be more important in creating couple cohesion than having large amounts of time together (e.g., that big once-a-year vacation) that occurs sporadically.

Altering Patterns

There are an infinite number of ways couples can alter problematic temporal patterns or create new ones. Here we will describe two interventions we frequently use to help busy couples connect more often during the day: the "decompression chamber" and the "60-second pleasure points."

The Decompression Chamber

This intervention is described in detail elsewhere (Fraenkel, 1998a). For couples, the transition between being apart during the work day and together in the evening can be a source of tension and misunderstanding.

Each partner may have different preferences for a sequence of activities in which they unwind from the day and reconnect with each other. One partner may wish to engage first in solitary activities (a shower, reading the paper, exercising) before engaging in conversation or other couple activities; the other may prefer immediate joint activities. When these needs are not clearly communicated and synchronized with the needs of the other partner, each can feel controlled or rejected. This exercise assists couples to negotiate this challenging transition.

First, suggest that this is a stressful transition for many couples. Introduce the notion of the "decompression chamber" as a metaphor for creating a period of time at the end of the day in which both partners' preferences for both joint and solitary activities are combined into a more complex but mutually satisfying sequence. Use Figure 4.1 to demonstrate pictorially what happens in this transition. Elicit the preferences of each partner, have them create a joint sequence and write it down, and suggest that they experiment with it over the next week.

The 60-Second Pleasure Points

This intervention, also described elsewhere (Fraenkel, 1996, 1998b), uses the malleable, subjective aspect of time perception to create a

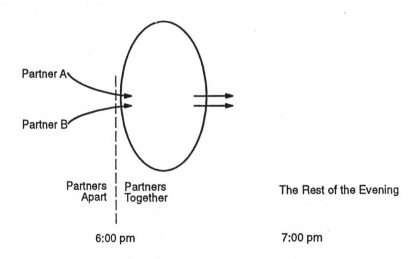

FIGURE 4.1. The decompression chamber. From Fraenkel (1998a). Copyright 1998 by Haworth Press. Reprinted by permission.

sense of greater couple connection with a relatively small investment of actual (chronological) time. Ask the partners to think of all of the fun, pleasurable, and/or sensual activities they could do with each other, in which each activity lasts only 60 seconds or less. Ideas collected from couples over the years have included a kiss, a hug, a foot (hand, neck) massage, feeding each other something, a quick dance, smelling a flower, saying a prayer together, looking at a sunset, telling a joke, reading a poem, tussling each other's hair, tickling, whispering sweet nothings, dressing the cat (!), stroking each other with a velvet mitt, and talking about what to do for fun when there's more time. Ask the couple to include in the list both activities that they can do when physically together as well as things they can do when physically apart (through use of the phone, e-mail, fax—putting technology to work for the relationship!).

The first benefit of this exercise is that the partners immediately see that there is a wide range of fun activities they can do even when quite pressed for time. In the next part of the exercise, ask the partners to imagine making six of these "60-second pleasure points" happen over the course of a day: for instance, two in the morning, one during the day while they're apart, and three in the evening. Use of a diagram such as that depicted in Figure 4.2 emphasizes the distribution of the points across the day. Now, ask the partners if either of them, as children, ever had a coloring book with dots, often with numbers next to the dots (virtually everyone has had such a coloring book); then ask

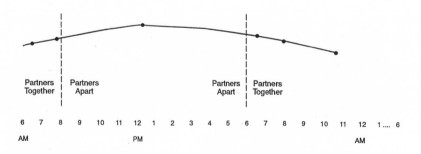

FIGURE 4.2. The 60-second pleasure points across the day creating an "arc of connection." From Fraenkel (1998b). Copyright 1998 by Haworth Press. Adapted by permission.

them what they did with these dots—invariably, the answer is "Connected them." Suggest that, just as they connected the dots in the coloring book, their minds will automatically, without effort, connect the "dots" of the 60-second pleasure points, and that as a result the 6 minutes or less of time devoted to these activities will create a sense of increased connection and pleasure (an "arc of connection") that far exceeds the time invested.

It is important to emphasize to couples that this technique is not meant to take the place of more extensive time together. But couples find it a helpful tool to enhance their sense of connection over the course of a day, and as a way to cope with exceptionally busy times when more extensive together time is not possible.

Activism

It is fitting that we end this chapter with the notion of "time activism." We predict that the time pressures resulting from overwork, exacerbated by the presence of work-related technology in the home, will reach such a crisis point in the 21st century that it will become the theme around which persons across classes join together to reshape the culture of work, and possibly also the consumer culture that contributes to people's willingness to work so much (Schor, 1991). As systemically oriented therapists, we may play a role in encouraging not only individual couples but communities of couples and families to join together to talk about their experiences and frustrations with the time pressures they face, and to generate solutions that may include taking a stand against companies that subtly encourage the ever greater permeability of the boundary between work and home. If the statistics are correct about who is working so hard, the hopeful thing about such a movement would be that, unlike union disputes that typically pitch the working class against management, this movement would include a healthy representation of managers, and maybe even some overworked corporation heads.

NOTES

1. The therapist in all case vignettes is Peter Fraenkel.
2. Of those who work more than 40 hours, 58% said they wanted more time with their partners, compared to 42% of those working 40 hours or less. Likewise, 64% of those working more than 5 days a week indicated they wanted more time with their partners, compared to 47% of those working 5 days or less. And of those working more

than 40 hours per week, 74% wished for more time with their children (Galinsky, Bond, & Friedman, 1993).

3. Recent data from the Current Population Survey (Bureau of Labor Statistics, 1997b), show that 12% of mothers and 18.3% of fathers worked regular nonday (evening or night) or rotating shifts. Other data (Presser, 1989) suggest that couples in which both partners work often have nonoverlapping work schedules—especially couples with young children.

4. Recent data from the U.S. Bureau of the Census (1997) show 25% of fathers in married couples with preschoolers provide child care while their wives are working, and 19% of fathers were the primary caregivers. This is particularly true for fathers who work evening or night shifts: they were almost twice as likely as men who work day shifts to take care of their preschool children (26% vs. 13%). However, there is an important class difference: poor fathers were almost twice as likely to provide child care as were nonpoor fathers (43% vs. 24%).

5. Data are not assembled exclusively on "commuter marriages," but the Census Bureau tracks the number of households in which a spouse is absent from the home for reasons such as employment or armed forces service. The increase from 1990 to 1996 quoted above (from 1.45 million to 2.1 million) is believed to be most likely due to an increase in commuter relationships (U.S. Bureau of the Census, 1996).

6. There are currently 22.4 million caregiving households for the elderly. These caregiving responsibilities result in 10% of workers giving up work, and 11% taking a leave of absence. Of those who continue to work, 49% of caregivers change daily work schedules because of these caregiving responsibilities: coming to work late, leaving early, or taking off time during the day (National Alliance for Caregiving & American Association of Retired Persons, 1997).

REFERENCES

Abelson, R. (1998, November 2). Part-time work for some adds up to full-time job. *New York Times*, Section 1, pp. 1, 18.

Belsky, J., Spanier, G. B., & Rovine, M. (1983). Stability and change in marriage across the transition to parenthood. *Journal of Marriage and the Family, 45*, 567–577.

Breunlin, D. C., & Schwartz, R. C. (1986). Sequences: Toward a common denominator of family therapy. *Family Process, 25*, 67–87.

Bumpass, L. L., & Sweet, J. A. (1989). National estimates of cohabitation. *Demography, 26*, 615–625.

Bureau of Labor Statistics. (1997a, March). *March supplement of the current population survey, 1997*. Washington, DC: U.S. Department of Labor.

Bureau of Labor Statistics. (1997b, May). *May supplement of the current population survey, 1997*. Washington, DC: U.S. Department of Labor.

Chapple, E. D. (1980). *The biological foundations of individuality and culture*. Huntington, NY: Krieger.

Crouter, A. C., & Crowley, M. S. (1990). School-age children's time alone with fathers in single and dual earner families: Implications for the father–child relationship. *Journal of Early Adolescence, 10*, 296–312.

Daly, K. J. (1996). *Families and time: Keeping pace in a hurried culture.* Thousand Oaks, CA: Sage.

Falicov, C. J. (1995). Training to think multiculturally: A multidimensional comparative framework. *Family Process, 34,* 373–388.

Families and Work Institute. (1995, May). *Women: The new providers. Whirlpool Foundation Study Part 1.* New York: Families and Work Institute.

Federal Highway Administration. (1997, September). *1995 nationwide personal transportation survey.* Washington, DC: U.S. Department of Transportation.

Fraenkel, P. (1989). *The Life Pace Questionnaire.* Unpublished manuscript, available from the author.

Fraenkel, P. (1990, October). *Relational time: Working with dyssynchronous couples.* Poster session presented at the annual meeting of the American Association for Marriage and Family Therapy, Washington, DC.

Fraenkel, P. (1994). Time and rhythm in couples. *Family Process, 33,* 37–51.

Fraenkel, P. (1996). The rhythms of couplehood: Using time as a resource for change. *Family Therapy Networker, 20,* 65–77.

Fraenkel, P. (1997). Systems approaches to couple therapy. In W. K. Halford & H. Markman (Eds.), *Clinical handbook of marriage and couples interventions,* (pp. 379–413). London: Wiley.

Fraenkel, P. (1998a). Time and couples, Part 1: The decompression chamber. In T. S. Nelson & T. S. Trepper (Eds.), *101 more interventions in family therapy* (pp. 140–144). New York: Haworth Press.

Fraenkel, P. (1998b). Time and couples, Part 2: The sixty-second pleasure point. In T. S. Nelson & T. S. Trepper (Eds.), *101 more interventions in family therapy* (pp. 145–149). New York: Haworth Press.

Fraenkel, P., & Wilson, S. (1998, June). *Time, work, and emergence from poverty: A qualitative study of time issues for homeless families returning to work.* Poster session presented at the 20th annual meeting of the American Family Therapy Academy, Montreal, Canada.

Galinsky, E. (1996, March 8–10). *Is the time famine real?* Unpublished paper prepared for *Our Time Famine: A Critical Look at the Culture of Work and a Re-evaluation of "Free" Time,* University of Iowa, Iowa City.

Galinsky, E., Bond, J. T., & Friedman, D. E. (1993). *The changing workforce: Highlights of the national study.* New York: Families and Work Institute.

Gleick, J. (1999). *Faster: The acceleration of just about everything.* New York: Panetheon.

Gonzalez, S., Steinglass, P., & Reiss, D. (1989). Putting the illness in its place: Discussion groups for families with chronic medical illnesses. *Family Process, 28,* 69–87.

Hall, E. T. (1983). *The dance of life: The other dimension of time.* Garden City, NY: Anchor Press/Doubleday.

Henderson, K. A., & Allen, K. R. (1991). The ethic of care: Leisure possibilities and constraints for women. *Society and Leisure, 14,* 97–113.

Hochschild, A. R. (1989). *The second shift.* New York: Avon Books.

Hochschild, A. R. (1997). *The time bind: When work becomes home and home becomes work.* New York: Metropolitan Books.

Hoffman, C. (1987). The effects on children of maternal and paternal employment. In N. Gerstel & H. E. Gross (Eds.), *Families and work* (pp. 362-395). Philadelphia: Temple University Press.

Kantor, D., & Lehr, W. (1975). *Inside the family*. San Francisco: Jossey-Bass.

Kluckhohn, F. R., & Strodbeck, F. L. (1961). *Variations in value orientations*. Evanston, IL: Row, Peterson.

Kraut, R., Patterson, M., Lundmark, V., Kiesler, S., Mukopadhyay, & Scherlis, W. (1998). Internet paradox: A social technology that reduces social involvement and psychological well-being? *American Psychologist, 53*, 1017-1031.

Lagerfeld, S. (1998). Who knows where the time goes? *Wilson Quarterly, 22*, 58-70.

Leete, L., & Schor, J. B. (1994). Assessing the time squeeze hypothesis: Hours worked in the United States, 1969-1989. *Industrial Relations, 33*, 25-41.

Levine, R. (1997). *A geography of time*. New York: Basic Books.

Lewis, S., & Cooper, C. (1989). *Career couples*. London: Unwin Hyman.

Markman, H. J., Stanley, S. M., & Blumberg, S. L. (1994). *Fighting for your marriage*. San Francisco: Jossey-Bass.

McGrath, J. E., & Kelley, J. R. (1986). *Time and human interaction: Toward a social psychology of time*. New York: Guilford Press.

McGuire, P. A. (1999). Worker stress, health reaching critical point. *APA Monitor, 30*, 1, 27.

Miller, D. A. (1981). The "sandwich" generation: Adult children of the aging. *Social Work, 26*, 419-423.

Moore-Ede, M. C., Sulzman, F. M., & Fuller, C. A. (1982). *The clocks that time us*. Cambridge, MA: Harvard University Press.

National Alliance for Caregiving & American Association of Retired Persons. (1997, June). *Family caregiving in the U.S.: Findings from a national survey*. Bethesda, MD: National Alliance for Caregiving.

Neal, M. B., Chapman, N. J., Ingersoll-Dayton, B., & Emlen, A. C. (1993). *Balancing work and caregiving for children, adults, and elders*. Newbury Park, CA: Sage.

Papp, P., & Imber-Black, E. (1996). Family themes: Transmission and transformation. *Family Process, 35*, 5-20.

Pasero, U. (1994). Social time patterns, contingency, and gender relations. *Time and Society, 3*, 179-191.

Presser, H. B. (1989). Can we make time for children? The economy, work schedules, and child care. *Demography, 26*, 523-543.

Pronovost, G. (1989). The sociology of time. *Current Sociology, 37*, 1-124.

Rayner, R. (1998, March 8). Nowhere, U.S.A. *New York Times Magazine*, p. 27.

Rosenbloom, S. (1998). *Transit markets of the future: The challenge of change* (Transit Cooperative Research Program Report 28). Washington, DC: National Academy Press.

Rowe, B.R., & Bentley, M. T. (1992). The impact of the family on home-based work. *Journal of Family and Economic Issues, 13*, 279-297.

Scharlach, A. E. (1994). Caregiving and employment: Competing or complementary roles? *Gerontologist, 34*, 378-385.

Schor, J. B. (1991). *The overworked American*. New York: Basic Books.

Silverstone, R. (1993). Time, information, and communication technologies and the household. *Time and Society, 2,* 283–311.

U.S. Bureau of the Census. (1996, March). *Marital status and living arrangements, March 1996* (Current Population Reports, P20-496). Washington, DC: U.S. Government Printing Office.

U.S. Bureau of the Census. (1997, October 8). *Economic conditions can influence married fathers' caring for preschoolers, Census Bureau reports*. Washington, DC: U.S. Government Printing Office.

Visher, E. B., & Visher, J. S. (1993). Remarriage families and stepparenting. In F. Walsh (Ed.), *Normal family processes* (2nd ed., pp. 235–253). New York: Guilford Press.

Voydanoff, P. (1988). Work role characteristics, family structure demands, and work/family conflict. *Journal of Marriage and the Family, 50,* 749–761.

Voydanoff, P., & Kelly, R. F. (1984). Determinants of work-related family problems among employed parents. *Journal of Marriage and the Family, 46,* 881–889.

CHAPTER 5

Infertility and Late-Life Pregnancies

Constance N. Scharf
Margot Weinshel

Infertility and late-life pregnancies bring increasingly important issues to couples. As more partners delay starting a family for professional reasons and women choose to have children later in life, a growing number of couples face the risk of struggling with infertility. Technological innovations in advanced reproductive technology (ART) have drastically changed reproduction, giving new hope to those facing infertility. In the early 1970s, fertilizing a sperm and an egg in a test tube to create an embryo outside the womb was only a fantasy. Today, *in vitro* fertilization (IVF) is a common reproductive technique, and the new applications of this procedure, as well as the ethical and moral dilemmas that they raise, are overwhelming. A man, through the use of intracytoplasmic sperm injection (ICSI), need only have one sperm to fertilize an egg. A woman can become pregnant at age 63, years after menopause, by receiving donor eggs from a younger woman. A dead man can "father" a child with his frozen sperm. An infertile woman can receive donor eggs from her mother, so that her daughter is genetically also her half-sister. The possibilities are daunting.

These astonishing technological advancements have provided the possibility for some infertile couples to have children who are genetically related to them. Yet few of these couples have been encouraged to think past the immediate interventions to address the complicated psychological and relational issues raised by these new practices. In this chapter, we will address the issues faced by modern couples as they encounter the devastating impact of infertility, and we will discuss therapeutic treatment approaches and strategies.

INFERTILITY: DEFINITION AND STATISTICS

The standard definition of infertility is *the inability to achieve pregnancy after 1 year of regular sexual relations without the use of contraception, or the inability to carry a pregnancy to live birth.* (*Merck Manual*, 1992). Infertility affects about 5.3 million people in the United States, which is approximately 9% of the population of reproductive age. There is a physical explanation for 90% of the cases of infertility: 35% is attributable to a male factor, 35% to a female factor, and 20% to an interactive factor between the female and the male, and 10% is unexplained (Menning, 1988). In late-life pregnancies, the most common cause of infertility in women is the advanced age of their eggs.

The age of the women is directly correlated with the success of achieving pregnancy per cycle. The following statistics are for unassisted pregnancies (Marrs, with Bloch & Silverman, 1997, p. 12):

At age 15: 40–50% success rate per cycle
At age 25: 30–35% success rate per cycle
At age 35: 15–20% success rate per cycle
At age 45: 3–5% success rate per cycle

In the United States today, 20% of women do not begin having children until the age of 35. Not very long ago, almost all women were finished having a family by the time they were 35 (Hodder, 1997, p. 61). Since maternal age is the largest factor associated with female infertility, one can see how there would be growing numbers of older women experiencing infertility.

THE MYTH OF WOMEN'S ETERNAL FERTILITY

"It's hard being 40 when you're a woman. You feel less feminine and not as sexy, so to find out you can't get pregnant easily is really a blow. I'm just so mad at my doctor, and I like him—he's my friend. I'm mad at the women's movement; I'm mad at society. I'm mad at everyone who made me think I could get pregnant whenever I wanted. Why didn't my doctor tell me if I wanted a baby I should get going? I thought I had endless amounts of time and now I've blown it. It's passed me by. I'm too old."

These words were spoken in a couple session at the Ackerman Institute for the Family's Infertility Project. They poignantly express the position that many women in their late 30s and early 40s find themselves in.

One of the myths for women is that they can have their own biological child whenever they choose to do so. Women are often not informed about the dramatic decrease in their fertility as they age. For women over the age of 39, there is a 7.6% chance of having a child with one's own eggs using *in vitro* fertilization; after age 47, there is essentially no chance of having a child with one's own eggs (Centers for Disease Control and Prevention [CDC] et al., 1997, p. 15). This fact places women at a distinct disadvantage to men, who have no age limit on their reproductive capabilities. For most professional career women, the time period in their life that is so critical for establishing professional success, their 20s and early 30s, coincides with the years when they are most fertile. Since many believe they can easily become pregnant in their late 30s and early 40s, they are shocked, bewildered, and angry to discover that they are having problems. A recurring refrain from these women is "If only I had known this information, I would have started earlier."

A 39-year-old nurse thought she was 100% fertile, and was shocked to discover she had serious fertility problems. Other women that we have seen, who are in their 40s, but who look youthful, have been surprised to find out they are infertile because of aging eggs.

It took until 1987 for the American Fertility Society (now the Society for Reproductive Medicine) to recommend to their member gynecologists that they should inform women about their statistical chances of becoming pregnant and explain the relationship between a woman's age and decreasing fertility. Unfortunately, when this practice is followed, some women experience such information from their physician as intrusive and disturbing. It may activate concerns about fertility at a time that neither she nor her partner or the relationship is ready for children.

COUPLES, LATER-LIFE PREGNANCIES, AND INFERTILITY

We can place older couples who come to treatment with infertility issues into roughly three different categories. The first are couples who are long married or cohabiting but have postponed starting a family until the woman's career was more established. These couples often come into therapy after they have learned that the woman cannot get pregnant on her own. They may not have tried any medical interventions or they may now be at the point where the woman is no longer fertile and their only options are an egg donor, adoption, or a life without children. Many are in shock since this is often the first time they have not been able to achieve one of their desired life goals. The second group consists of couples who easily conceived when the women were in their late 30s, but now that they are in their 40s they have been diagnosed with secondary infertility.

> "I feel Mother Nature played a terrible trick on us. If we had had trouble the first time, we would have started much earlier to try again." Debbie and Steve are a couple in their early 40s. She was 40 when she became pregnant on their first try. They decided to wait until she was 43 to have a second child, and after many attempts were diagnosed with secondary infertility.

The last group are couples in their late 30s who have recently met and married, and have immediately tried to become pregnant because of the woman's "biological clock." These latter couples face an additional issue since they have not had sufficient time to develop their relationship within the marriage. The relationship tasks are compressed into a shorter time frame as they move immediately from marriage to trying to conceive. They may also have differences in their desire to become pregnant. However, if the couples experience infertility, then they are forced to struggle with extremely difficult decisions, including the steps they may need to take to overcome infertility, both medical and financial, that can stress the relationship before it has become solidified. For some, however, this process can actually strengthen and affirm the relationship.

> Roseanna, age 37, a lawyer, and Jimmy, age 34, a reporter, came into couple therapy because of a conflict about their difficulties

in becoming pregnant. They had recently met and married. Because of Roseanna's age, she pressured Jimmy into trying to become pregnant and he "agreed." However, on the days when she was fertile, he often became angry with her and refused to have sex. He said he was concerned about their relationship and wanted more time to get to know her before having children. Roseanna said she wanted a child no matter what happened to the relationship.

Julia, age 40, and Richard, age 45, recently married and started a new business. Richard became severely depressed, and the plan to start a family was initially put on hold until he recovered from his depression. When a year had passed, Julia convinced Richard to try to have a child. After several failed attempts, Julia was diagnosed with infertility because of aging eggs. Donor eggs had been suggested, but Richard was still ambivalent about children and also worried about the possibility of multiple births if they used donor eggs. They came for couple therapy with severe conflicts about the decision to use donor eggs.

Many couples think the only problem in older couples is the woman's fertility. Thus they may be shocked to discover that it is the man who is infertile. It is only in the last 5 years that infertile men had any option other than the use of sperm from another man. Now, for men, it is possible, with the use of ICSI, to take one viable sperm and, through IVF, to inject it into the woman's egg.

IMPACT OF INFERTILITY

The impact of infertility on couples can be profound. It is usually experienced as a traumatic crisis and can have a demoralizing effect on the infertile individual's sense of self and the couples sense of their integrity as a healthy unit. It frequently evokes feelings of defectiveness, shame, and devastation. To make matters worse, the couple's experience is usually little understood and not valued by their family and friends (Meyers, Diamond, et al., 1995, p. 227).

Each member of the couple may experience the event differently. These differences can be attributed to gender issues, coping styles, and differences in one's desire to have a child. Women particularly experience the heartbreak of infertility. Research has found that women with infertility have the same levels of depression as those with cancer, heart disease, or HIV infection (Gill, 1998, p. 171). Independent of whether the man or the woman carries the infertility factor, women continue to exhibit greater distress than men: 50% of women and only 15% of men report that infertility is the most upsetting experience of their lives (Freeman, Boxer, Rickels, Tureck, & Mastrioanni, 1985).

A major gender difference is that men prefer to avoid conversation and pursue action, while women prefer to talk (McEwan, Costello, & Taylor, 1987). Interestingly, talking about the problems often made men feel worse and women feel better. In addition, women seem to have high levels of distress about the infertility, whether they or their partner carry the infertile factor. Men seem to have lower levels of distress, except when the man himself is infertile, in which case men's levels of distress are as high as women's (Nachtigall, Becker, Wozny, 1992).

> One man we saw defined his infertility this way: "The term that comes to my mind is that of identity—self-identity: How do men define themselves? Through the ability to have children, and through work. Those are the two big ones. My world is fundamentally shaken by this. It makes me ask, Who am I, Where am I, How did I get here, What do I do with myself with this realization that one of the defining factors in my life isn't there?"

Women often protect men and take on the infertile identity.

> With one couple we treated, the man was infertile. Their cultural background was Italian American, and his virility had been strongly affected by his diagnosis of male infertility. The wife, in order to shelter her husband from other people's reactions, told her family and friends it was she who was infertile. At a family barbeque, the wife's father approached the husband and said he and his family would understand if the husband wanted to divorce his daughter because she could not produce any children.

Pressures from society, family, and friends to become a parent add to the couple's experience of being marginalized, feeling different, and out of step with other couples who are starting their families.

We have found that the crisis of infertility can make a couple's interactions appear highly problematic and dysfunctional at first sight. However, we have learned that this is typical of couples struggling with infertility, and not indicative of the couple's strengths and potential coping abilities.

LOSS AND MOURNING

Loss and mourning are the leitmotifs of infertility. Loss of the experience and joy of an easy conception, loss of the privacy (without medical intervention) of conception, loss of the expectation to have a shared biological child, loss of the expected continuation of one's family lineage—these are just a few of the losses. These losses need to be recognized and validated, and couples need to be helped to mourn.

ASSISTED REPRODUCTIVE TECHNIQUES: *IN VITRO* FERTILIZATION AND DONOR EGGS

In vitro fertilization (IVF) is a medically assisted conception in which eggs are vaginally retrieved from ovulating females and combined with sperm in a petri dish. If fertilization occurs, the embryos are then inserted, after 2 or 3 days of development, in the uterus through the vagina via the endocervical canal. Embryos may also be cryo-preserved for future use. In 1995, 59,142 ART cycles were done in the United States (CDC et al., 1997, p. 6). The live birth rate per cycle, which includes all women trying IVF, was 19.6% (CDC et al., 1997, p. 6). Success rates decline as women's ages rise, from 25% among women aged 34 years and younger to 17% for women ages 35–39. Over age 39, the rates decrease from 7.6% to zero for women 47 and older (CDC et al., 1997, p. 15). Statistics are slightly higher for gamete intrafallopian transfer (GIFT) and zygote intrafallopian transfer (ZIFT), but because they are invasive procedures many clinics have stopped using these techniques. One standard IVF attempt, depending on whether drugs are part of the protocol, costs between $7,800 and $12,000. IVF clinics recommend three or four cycles to try to achieve a pregnancy (CDC et al., 1997, p. 12).

With IVF, the ovaries are stimulated with follicle-stimulating drugs to increase the number of eggs produced, thereby improving the odds of conceiving. While most fertility clinics limit the number of implanted zygotes to four, multiple zygote transfer increases the chances of multiple births. In fact, ART pregnancies result in multiple births 37% of the time as compared with 2% of the time in the general population (CDC et al., 1997, p. 14). Multiple births pose medical problems for the babies. The children tend to be born prematurely with a lower birth weight, which puts them at risk for serious medical, developmental, and learning problems.

The advent of donor eggs has radically changed the age at which women can become pregnant. The oldest known recipient to carry and deliver a child conceived with a donor egg was a 63-year-old woman in 1997. Most fertility clinics have a cutoff age between 47 and 55. Mark Hornstein, director of the IVF program at Brigham and Women's Hospital in Boston, stated:

> "Women in their forties are of advanced reproductive age but they're still of reproductive age. But the California woman who gave birth at 63 is another story. Her life expectancy is 16 years or so. If her husband is the same age, it is statistically unlikely that both parents will survive long enough to see that child into adulthood. I have a problem with that." (cited in Hodder, 1997, p. 98)

Linda Blum, a sociologist and women studies specialist at the University of New Hampshire, views this as just another double standard:

> "When a man in his sixties—or even older—has children, we admire his attainment of a better moral orientation, since he was too career-oriented before. But now, a woman in her sixties has done the same thing; there's a blatant cultural revulsion that a woman who's supposed to be all 'dried up' has the audacity to claim this right." (cited in Hodder, p. 98)

As technology has become more sophisticated, the use of donor eggs has increased. The technical capacity to use donor eggs has been available since the mid-1980s but the number of children born from donated eggs has jumped from 112 babies in 1989 to 1,240 in 1994 (CDC et al., 1997, p. 14). In 1995, donor eggs were used in 8% of all ART cycles. Since the donors are young women with healthy eggs, the success rate for the use of donor eggs across all female recipients ages 22–50 is 30%. The cost of the donor egg procedure, which must be added on to the cost of IVF, can range between $1,000 and $5,000. Donor egg procedures are becoming more prevalent among women age 36 and older since they are more likely to have success using this technique than by using their own eggs.

Besides the issue of cost, the egg donation process is much more difficult than sperm donation. In order to coordinate her period with the donor, the recipient is put on medication that has unpleasant side effects, including menopausal symptoms. In addition, the donor must inject herself with hormones for about 2 weeks, making her ovaries swell until they grow, in some cases, to the size of grapefruits. During that time, she needs to undergo frequent blood tests and ultrasound examinations to assess the ripening clusters of eggs in her ovaries. Finally, she must visit a medical center so her eggs can be "harvested." In this process, a thin needle is inserted through her cervix to her ovaries, and eggs are suctioned out.

Although the overwhelming majority of egg donors suffer no untoward consequences, there can be medical risks. Hyperstimulation of the ovaries can occur, causing the woman's ovaries to keep producing eggs. In rare cases, the woman can go into renal failure. Another risk donors face is the long-term effects of ovulation-producing drugs. There is some evidence that these drugs, particularly for donors who do not experience the 9 nonovulating months of pregnancy, increase their risk of ovarian cancer by a factor of 3. It is important to note that there is no research on the long-term effects of ovulation-stimulating drugs, since egg donation has only been used since 1984 (Rossing, Daling, Weiss, Moore, & Self, 1994, p. 776).

IMPACT OF THE USE OF DONOR EGGS

One of the men in our project spoke about his experience in using donor eggs. "I mean to me it's almost an abstraction. I've never even met this woman. I've never had a cup of coffee with her. I've never heard her voice. I mean this is an arrangement made by fax and phone."

The concept of donor eggs can astound the imagination. Most couples, at first, firmly reject the idea as unacceptable. However, as failures accumulate from unassisted and assisted reproductive attempts, the idea slowly begins to become more appealing because it gives the woman a chance to experience pregnancy and the man the chance to have his own genetic child. Most physicians treat the donor egg procedure primarily as another step in the infertility ladder, a medical advancement using IVF technology. Since donor sperm has been used for more than 100 years, donor egg is now treated as donor sperm had been previously treated by the medical community. The usual presentation is that, once pregnant, there is no difference between the use of donor gametes or one's own gametes during pregnancy and parenting. In our experience, while this approach is an effort to normalize a pregnancy for infertile couples, it minimizes the meaning and impact of the use of a donor gamete on the couple, the family, and on society as a whole. According to clinical geneticist Susan Parker,

"[ART] has gone beyond assisted reproduction to manipulations that
we certainly didn't dream of twenty years ago. We're getting away from
the natural selective process of people being attracted to each other,
one of whom had eggs, one of whom had sperm and the male bearing
the sperm to the site of ovulation. Our society is not prepared for the
families that will result from these interventions." (cited in Hodder,
1997, p. 62)

We have found a number of issues central to the use of donor gametes that couples need to explore. These issues are equally important
whether the couple uses donor eggs or donor sperm. Often, because
many of these couples have already been through multiple infertility
treatments, and have reached the point that a donor gamete is their
only option to have one partner's biological child, they may not take
the time to think fully about the ramifications of having a child that is
genetically related to only one partner. They may not have thought sufficiently about the many issues raised by donor gametes, for the couple,
for the man and the woman individually, and for the child.

The first decision to make in using donor eggs or donor sperm is
whether to use a known or an anonymous donor. Known donors are
usually siblings, relatives, or friends. With donor sperm, a sibling is less
frequently used; with donor eggs, sisters are often the most common
choice. However, this choice can potentially create complex and negative consequences and needs to be thought out very carefully. It can
have impact on the relationships among the two sisters, the sisters and
their own husbands, the sisters and their sisters' husbands, the two husbands, as well as the relationship of each adult to the child.

The decision to use an anonymous donor leads to another decision: Who chooses the donor, the couple or the fertility clinic? This, in
turn, raises the issue of closed or open information about the donor
that is available to the couple. With a closed match, the fertility clinic
chooses the donor and will supply the couple with varying amounts of
information about that donor. Usually, the information is very sparse,
offering little more than a brief description of the donor. With an
open-choice egg donation, the couple chooses the donor themselves by
looking through a catalogue that includes pictures of the donors, descriptions of their lives and families, and handwritten statements about
their wishes and reasons for volunteering to be a donor. Open-choice
donation is done primarily in California, although a few other states
are also beginning to use this approach. Sperm donation, too, has become more open, so that today more detailed information about the
donor is available to the couple.

This process can become a Rorschach test for each partner concerning what attributes she or he likes or does not like about her or his partner and herself or himself. Some couples choose physical attributes they wish their partner had, while others try to match the donor's traits to their partner's traits as closely as possible.

As one couple described how much they liked the donor, the husband said his only complaint was that she was short. The wife laughingly turned to her husband and said, "But I'm short." She continued, "I realized as we went through the catalogue together that you probably would not have chosen me to be our donor!"

The use of a donor gamete brings the couple and the donor together in a highly intimate way that is very apparent during the medical process. Traditionally, with a sperm donor, the couple has no knowledge of or contact with the donor (unless he is a known donor), and the insemination can be done at any time if frozen sperm is used. With an egg donor, the donor and recipient's menstrual cycles have to be coordinated, which sets in motion a powerful connection between the two women. At the time of fertilization the man has to be present to produce his sperm sample while the donor is having her eggs harvested. This experience can create a bond between the man and egg donor. One of the men in our project described this connection:

"Suppose somebody put you in a room and they said that in the next room is the woman you will have a child with and you have never met her. That process is already started and you haven't even seen this woman. She is breathing and living and existing in the next room and probably thinking of you. You are going to have a child together. That child will grow up and probably live long after you. What happens to you? I mean, unless you are numb or dead, you have to be having feelings that are stirred in you, and they certainly were in me."

Who to Tell and What to Say

The couples need to decide the level of openness regarding whom to inform about the donor gamete. In addition, the couple has to decide whether to tell the child about the use of a donor gamete. This opens up the issue of secrecy and privacy. We use the distinction between secrecy and privacy that is used in the adoption literature. *Secrecy* is defined as having information that would affect the well-being of another that is not told to her or him and therefore can hurt her or him; *privacy* is defined as putting boundaries around information that is personal and does not affect the person who is not being told (Schaffer & Diamond, 1993, p. 109).

Because these issues are still so new, there is very little research or literature to guide couples in telling family, friends, and the child. The medical community still believes in secrecy. In the past, physicians always advised patients to keep the use of donor gametes a secret; traditionally, this was the way donor sperm was handled. Women, in general, want to be more open about the use of donor egg than men in the past have been about using donor sperm. Women do feel better when they talk, and initially often feel helped by their conversations with others about the dilemma of whether or not to use donor eggs. However, when the couple eventually decides to use donor egg, they then may feel that they have been too open in revealing their problem and may subsequently want to keep the information more private. A customary statement couples often make to families and friends at this time is that they are trying IVF one last time with a different fertility center whose personnel are more optimistic for them. The woman becomes pregnant, but by donor egg. Unfortunately, while this statement recaptures privacy for the couple, it can have an unfortunate effect on other female friends who also are struggling with infertility and with whom they have shared this struggle. Knowing someone who has gone through multiple IVF cycles and then "miraculously" becomes pregnant can have the effect of influencing the friends to do additional cycles before considering donor eggs.

> One couple we were seeing in our project had four IVF cycles and were trying to decide whether or not to have a fifth cycle, which was recommended by their clinic. They were emotionally exhausted by the failures and financially strapped. One factor that was strongly influencing their decision to go ahead was the knowledge that their 47-year-old friend had finally gotten pregnant in her fifth cycle. Unbeknownst to our client, her friend was also being seen in our project and had become pregnant using a donor egg but had decided to keep this private.

To tell or not to tell the child is one of the major decisions a couple needs to make in using donor gametes. In the beginning, the decision to use donor gametes can be overwhelming to the couple. Often there are differences between them about whether to tell the child. As the experience becomes more integrated, couples are able to focus on this issue. In our experience, although each partner may have a different belief about whether to tell, through treatment, the couple often decides to share this information with the child.

Does the Child Have the Right to Know?

There is controversy in the professional community about whether a child "needs to know" or "has the right to know" about her or his biological heritage. Currently, physicians differ about whether or not a parent should disclose the use of a donor egg to the child. Many physicians still counsel couples to keep this fact a secret, even from their child, but more and more infertility clinics are recommending disclosure to the child because of the need to know one's genetic roots.

Since the first egg donation was done in 1984, there has been very little long-term research on the effect of donor eggs on the child and family. This contrasts with adoption, where there is an excellent body of expanding knowledge. In adoption, the current thinking is that the child should know about her or his biological parents and their heritage. But with donor gametes disclosure is still controversial.

We borrow from the adoption experience. When a couple is planning to use a donor egg, we ask them to consider the donor story they will tell to their child. We do not know what is going to happen as the child gets older about her or his desire to know her or his genetic mother. However, we advise the couple that there is no better time that they will have access to information about the donor than when they are choosing her. We suggest that they learn as much as possible about the donor's background, her family, and her medical history. They may never use this information, but it is important to know it. This approach is uncharted territory, and it is not known yet whether children born from donor gametes will follow the same path that adopted children have in wanting to search for their biological parent, but we have no reason to believe these children will be different from adopted children in their desire to know about their genetic parent.

Psychological Impact of the Donor

The psychological fact of the donor can create a triangle among the donor, the genetic parent, and the nongenetic parent. Although it may recede into the background of everyday life, it can also arise in any number of ways: a fleeting hand movement that neither parent can claim as theirs or a talent in a particular area that is not part of the heritage. It can also become a major factor in a medical history with a hereditary illness. Significant life events—birthdays, graduations, weddings, the birth of the adult child's own children—may also evoke the donor's presence.

The use of donor gametes may affect the balance of power in the marital relationship, since one parent is genetically related to the child and the other is not. The meanings that get connected to this need to be fully explored, in connection to the marital relationship as well as to the parental relationship. There have been situations where the biological parent may feel he (or she—if donor sperm is used) has more of a legitimate bond to the child than the nonbiological parent.

> During an acrimonious fight between a couple with a donor-egg child, the husband threatened that if they were to divorce, he would claim custody of their child since it was his biological offspring, and not hers.

The experience for the woman during her pregnancy with a donated egg also needs to be explored, with particular attention given to any problems with attachment.

> A woman in our project, 7 months pregnant with twins from donated eggs, described her feelings: "I feel very detached in a lot of ways. I mean, we went through a very upsetting weekend because we gave our dog away, and I feel we have nothing to show for this. We did it for the anticipation of the children, but they're not here yet. Nick says they are—they kick, they're large little people at this point. But I just don't think that way. They're an abstraction to me. I haven't bonded with them yet. I feel like the twins are somehow responsible for all this pain, for us having to give our dog up for something that's just an anticipation."

> Another woman impregnated with donor eggs described feeling as though aliens were inhabiting her body.

As therapists we become concerned if there are problems with attachment during pregnancy, for this may affect the attachment to the child after birth. We try to explore the meaning and impact of the infertility, the donor egg, and the woman's and man's own experience in being parented. We try to track the feelings about being the non-genetic parent with family-of-origin work (if needed) that will help the mother and father feel freer to attach. It is important to validate the feeling of inauthenticity that the nongenetic parent may feel, but also to do preventive work to strengthen the connection to the fetus.

TREATMENT CONCEPTS AND TECHNIQUES

As therapists, we see couples in many different phases of the infertility process, from their first recognition of the problem to the long-term legacy. The concept of the phases of infertility and treatment techniques for the phases has been developed fully in our book, *Couple Therapy for Infertility* (Diamond, Kezur, Meyers, Scharf, & Weinshel, 1999).

Assessing the Couple's Relationship

Infertility creates its own set of problems irrespective of the couple's dynamics. It is important that the therapist knows the impact that infertility can have on a couple's relationship. However, it is also necessary to get a history of how the couple has handled earlier difficulties in their marriage. We ask questions to track their problem-solving abilities, to examine the pattern of interaction around problematic issues, and to explore family-of-origin themes and beliefs. We also highlight the couple's strengths and resources.

The therapist has to be able to follow two tracks simultaneously: the specific issues of infertility, the couple's own relationship issues, and the impact of one set of issues on the other. Without specific knowledge concerning infertility issues, many therapists are unable to separate out infertility issues from the couple's own unique problems and thus tend to view the couple's functioning in a more negative pathological way. The primary goals of therapy are to highlight the infertility as a *couple's* issue: to validate the intensity of their pain, to strengthen the couple bond, and to help the couple handle the challenges of infertility.

Being Knowledgeable about Infertility

It is vital that a therapist treating infertility be well versed in the medical techniques and their acronyms. Couples want to feel you are knowledgeable not only about the medical issues, but also about the impact and experience of infertility.

With one couple we saw, the woman was describing her journey with infertility. In the middle of the story, she looked at the therapist and said "You know the lingo, don't you?" When the therapist responded, "Yes," the couple nodded their heads and the woman said, "Thank God! I had to explain everything to my last therapist. It made me feel she would never understand what we were going through."

Other couples have reported that our knowledge of infertility, as contrasted with the ignorance of their previous therapists, helped them focus on the essential dilemmas they were trying to solve.

Coaching Couples to Be "Educated Consumers"

We want to know how our couples are dealing with the medical system. We encourage them to become informed consumers of the medical procedures, for example, by learning about the rates of success for each new procedure. Often couples are afraid to ask their doctors hard questions because they fear that the doctors may get annoyed and withhold treatment. We help them to ask any and all questions and to advocate for themselves. Because the site of most infertility treatments is the woman's body, the woman in a couple may go alone to the medical appointments even though the problem may be the male factor, or an interactive factor. We encourage couples to go together to all medical appointments and to hear the results of the medical tests and procedures while they are together. When they are unable to do that, we encourage them to tell each other the results of the consultations as soon as possible, so it becomes a shared experience, and does not remain solely the responsibility of the woman.

Asking Couples to Tell Us Their Story

When we first see a couple, we start by asking them to tell us their story about infertility (Meyers, Weinshel, et al., 1995, p. 235). We are interested in their experiences with infertility and where they are in the process. This is an open-ended discussion, in which we encourage the couple to take the lead. From the outset, we track the interactional patterns of the couple, including their communication patterns. We also map the couple's relationships with family and other networks, including the medical system. We attend to the paradigms and beliefs that color each partner's experiences of the infertility process.

Exploring the Meaning of Infertility

We ask couples to describe the impact of infertility and how it has affected their perceptions of themselves, their partners, and their relationship (Meyers, Weinshel, et al., 1995, p. 226). Through an exploration of these descriptions, we highlight each partner's unique premises related to sexuality, gender roles, and parenthood. Through our use of explicit questions, we identify couple's beliefs and assumptions.

- What does infertility mean to you?
- How has infertility shaped the way you see life?
- How is infertility connected to your view of yourself as a woman (as a man)?
- How has your partner's infertility affected how you view him/her?

Recognizing and Validating the Grief, Loss, and Mourning

It is essential for therapists to recognize the losses in all the stages of infertility, from a woman's disappointment when she gets her period, to negative lab results, failed treatment protocols, and miscarriages. These losses need to be mourned by the couple. Otherwise, they can profoundly affect both the individuals and their couple relationship. Often the therapist needs to slow the couple down, to put a brake on their desire to move on to the next treatment in order to allow them to deal with these losses. When use of donor gametes is part of the process, the therapist should be aware of the couple's need to mourn the loss of their dream of having a fully genetically related child.

The use of rituals to facilitate mourning is very helpful. We try to help couples design their own rituals that feel comforting to them.

> One couple designed their "Bed and Chocolate Ritual." After each treatment failure, the husband would bring home videos and special chocolate candy they both loved. The couple would get into bed, cuddle, and watch the videos.

This ritual met this couple's need to be physically and emotionally close in sharing the sadness, without having to explicitly talk about the treatment failure.

Exploring the Value and Meaning of Children

We ask questions to help each partner explore and identify his or her own beliefs about children and parenting. We look not only for their own beliefs, but for those messages from their family of origin and assumptions drawn from their cultural context and the larger society that have influenced their thinking and feelings. Some of the questions we ask are the following:

- What are your thoughts and feelings about not having/having children in your life?
- How has not being able to get pregnant affected your view of yourself as a woman or man?
- How far is each of you willing to go to have a genetically related child?
- Is it a "child at all costs" or are there limits?
- What is it like for each of you to know you are not going to have a child that you create together?
- How will it be different if your child is not from your genetic material?
- Will it be worth all that it may take (physically, emotionally, and financially) to have a child that is fully related to both of you genetically?
- What will you do if you are not successful in getting pregnant?
- What is more important, giving birth to a child or being a parent?
- Have you always assumed that becoming a parent was not a matter of choice?
- If you choose not to have children, what challenges do you think you might face in regard to your family and friends? What about society at large?

Exploring the Consequences of Using a Donor Gamete

Often the use of donor gametes can be presented by the physician as just another treatment in the infertility protocols, with too little consideration to the meanings it may have for the couple. We try to slow down the process of moving rapidly to this new step by asking couples to take some time to consider the ramifications of using donor gametes. We raise the following questions for the couples to discuss:

- How will each of you feel if the child is genetically related to only one of you?
- Do you imagine that this will cause friction between you?
- How will one partner feel toward the other if he or she is the nongenetic parent?
- Do you imagine there will be a difference in your feelings toward the child about bonding, attachment, unconditional love, acceptance of difficulties and differences?
- How will each of your families of origin feel about the non-genetically related child? Will it affect their connection? Will the family of the genetic partner feel they have more of a claim to the child? If so, how will each of you respond to them and how will it affect your relationship to each other?
- What do you anticipate it would feel like at significant events such as birthdays, graduations, weddings, and the birth of a grandchild? Will you think about the donor at that time? Do you think such thoughts would alter your shared experience?

For the next group of questions, we ask Do you feel similarly or differently? Can you both discuss the issues? What effect do you feel the differences will have on your relationship?

- Do you plan on telling your child?
- At what age would you tell him or her?
- If your child has a physical problem, an emotional problem, learning problems, or social problems, how will you feel then about the use of donor?
- Do you plan on telling your family and friends about the use of donor at this time?
- How will you feel about your openness with others once your child is born?
- Do you think you might regret your openness at that time?
- What if the donor contacts you and wants to stay involved?

These questions are a starting point for the therapist to open up discussions to help couples anticipate and prepare for the emotional landmarks of using donor gametes.

Our Infertility Project does have a position about whether or not to tell a child. We do explore with couples what they think, but if asked, we will say that we lean toward being open and telling their child about the use of a donor gamete. Unfortunately, there is no research on what happens to children who are told or not told about donor origins. Since there is an actual pregnancy consequent to the use of donor sperm or egg, it can be easy to keep this fact a secret. But we believe that the child will eventually notice the secret in his or her parent's comments, and this can influence how the child views the world. Also, the adoption literature tells us that children who learn of their adoption at older ages often feel betrayed by and distrustful of their adoptive parents.

There are also conflicting opinions about the best time to tell a child. Annette Baran and Ruben Pannor (1980) think the ideal time to tell a child is when she or he is 10 and can understand the mechanics of reproduction. Carol Lieber Wilkins (1995) suggests telling a child at age 3, or when the child starts to ask about her or his birth story. We agree with Lieber Wilkins and think it may be easier for the child to accept his or her origins if this idea is introduced at an early age, as part of the birth story. It is also important that partners feel comfortable with the use of a donor gamete and that each has achieved some peace with the infertility. One explanation we suggest for using a donor egg is: "Mommy and Daddy weren't able to make a baby grow inside Mommy because she didn't have enough eggs. A nice woman gave us some of her eggs so we could make a baby." The degree of disclosure can increase as the child gets older and asks more questions. Therefore, the more details one can amass about the donor, the more information you can offer the child. Moreover, the child will appreciate that the parent is interested in giving him/her this vital information.

Another reason to speak openly about the donor is the explosion in genetic research, the increased knowledge about genetic diseases, and the importance of knowing one's genetic background.

> One woman we saw who was considering using donor eggs had a history of breast cancer in her family. Her mother had just died from breast cancer and so her sister had decided to have a prophylactic double mastectomy. A daughter from a donor egg would not have the same genetic background and would need to know that she was not likely to develop breast cancer and would not be facing the same choices.

Holding Separate Sessions to "Speak the Unspeakable"

We routinely offer separate individual sessions, along with the couple sessions, in order to explore topics each has kept secret from her/his partner. In these sessions, we question the problematic premises on which the secrets are based in order to free partners to discuss them with each other. We also focus on the future consequences of talking or not talking with one's partner, talking only with one's individual therapist, or remaining silent. Focusing on a future perspective with the use of future questioning (Penn, 1985) helps to make the constraining secrets more conspicuous and enables partners to share them. We call this process *"speaking the unspeakable."* We ask each individual what they are not telling their partner about their feelings and beliefs about the infertility, and what the consequences would be of saying or not saying them.

> One woman told us in a separate session that she did not want to have sex with her husband because he was sterile, and she no longer found him sexy. Sex was a painful reminder of his infertility. She preferred faking her sexual response rather than telling him, because she feared it would hurt him and hurt their relationship. She felt these things were best shared only with her individual therapist. We asked her, "If the situation were reversed, would you want him to tell you?" She replied: "Absolutely not!" We then asked her, "How do you imagine your marriage will be in the future if you take all your painful issues to an individual therapist rather than to your husband?" At the next couple session, the wife said she had thought about what had been said and decided to speak with her husband. She was amazed to discover that he too was finding sex painful and a sorrowful reminder of what they could not do together—make a baby.

Using "Time In" and "Time Out"

Because infertility can be so consuming and omnipresent, we have found it is important to help couples learn how to take a "break" from this constant focus. We have drawn on the strategy of a *"time in and a time out"* from the world of infertility. We give couples the task to schedule a *"time in,"* to talk about the infertility, and a *"time out,"* not to talk about the infertility, and to do something pleasurable during the time out when the infertility is not discussed. A time in and a time out can also be used with sex: time in for sex for baby making, and time out for sex for fun.

> A couple we saw was having sexual problems due to his impotence, which only occurred when she was ovulating, and therefore they needed to have scheduled sex. We emphasized that they should

not expect their baby-making sex to be passionate or even enjoy-able. They just needed to do it. We suggested that at other times during *the* month, without the pressure of baby-making, they try having sex for fun.

CASE EXAMPLE

Sara and Barry, both 39 years old, married for 2 years, were seen in the Infertility Project. Since Sara had had an abortion and Barry had been told he had impregnated his former girlfriend, both assumed they would have no trouble conceiving. They moved from an apartment in the city that was convenient for work to a house in the suburbs which they chose as a place to begin their family. They picked the neighbor-hood for its good schools and family community. They tried to become pregnant, but after a few months without conception Sara became sus-picious that there might be a problem. Her gynecologist would not take Sara's concerns seriously. Without even asking if she had a job, he sug-gested that she was a bored housewife, and indicated that if she had more to do, she would not worry so much about becoming pregnant After a year of trying to conceive, the couple went for an infertility con-sultation and discovered that Barry had practically no sperm and was infertile. At this time, ICSI was still in the experimental stage. There-fore, the only options open to the couple were donor sperm or adop-tion. Either way, Barry would not be able to have his own genetically re-lated child. He was devastated. Both Barry's father and brother offered to donate sperm. For Sara, sperm from Barry's father was unthinkable; sperm from Barry's brother involved telling his wife, and the couple wanted to keep this a secret from her. Sara also worried about the fu-ture consequences of using Barry's brother's sperm. Sara admitted, however, that if she had been the infertile one, she would have had no problem in receiving an egg from her sister, and Barry agreed.

They came to see us after Sara discovered that Barry had gone to a meeting about adoption without telling her. The couple was devastated about the infertility and out-of-synch with each other about the next step to take. Sara's choice was donor sperm, and she was upset that Barry had jumped to adoption without discussing it with her. In the first interview, we asked them to "tell us their story." What came across were their feelings of overwhelming pain and sadness and their sense of isolation from their family and friends, who were impatient with their reactions and could not understand the extent of their grief.

At the end of the session, we posed a series of questions for the couple to think about to help them focus on their next step. We asked Sara, "What is your worry if you tell Barry all the feelings you have about your egg and his sperm not being able to meet?" We asked Sara and Barry, "Which option, donor sperm or adoption, would each one of you prefer? Which do you think would be your partner's choice? What do you imagine it will be like to tell people that you will be using donor sperm? At what point would you tell them? With the implantation? When you become pregnant? Who will you tell, and who will you not tell? What are the implications of keeping it a secret or being open? What do you think your family's response will be to donor sperm? to adoption? How do you think you will respond to your family's reactions? What do you each imagine the other will feel if you have a baby with donor sperm? With adoption?" We told the couple to think about these questions, and also told then that although they did not need to discuss them all before the next session, their answers would determine their next step.

At the next session, they started by saying how important the questions had been for them. They felt we had given them permission to talk and this had opened up a level of communication that had been blocked before because each was worried about hurting the other. They spoke about how the infertility had affected their own sense of their masculinity and femininity. They had decided to go ahead with donor sperm but were still very sad about their inability to have a child together. Barry described his infertility: "The images of infertility are devastating. It's like literally the end of the line." Poignantly, Sara opened up and said to Barry:

> "What I want you to understand is that I, too, have been in pain for you and for myself. The last time we were here, I was very upset because I felt you had shared your pain with me, as you should have, but I had only been able to share with you my sadness for you. I felt you were not able to understand that I have my own sadness and loss and for some reason, it is very important for me to have you validate that. Family and friends have said that your loss is a tragedy and I shouldn't even cry in front of you because it will make you feel guilty. But, it's a loss for both of us—and a loss for you, and a loss for me. I know that your loss, Barry, is profound and unthinkable, but I too feel a profound sense of loss. I don't want to just have a baby. I want *your* baby."

At the end of the session, the team shared its thinking about the couple's situation. We told Barry that the men in the group understood his feelings of loss. We told Sara that the women in the group understood that she would have feelings about not having a child with Barry and having anonymous sperm inside of her. We thought that Sara had taken a risk to tell Barry her feelings and it had given Barry a chance to comfort her (which he had done in the session). Up until now, it had been Barry's loss and Sara had had to be sympathetic to him. We said they were in different places: for Barry, the pain was in the present, and he was mourning his infertility. For Sara, the moment of extreme sadness would be at conception—which was in the future. Sara then started to sob and said "Thank you for saying that." Barry added, "I look back with anxiety, she looks forward." When she finished sobbing, Sara said: "I didn't think anyone else would ever understand that. I'm not sure that anyone else ever will—outside of this room."

This session freed the couple to stop protecting one another and they moved forward to make mutually acceptable decisions about the infertility. They chose donor sperm and decided to be open about their decision before and after the child was born. We continued to see them throughout the inseminations, the pregnancy, and the birth of their son. On a follow-up visit, they were doing well. They did not want their son to feel different about his origins so they had organized a group of parents with donor offspring that had become their social network.

THERAPISTS' ASSUMPTIONS

It is very important for the therapist to be aware of his/her own assumptions. These include how he/she thinks about the need for a couple to have children; his/her own personal beliefs about using reproductive interventions for infertility, donor gametes, and adoption; and how he/she feels about a couple choosing not to have children.

Using donor gametes and adoption can induce powerful feelings in therapists. It is crucial that those feelings do not get conveyed to the couple and influence the couple's own decision making. The therapist, as in all therapy, is there to help the couple come to *their own* decisions.

FAMILY THERAPISTS AND INFERTILITY

Infertility can be a devastating problem for couples who struggle with it, but often this struggle remains invisible to the outside world. The loss of an imagined fully genetically related child has been minimized by society and consequently by those close to the couple. The advent of advanced reproductive technology combined with the baby boom generation's belief that the only limits to achievement are one's own drawbacks made pregnancy seem possible to everyone. However, for many older women whose fertility has decreased the only possibility of having a pregnancy is through the use of donor eggs. ART has opened up choices that will affect the couple for the rest of their lives, as well as pose ethical and moral dilemmas for their relationships with each other and with their child.

When seeing couples and getting a history of their relationship, therapists need to be alerted to the possibility of infertility. In the case of adoption, infertility is usually clear. However, if a couple has no children, the question of whether this is a voluntary or involuntary decision needs to be asked. If there is a gap between the couple's getting together and having children, or a large space between the ages of the children, questions about infertility need to be addressed. Even if a couple has two children (which is the current culturally accepted number), the therapist should ask if the couple has the number of children they wanted.

The legacy of infertility is powerful. It can be the onset of ongoing sexual and couple concerns that may continue long after the infertility has presented as a problem. It can affect all aspects of the couple's sense of themselves as individuals and of their relationship. Therapists need to respect infertility's power and work with the couple to strengthen their relationship so they can cope together with the many challenges of infertility.

ACKNOWLEDGMENTS

The ideas in this chapter come from the combined work of the Ackerman Institute's Infertility Project. The other members include Ronny Diamond, David Kezur, and Mimi Meyers, whom we thank.

REFERENCES

Baran, A., & Pannor, R. (1989). *Lethal secrets.* New York: Warner Books.
Centers for Disease Control and Prevention (CDC); National Center for Chronic Disease Prevention and Health Promotion, Division of Reproductive Health, Atlanta, Georgia; American Society for Reproductive Medicine, Society for Reproductive Technology, Birmingham, Alabama; & RESOLVE, Somerville, Massachusetts. (1997). *1995 assisted reproductive technology success*

rates: National summary and fertility clinic reports: Vol. 1. Eastern United States. U.S. Department of Health and Human Services, Centers for Disease Control and Prevention, & National Center for Chronic Disease Prevention and Health Promotion.

Diamond, R., Kezur, D., Meyers, M., Scharf, C. N., & Weinshel, M. (1999). *Couple therapy for infertility.* New York: Guilford Press.

Freeman, E. W., Boxer, A. S., Rickels, K., Tureck, R., & Mastrioanni, L. (1985). Psychological evaluation and support in a program of in vitro fertilization and embryo transfer. *Fertility and Sterility, 43,* 51.

Gill, M. S. (1998, May). Fertility goddess. *Vogue,* pp. 171–173.

Hodder, H. F. (1997, December). The new fertility. *Harvard Magazine,* pp. 61–98.

Lieber Wilkens, C. (1995). *Talking to children about their conception: A parent's perspective.* Paper presented at the 51st annual meeting of the American Society for Reproductive Medicine, Seattle, WA.

Marrs, R., with Bloch, I. F., & Silverman, K. K. (1997). *Dr. Richard Marrs' fertility book.* NY: Delacorte Press.

McEwan, K. L., Costello, C. G., & Taylor, P. J. (1987). Adjustment to infertility. *Journal of Abnormal Psychology, 96,* 108–116.

Menning, B. E. (1988). *Infertility: A guide for the childless couple* (2nd ed.). New York: Prentice-Hall.

Merck manual (16th ed.). (1992). Philadelphia: National.

Meyers, M., Diamond, R., Kezur, D., Scharf, C., Weinshel, M., & Rait, D. (1995). An infertility primer for family therapists: I. Medical, social, and psychological dimensions. *Family Process, 34,* 219–229.

Meyers, M., Weinshel, M., Scharf, C., Kezur D., Diamond R., & Rait, D. (1995). An infertility primer for family therapists: II. Working with couples who struggle with infertility. *Family Process, 34,* 231–240.

Nachtigall, R. D., Becker, G., & Wozny, M. (1992). The effects of gender specific diagnosis on men's and women's response to infertility. *Fertility and Sterility, 57,* 113–121.

Penn, P. (1985). Feed-forward: Future questions, future maps. *Family Process, 24,* 299–310.

Rossing, M., Daling, J., Weiss, N., Moore, D., & Self, S. (1994). Ovarian rumors in a cohort of infertile women. *New England Journal of Medicine, 331,* 771–776.

Schaffer, J. A., & Diamond, R. (1993). Infertility: Private pain and secret stigma. In E. Imber-Black (Ed.), *Secrets in families and family therapy.* New York: Norton.

CHAPTER 6

Gender Differences in Depression

His or Her Depression

Peggy Papp

Depression is the psychiatric disability of our time. During the past decade there has been a sharp rise in the incidence of depression around the world. According to a report from the World Health Organization the second leading worldwide cause of disability in 1990 was unipolar major depression (cited in Grinfeld, 1996). In the United States more people are hospitalized for depression than for any other psychiatric condition.

This rising tide of depression has resulted in a river of information that has flooded the mass media and professional literature. Key professional journals have devoted whole issues to the evaluation and treatment of depression, guidelines have been published in medical journals for the use of antidepressants, and articles appear daily in newspapers and magazines describing symptoms and treatments. Antidepressants were initially hailed as the great pharmacological discovery that was to wipe out depression just like the Salk vaccine had eliminated polio. Prozac was featured on the front page of *Newsweek*, and the accompanying article was filled with stories of instant transformation. Peter Kramer's (1993) book *Listening to Prozac* became a bestseller, Prozac Anonymous groups sprang up around the country, and depression became a "hot" topic on the talk shows.

In our society's zeal to find simple solutions to complex problems, depression was defined primarily as a biochemical disease to be treated medically. Thus this complex condition with all its emotional, psychological, cultural, and biological elements was disconnected from life events and human circumstances and reduced to a mere genetic defect.

Over the years, in the search for a solution to this mysterious and unpredictable condition, treatment approaches have undergone many variations that mirrored the therapeutic trends and climate of their times. The early Freudian models looked for intrapsychic causes associated with repressed anger and early childhood deprivation and losses. Depressive symptoms were viewed as the result of unconscious conflicts with the transference relationship, a key feature in treatment. The most recent development in the Freudian approach is a time-limited psychodynamic therapy created by Strupp and Binder (1984), who have published a training manual based on their method of changing personality and character structure.

In the middle of the century, time-limited short-term approaches came into vogue, such as cognitive, behavioral, and interpersonal therapies. The behavioral approach introduced by Ferster (1965) postulates that depression is caused by a loss of positive reinforcement due to separation, death, or sudden environmental change. Behavioral techniques such as self-monitoring and self-reinforcement are employed. Jacobson (1984) has published widely on marital therapy for depression based on the behavioral approach.

The marital discord model of Beach, Sandeen, and O'Leary (1990) expanded the behavioral model to address both cognitive and affective aspects of the couple's relationship. Tasks are given to promote marital support and intimacy while also attending to individual vulnerability and self-esteem.

Cognitive therapy, developed by Aaron T. Beck and his colleagues (Beck, Rush, Shaw, & Emery, 1979), attributes depression to faulty cognitions, or patterns of thinking. The depressed person is seen as having unrealistically negative views of the self, the world, and the future. The goal of cognitive therapy is to correct this distorted thinking.

Teichman and Teichman (1990) integrated cognitive marital therapy with a systematic perspective incorporating cognitive, emotion, behavior, and environmental context. Michael Yapko recently combined a cognitive with a family systems approach in his book *Hand-Me-Down Blues* (1999).

Coyne's model of strategic marital therapy (1995) is based on the assumption that depression is maintained by the ineffective coping style of the depressed person and by the resulting negative interactional sequence between the marital couple. Treatment is focused on interrupting this negative sequence and increasing the coping capacity of the depressed person.)

Interpersonal therapy, developed by Klerman, Weissman, Rounsaville, and Chevron (1984), is based on the assumption that interpersonal difficulties are the cause and/or consequence of depression. Clients are seen individually to help them deal more effectively with their interpersonal problems.

The systems model, the cornerstone of family therapy, is based on examining and treating problems within their relational and social contexts. This means looking at the various systems that impact a depressed person's life, including family, work, cultural, interpersonal, and biological systems. The emphasis is on the *connection* and *interplay* between inner experiences and these outside systems that perpetuate depressive symptoms. Among those noted for bringing a systems perspective to treatment of depression are Papp (1997), Real (1997), Braverman (1986), Moltz (1993), Howard and Weeks (1995), Taffel (1991), and Yapko (1999).

With the introduction of a biological explanation for depression and the development of antidepressants in the 1980s and 1990s psychotherapy of all kinds was relegated to the back burner. The typical treatment for depression was pharmacological, consisting of a 15-minute session once a month with a psychiatrist who prescribed and monitored antidepressants. Psychotherapy as a legitimate treatment was considered passé. However, it soon became clear that the early descriptions of sudden personality transformations from taking antidepressants were exaggerated and misleading. Only a very few depressed people experienced such dramatic results. For the vast majority, improvement from antidepressants ranged from significant to moderate to no improvement at all. Although antidepressants have undeniably made a substantial and sometimes lifesaving contribution to controlling the symptoms of depression, they do not eradicate its complex causes. Depression for most people is related to more than brain chemistry.

A turning point in this medically oriented climate came in 1995 when the Consumers Union issued the results of a study showing that psychotherapy is as effective or more effective than drugs for treating depression, with no side effects and lower rates of relapse. This report confirmed what most therapists have long known: that depression takes place in an interpersonal context and is profoundly influenced by close intimate relationships. Subsequent research and personal histories supported the Consumers Union report and led to the current consensus that a combination of antidepressants and psychotherapy is the most effective treatment for depression.

We are still in the dark as to just how the complex interaction between serotonin levels and life experiences takes place. So far the majority of studies linking depression to abnormal serotonin levels in the brain fail to take into account that the mind–body connection runs in both directions and that our thoughts can make us depressed. Researchers Henn and Edwards (cited in Real, 1997) produced all the symptoms of a "depressed brain" in rats by giving them electric shocks from which they could not escape. The rats eventually gave up trying to escape and thereafter exhibited all the signs of severe depression, including altered chemical levels in their brain. After the researchers taught the rats to escape their helplessness by pressing a lever to end the shock, their depression subsided and so did their brain abnormalities.

At this point in time what is needed is more research that will illuminate the interplay between the biological and psychological theories of depression. These conflicting theories make this condition one of the most confusing and difficult to treat. Therapists are left to wonder, "Is this person's depression due to a chemical imbalance or an unhappy marriage, a death in the family, a job failure, a painful divorce, or a chronic illness?" There are a wide range of factors that may be contributing to depression. The triggers that set it off at any particular time will be different for each person, and consequently the solution will be different for each person. To adequately treat depression it must be understood within a person's total life situation.

The Depression in Context Project of the Ackerman Institute was set up to develop a multidimensional approach to depression, one that would take into account its biological, psychological, interpersonal, social, and gender aspects. The impetus for the project came from a number of research studies showing a connection between depression, marriage, and gender that have been largely overlooked by our field. We decided to address this omission by paying particular attention to this connection.

It has long been recognized that twice as many women as men suffer from depression. Numerous theories have been advanced in attempting to explain this higher incidence of depression in women, including biological differences, lower socioeconomic status, developmental and temperamental differences, and stereotypical sex role expectations, but so far no research is conclusive and all these theories remain speculative.

We do know that the most stressful life event that precipitates depression is that marital conflict and marital conflict is the single most predictable indicator of relapse. It has also been established that marriage serves a protective function for men but not for women in terms of depression. Married men are the least subject to depression as compared to single men or married, single, or divorced women. Other studies show that the reaction of a depressed person's spouse to her or his depression is of primary important in her or his recovery and is more highly correlated with relapse after hospitalization than with the original degree of depression.

We believe these statistics have profound implications for the diagnosis and treatment of depression. We set up the Depression Project to address the following questions:

- Do men and women get depressed for different reasons?
- Do they react differently when depressed?
- What part do traditional sex roles play in depression?
- Is the adaptive behavior of men and women to a depressed spouse different?
- Are there stereotypical gender beliefs and expectations that predispose both men and women to depression?

We decided these questions could best be addressed by treating couples in couple therapy because gender beliefs and expectations are played out on a daily basis in an intimate relationship.

GENDER, SELF-ESTEEM, AND DEPRESSION

Women's Self-Esteem

Depression is universally described as *a profound disturbance of mood connected with a negative view of one's self-image.* Terms such as "lack of self-esteem" and "low self-image" are used over and over in the literature on depression. It is impossible to separate one's self-image from one's identity as a woman or a man. The self does not exist in a vacuum but in a relational and social context. This context is profoundly influenced by the gender norms and expectations that prescribe how we are supposed to behave as women or men. Failure to live up to these expectations can be damaging to our self-esteem. As Virginia Goldner (1985, p. 21) so aptly states, "Personhood and gender identity develop together, co-evolving and co-determining each other. As a result, one could no more become de-gendered than de-selfed." Much of the diagnosis and treatment of depression is "de-gendered."

In exploring the connection between gender and self-esteem, we first considered the different ways in which women and men assess and maintain their self-esteem. Women's self-esteem is still built largely around relatedness and emotional connections in their professional as well as domestic life. Their self-worth is associated with being responsible for and giving to others. This often requires them to put their own needs second, suppress their anger, take responsibility for the physical and emotional well-being of those around them, and blame themselves if anything goes wrong. Women usually get depressed because of a cut-off or disruption in a close relationship.

In *Silencing the Self* (1991, p. 168), Dana Crowley Jack describes depressed women as experiencing a divided self, "an outwardly conforming, compliant self, and an inner, secret self who is enraged and resentful." According to Jack, by silencing their voices, the women kept themselves from expressing their anger openly and their mates were unaware of its source. Jack concludes that the women had silenced their voices and become depressed not because they were "passive and dependent" but because they didn't trust their perceptions and feelings and were afraid of isolation or reprisal if they expressed them openly.

Depressed women are nearly always acutely aware of an emotional distance in their marital relationship, and so they reach out for more contact and closeness. When they feel safe enough to express their underlying feelings we hear statements such as "I feel I'm living on an emotional desert." "He's not interested in my feelings." "We never talk to each other."

Men's Self-Esteem

Men's self-esteem remains largely performance-oriented, that is, it involves achievement and success in the workplace, earning money and accruing status and power, excelling in sports, performing sexually; taking part in other externally socially validating experiences. In order to live up to these masculine standards, they are required to deny dependency, repress personal emotions, guard against intimacy, and avoid any feelings that incapacitate them or make them feel weak and helpless. Men are prone to depression when they fail to live up to these cultural expectations and cut themselves off emotionally from intimate relationships.

Unlike depressed women, most depressed men seem unaware of their need for intimacy and have a hard time reaching out to their partner for comfort or more contact. They rarely connect their depression with any aspect of their relationship—even though when they are able to develop a more open and supportive relationship with their partner they are better able to handle the stress and competitiveness in the workplace. Many men are reluctant to share feelings of disappointment, anxiety, anger, and frustration that are generated at work. We often hear remarks such as "I don't want to bring problems home" or "I've always believed in handling my problems myself." By doing so they deprive themselves of the support and comfort they might gain from their partners and at the same time deprive their partners of an opportunity to share their lives.

DIFFERENCES IN CARETAKING

There is a marked difference in the caretaking practices of men and women. Again, these often fall into stereotypical gender patterns. When women are depressed, men typically try a problem-solving approach replete with talk of "fixing it," "analyzing the situation," "coming up with a constructive solution," or "mapping out a plan of action." The depressed women generally experience these efforts as dominating and controlling. Instead of advice and suggested solutions, they want more verbal exchange and a sharing of feelings. The men have great difficulty understanding what it is the women are asking for since they experience themselves as having made every effort to "help" them. An exasperated husband, after a weekend of unsuccessfully trying to raise his wife's spirits, exclaimed, "I took you boating, didn't I?," to which his wife sadly replied, "Yes, but you never talked to me."

Women react differently when men are depressed. They tend to protect, placate, and appease. They cater to their moods, shield them from intrusive telephone calls, keep the children away, and protect them from their extended families. Although the men rely on their caretaking, they often resent it because it makes them feel dependent and controlled.

Despite all the changes that have taken place in traditional male/female roles, stereotypical beliefs and patterns still tend to dominate couples' lives in important ways and are intricately interwoven in the patterns of depression. Of course, depression is an individual response to these traditional beliefs and expectations. After all, everyone who holds such beliefs does not automatically become depressed. However, we think it is important to become aware of the different ways in which they might be contributing to a person's depression.

TREATMENT APPROACH

We view the couple relationship as a potential source of healing and future prevention. Thus we involve the nondepressed partners in the recovery process from the very beginning of therapy. We learned early on the importance of acknowledging the effect of the depression on the partners, who not only feel left out and rejected by their depressed mate, but also feel ignored by the mental health system in which they are typically excluded from treatment plans. They are bewildered and frightened by the ambiguous loss of a partner who is there in body but not in spirit. Their frequent attempts to rescue their partner from the black pit of despair have failed and they are left alone to cope with their feelings of frustration, anger, helplessness, and guilt. We convey a sense of confidence in their ability to do something that will make a difference, while also sympathizing with their despair and acknowledging their fortitude and commitment.

The first stage of therapy is focused on identifying the precipitating event that led to the most recent episode of depression, dealing with the aftermath of the hospitalization, and exploring the effect of the depression on the couple's relationship over the years. This is usually the first opportunity either partner has had to express their pent-up feelings of anxiety and confusion in a safe setting.

We cast a wide net in searching for the experiences or situations that may be creating a depressed person's sense of hopelessness. Is it interpersonal relationships work, extended family, or past history? We look for the triggers in the couple's interaction that may be affecting the degree of depression, and we examine the expectations and beliefs behind these daily interactional patterns. We pay special attention to those beliefs involving power, dominance/submission, equality, and responsibility and the effect of those on the couple's decision making around crucial issues such as sex, money, work, and parenting.

The links among each partner's beliefs and those of their family, culture, and religion are explored. Each spouse's functioning, as a marital partner and in other roles—daughter, son, mother, father—is examined. This is based on our observation that conflictual relationships with parents or children can contribute substantially to depression.

Our referrals come primarily from psychiatric hospitals. Most of the depressed spouses we see have a long history of depression, with numerous hospitalizations and some serious suicide attempts. All of the depressed partners take antidepressants that are being monitored by an outside psychiatrist with whom we maintain a collaborative relationship. The antidepressants have initially provided varying degrees of symptom relief but have had little or no effect on the couple's relationship. In our experience antidepressants are helpful in alleviating the most severe symptoms of depression and enabling people to begin to *face* life's problems but they don't *solve* life's problems.

The members of the project staff—Jeffrey Seibel, Gloria Klein, Paul Feinberg, Sanja Rolovic, and myself—work in male–female cotherapy teams. While one team interviews the couple, the other team observes behind the one-way mirror and serves as a consultation team.

BEING HEARD

A sense of emotional connectedness is essential in alleviating depression in both men and women. But just as the source of the disconnection is generally different for men and women, the approach to reconnecting should be tailored to their individual needs.

Whatever else is bothering the depressed women, their major complaint is not "being heard" by the men they live with. The men often feel overwhelmed by the women's complaints and either dismiss them as part of their "sickness," invalidate them with defensive justifications, or become angry and leave the room. The sessions provide a safety zone for raising and discussing these forbidden subjects.

In one situation, a depressed wife was able to speak for the first time about how she felt abandoned every night when her husband went into an alcoholic stupor. This was a taboo subject that she had never been able to broach without a heated argument. The husband who, until now, had blamed all their problems on the wife's depression was initially enraged when she introduced what he considered to be an irrelevant subject. When the wife became intimidated and started to withdraw, we encouraged her to continue to express what was bothering her. In the discussion that followed the husband was finally able to admit he was "not really there" when he drank and revealed his own secret fear that he would become an alcoholic like his mother. He agreed to start limiting his drinking and promised to go to AA if he could not control it. This made an enormous difference to the wife, as she felt her husband had "heard" her and that he valued the relationships enough to do something that was difficult for him. Her feelings toward him, cut off and withheld for many years, began to return. As a result of her new insight that her "illness" was *not* responsible for all their problems, her depression lifted to the point where she was able to get out of bed and resume functioning.

In another case, a wife's desire to throw herself out the window arose from her despair over her inability to "get through" to her husband concerning a desperate financial situation. Every time she attempted to bring it up, her husband diverted the conversation into complaints about their sex life. Finally, trembling and crying, she announced that she could no longer remain silent about what was happening in their life. She then revealed that her husband, who had been fired from his job and had not worked for many months, was involved in illegal activities. She lived in constant fear of his being caught because this would implicate her and jeopardize her job. Her husband had refused to discuss these issues because he said his wife became "irrational" and "hysterical." He believed her worries to be "excessive" due to her "illness." The wife was left with no recourse and felt trapped in an intolerable situation. Once her fears were out on the table and validated as "real" by the therapists, her husband could no longer dismiss them as "excessive." He eventually conceded that there was some risk involved for his wife and family in the present situation and agreed to take responsibility for working out a different financial plan. When the wife felt "heard," her hope returned and she saw other alternatives to throwing herself out the window.

BECOMING CONNECTED

Since men's identity is closely connected with their work, we consider it crucial to explore the meaning of work in their lives and particularly the impact of their work on their self-esteem. It is not unusual for them to suppress their unique abilities and talents in order to conform to the societal mandate to achieve status and make money, or in some cases, simply to make a viable living for themselves and their families. They often find themselves locked into jobs they dislike, which they perform routinely without enthusiasm or hope. Thus life becomes meaningless and drab. As their dreams go down the drain, their sense of identity and purpose goes with them. Whenever we discover that a man's work situation is a factor in his depression, we ask him to examine his priorities, values, and options and, in some circumstances, we encourage him to consider a different life plan.

Prior to entering our project, one husband had admitted himself to a psychiatric hospital after having been promoted to a managerial job. In the first session we discovered he had become depressed several times before as a result of a promotion. He had been told by a succession of previous therapists that he was "afraid of success." These therapists had persuaded him each time to return to his new job and "face his problem."

In exploring his work experience, we discovered that he had valid reasons for not wanting to be promoted. He loved the hands-on work on the lower rungs of the ladder and felt awkward and uncomfortable in the role of manager or supervisor. In his most recent supervisory position he was required to side with management on employment practices that he believed to be exploitive. He had accepted the promotion because "that's what a man is supposed to do—climb the ladder, be ambitious, get ahead, make more money." He was convinced that his inability to conform to these values was a "fatal flaw."

We offered an alternative explanation to the previously offered "fear of success." Rather than seeing it as a "fatal flaw," we saw his panic and depression as a natural reaction to his going against his innate values and integrity and trying to wear a mantle for which he was unsuited. One of our therapists told the story of a famous acting coach who, after sitting through a painful rendering of a scene from *Medea*, turned to the student and said, "If Frank Sinatra had tried to sing opera he would have been a dismal failure. Stick with what you do best." The husband then hinted, somewhat embarrassedly, that he would really like to return to his old job, but felt his wife would object because it would mean a lower income. His wife, who had been listening intently, confessed that until now she had never understood the meaning of his promotions, and had always assumed that his running away from them was a sign of weakness. Her new understanding enabled her to support him in his decision to return to his old job—she felt it was a small price to pay for his mental and emotional well-being.

This case points up the importance of having the partner participate in the treatment. Had the wife not been present, she may never have understood the connection between her husband's depression and his not being able to devote his life to the kind of work he loved and was best suited for.

CHANGING BELIEF SYSTEMS

When two people come together to form an intimate relationship, they bring with them a whole set of beliefs regarding love, marriage, intimacy, sexuality, gender roles, and the way men and women should relate to one another. They are generally unaware of the way that these beliefs, which are implicit rather than explicit, govern their lives and relationships. We believe it is important to understand each partner's belief system and the way in which these interlock to form the foundation of the couple's relationship. When these belief systems are better understood, they can be used as a code for deciphering the interactions that set off episodes of depression.

The following three cases are examples of the way in which we identify and challenge the underlying beliefs of each partner on several different levels, including their beliefs around work, extended family, and stereotypical cultural myths.

"I Don't Want a Father Figure"

Upon her release from the hospital, where she had spent a month for a severe depression, Sonya, a 40-year-old European woman, requested marital therapy but was told by the hospital staff that she needed individual psychiatric treatment. She complied with the hospital's assessment and saw a psychiatrist for the next 6 months. However, she continued to feel her depression was connected with marital problems and finally left the psychiatrist and applied to our institute for couple counseling.

During the first session it became clear that she was extremely dependent on her husband, Tom, for approval, which she sought constantly but failed to attain because he was extremely critical. Tom saw his criticism as "helpful advice" in the service of "straightening her out" and "keeping her from going down the tubes." In response to his criticism, Sonya felt defeated and withdrew to her room to cry for hours.

In the following dialogue we are exploring Tom's belief that the best way to help his wife is to constantly criticize her.

THERAPIST: (to Tom) Do you understand, Tom, what she means when she says she feels dominated by you?

TOM: No, I don't understand. She's a dominant woman and I let her be dominant. All I do is give her helpful advice and she thinks it's criticism.

THERAPIST: (to Sonya) Do you want his advice?

SONYA: No.

TOM: I know she doesn't, but I give it to her anyway because I can't stand to see her going down the tubes the way she's going. The thing is, I feel if I give her the tweak which is the advice and she reacts violently, then she will see the error of her ways. What I'm trying to do is let her see her own mistakes.

Sonya then tells of a recent incident in which Tom was the one who made the mistake and screamed at her for something she hadn't done. Tom admitted he made a mistake but refused to apologize. In explor-

ing the belief behind his refusal, the therapist uncovers his deeply ingrained belief that compels him to keep criticizing her.

THERAPIST: You would never apologize even though you knew you
made a mistake?

TOM: Not if I'm going to help her. Because then she's going to think
I'm weak and not capable of taking care of her.

THERAPIST: I see. You think if you apologize then you—

TOM: She would not accept my criticism then.

THERAPIST: So you feel you have to remain very stern and like a father?

TOM: Yes.

SONYA: Wow! I never knew that.

TOM: If I weaken she's going to go ahead and do all this stuff.

THERAPIST: (*to Sonya*) What do you think? If he had said he was sorry
would you—

SONYA: I would have cried out of happiness realizing how strong he is
that he has grown to understand how to relate to a woman.

THERAPIST: I see—so you would think he was strong if he did that?

SONYA: Of course!

THERAPIST: (*to Tom*) You thought she would think you were weak?

SONYA: It takes strength to admit something that didn't go quite right.

THERAPIST: Did that ever occur to you—that she might think you were
strong to do that?

TOM: (*after a long pause*) No.

THERAPIST: How does that sound to you now?

TOM: Would you accept my criticism if I apologized?

SONYA: I wasn't asking for criticism.

THERAPIST: Do you think she needs your criticism or your support?

TOM: She needs my help. I think it's support. I don't see anything
wrong with it.

THERAPIST: (*to Sonya*) What do you think is wrong with it? What would
you rather have him do?

SONYA: I'd like to have an adult discussion with him person to person.

I don't want a father figure. I don't want a police figure. I don't want a superior figure talking to me.

Sonya is able to state her need for an "adult" relationship involving support, equality, and understanding. This conflicts with Tom's belief that coercion and criticism equal strength and empathy and support equals weakness. He is reluctant to relinquish his expert position for fear he will lose Sonya's respect, and thereby his control over her. The idea that she can respect him as anything but a stern authoritarian father figure is new to him.

Tom's practice of using intimidation to exert control was learned early in his life. As the eldest son, he felt compelled to control a "crazy and chaotic" family. The only option that seemed open to him was to use strong-arm tactics. This practice served him well as a teenager growing up in a tough neighborhood and was later reinforced in the business world where it brought him status and money.

Eventually Tom was able to see that there were better ways of helping his wife than his strong-arm tactics. He learned to tolerate the anxiety that accompanied his letting go of the expert position as he experienced the rewards of a closer relationship with Sonya.

Sonya's desire for an "adult" relationship required a continuing effort on her part to avoid lapsing into the helpless victim position. This was difficult for her to do as she had no model of an assertive woman. She saw her mother as weak and passive for succumbing to her father's abusive and domineering behavior. She blamed her mother for not saving her from her father's physical abuse, and paradoxically favored her father despite his abuse.

It is common for depressed women to have contempt for their mothers, whom they see as disempowered second-class citizens, while respecting the power and authority of their fathers—even when it is turned against them. This gender-biased view is bound to effect their feelings about themselves as well as their relationship with the opposite sex. Sonya's contempt for her mother was mirrored in her contempt for herself and led to feelings of despair whenever she experienced the sense of following in her footsteps. An important part of our work lay in helping her to perceive her mother differently and reconnect with her on a new basis.

She had not spoken to her mother for 2 years because of an argument on her last visit home. Although she claimed she wanted nothing more to do with her and had written her off as "cold and uncaring," she became despondent every Mother's Day.

In order to learn more about her mother's social context, we began asking Sonya questions about the culture of her country and women's place in it. She stated that men ruled the home and were considered to have the final authority. As we continued to explore the conditions of her mother's life, she began to realize it must have taken a great deal of strength and courage for her mother to survive under such oppressive conditions. She concluded, "I see I have not given her enough credit." We encouraged her to let her mother know this, so she sent her a card on Mother's Day. Her mother surprised her with a long-distance telephone call to say how happy and relieved she was to hear from her.

Through the exchange of letters that followed, Sonya forged a new relationship with her mother. She developed a kindlier, more forgiving attitude toward her, and thus toward herself. She stated tearfully, "For years I have had this nightmare of standing over my mother's grave and feeling sad and guilty. Now I know I won't have to do that and it is such a relief!"

As a result of no longer feeling cut off from her husband and mother, Sonya was no longer depressed and was able to turn her attention and energy to her business pursuits. These comprised the central focus of the last phase of the therapy.

"I Wanted to Have More and Be More"

At the beginning of therapy, Henry seemed to be living in a vacuum, out of touch with his own feelings as well as those of others. He was unaware of what led to his hospitalization. He did not associate his suicide attempt with either losing his job or his wife threatening to leave him.

His 10 years of marriage had been plagued with financial difficulties. He had changed jobs frequently, run up debts, and lied about his commissions. He credited his overspending to his wanting to "have more and be more." Henry was a salesman who lived on "a shoeshine and a smile." His life was selling dreams, and therefore he had to believe in them. His problem was distinguishing between where the dream ended and reality began.

Selma, his wife, had been left to pick up the pieces when the dreams fell apart. Since the beginning of their marriage, she had played a motherly protective role, bailing him out of difficulties, seeing him through his depressed moods, and taking responsibility for paying off their debts. She was now torn between her concept of a good supportive wife—"When people are in trouble, people who love the people in trouble are supposed to help them"—and her own survival: "I feel I'm on the verge of a nervous breakdown." Besides working full time and running the household, she was making daily visits to her dying mother in the hospital.

Henry was guilt-ridden about squandering their money and felt like a failure not only in business but as a husband. As she reviewed their marriage, Selma began to realize how unreal their life had been. She felt she had been fooled by Henry's promises and dreams: "Henry was never really there for me." But she quickly added, "But of course he couldn't be. He wasn't there for himself." Henry agreed: "I wasn't there for myself, how could I be there for anyone else?"

We challenged this couple's shared assumption that Henry couldn't be there for Selma until he was there for himself with the reverse assumption that the best way for Henry to be there for himself was first to be there for Selma. In our experience, it is sometimes more important initially to enable depressed men to get in touch, not with their own feelings, but with those of others. Responding to others activates that part of themselves they have learned to shut down, the caring emotional part. It gives them a way to become involved that is tolerable because it is active and they are in charge.

When Selma despairingly said she felt like she was "buried under a sandstorm of unsolvable problems," we listed the problems on the board and asked Henry if he felt he could muster enough strength to relieve her of some of them. We expressed concern over her critical emotional state and stressed the importance of her being able to rely on his strength and support at this time. He said it would be difficult given the state he was in, but he agreed to take over several household tasks and to accompany her on a visit to her dying mother.

During one of the trips to the hospital Henry discovered a new facet of himself when he reached out and comforted his wife and father-in-law. This was the first time in his life he had ever comforted anyone. "I'm the kind of person who's always kept everything inside. I felt I wasn't worthy of letting anything out. If I did, whoever I was letting it out to would think I was stupid or something like that. So in order to shield myself I put up this barrier. Now I feel there are people who might be able to depend on me. It's a good feeling."

Putting Henry in the caretaking role mobilized his available energy and resources and gave him concrete ways of alleviating his guilt and winning back his wife's trust. It was a validating experience that made him feel needed and competent in an area in which he generally felt incompetent.

After this experience Henry became more emotionally and physically available and began looking for work. Gainful employment was an extremely important aspect of regaining his self-esteem. We explored his doubts and anxieties as a middle-aged man with an irregular work history seeking employment in an uncertain job market.

In order to better understand the meaning of work and responsibility in relation to his self-esteem, we drew an outline of his work history on the blackboard highlighting his most satisfying and successful work experiences. He described feeling best about himself when he was using his special skills as an English teacher. This boosted his confidence because he was considered an excellent teacher. After several years, he left this line of work to become a stockbroker, with an eye to making big money. He was never happy or comfortable in this line of work; his mood soared or plummeted with the stock market. His father and two uncles had been gamblers who had subjected their wives and families to tremendous hardships. He resolved not to follow in their footsteps. After this session he decided he would go back to teaching where he had felt skilled and competent and could depend on a steady income.

As he began actively looking for work, Selma found it difficult to let go of feeling responsible for him. She cut out want ads, kept giving him advice, questioned his motivation, and pushed him to do more. We noticed that Henry reacted with visible annoyance to her constant involvement, but rather than voicing it openly, held it in and withdrew. In the past this interaction would have been the trigger for a new bout of depression. We encouraged Henry to let Selma know when he wanted her help and when he wished to make his own decisions. We encouraged Selma to trust him enough to allow him this prerogative. This required a leap of faith on Selma's part given Henry's past history, but she soon discovered the more responsibility she relinquished, the more Henry took on. Letting go of responsibility is a common problem for women who have spent their lives taking care of the needs of others and don't know how to let others take care of themselves. It requires practice and constant self-vigilance. On one occasion when she was too exhausted to do their taxes, a job she had routinely assumed, she was surprised and relieved to discover that Henry had taken it upon himself to do them.

Within a short period of time Henry obtained a teaching job. He reported feeling good about himself because "I'm helping children and that's a good feeling." Having meaningful work and feeling connected with his wife, Henry no longer had to "have more and be more."

"Performing Romance"

Depression and antidepressants can have a dampening effect on the libido, often resulting in decreased sexual desire or even impotence. It is sometimes difficult to untangle the side effects of the medications from the couples' long-standing interactions around sex. It is not uncommon for the couple and therapist to blame the sexual dysfunction entirely on the effect of the antidepressants rather than addressing the relational problems that contribute to it.

Masculine and feminine identity is never more vulnerable than in the bedroom where the meaning of a "real man" or a "real woman" is thrown into sharp relief and enacted in both symbolic and graphic terms. Male and female sexual needs, fantasies, desires, and expectations crisscross in a complex dance that can lead either to a blissful fusion or to alienation, frustration, and disappointment.

Such a dance had been going on for 47 years with Ben and Ruth when Ben was hospitalized for depression at the age of 73. He believed his depression was primarily due to his unsatisfactory sex life. He had always equated his masculinity with sexual potency. He had had problems with impotence during their entire married life but his impotence had increased after a prostate operation a year earlier. Sex had always been extremely important to him but he complained that his wife had never been interested in sex: "She is like a refrigerator. I feel I'm only getting the appetizer out of a possible big meal." Ruth, his 71-year-old wife, complained that Ben wasn't affectionate or romantic. "I might as well be a hole in the wall. There's never any kissing, touching, talking. I feel lonely and unloved."

According to Ruth, despite her feelings of deprivation, she had put her own needs aside and devoted herself to trying to turn her husband on. She brought home erotic literature, rented pornographic video tapes, read every sex book she could get her hands on, and tried every sexual technique, but Ben had remained dissatisfied and she was left with a great sense of failure. Asked where she got her idea that she was responsible for her husband's orgasm, she said, "I suppose from movies, television, women's books and magazines, Marilyn Monroe—a real woman knows how to turn a man on."

Ben said he understood what Ruth needed when she complained about his lack of affection but felt unable to meet her needs because he had never been good at "performing romance." He felt guilty and inadequate and often thought she should find another man who knew better than he did how to give her what she longed for.

Sex had now become the symbol around which their whole relationship revolved. For Ruth it represented 47 years of frustration trying to satisfy and please her husband and for Ben 47 years of feeling incompetent in the relationship and impotent in bed. Neither was living up to the myth of what a "real man" or a "real woman" should be.

The major thrust of our therapy was in dispelling these myths. We suggested to Ruth that rather than trying to turn her husband on she might focus instead on her own enjoyment and pleasure. We challenged Ben's notion that he was unable to "perform romance." We discovered he had been an actor when he was young, that he had played romantic leads, that he was still involved in amateur productions, and that he took great pride in his acting ability. Focusing on this area in which he saw himself as a romantic figure, we wondered if he might use his acting ability to "perform romance" with his wife. We invited him to envision himself as a leading man in a scene in which he seduced his wife. How would he go about doing it? There was much humor and laughter in imagining all the various possibilities.

The couple entered the session a few weeks later smiling coyly. Ruth reported that Ben had surprised her on their anniversary by arranging a "romantic" weekend in a country inn, replete with a candlelight dinner, soft music, and roses. They giggled and blushed as they described their romantic tryst in which Ben had "performed romance."

Ruth said it was not so much the roses and candlelight that made her feel loved and sexual but the fact that Ben had stopped at a mall on the way to the country and sat in the car and waited for her while she went shopping. Previously, he had refused her request to stop, leaving her feeling everything was always centered around him and his needs. His willingness to wait for her to do something she wanted to do was experienced by her as an act of love and caring. As a result sex became a pleasurable experience for her rather than an ordeal. Ben, perceiving her pleasure, responded with masculine verve.

This experience allowed them to envision different possibilities in their relationship. Ben was no longer in the passive role of waiting for his wife to turn him on and then blaming her when she didn't succeed. Ruth, no longer shackled by a sense of duty and responsibility, was able to relax and respond to her own bodily desires. Following this, Ben began taking more initiative in other areas of their relationship, suggesting walks, making dinner arrangements, buying concert tickets, and visiting friends. As a more open communication developed between them, he was able to bring up some touchy issues that had been upsetting him for a long time but which he had been reluctant to broach. He was able to tell Ruth about his hurt and resentment over her excluding him from important decisions regarding the children. Ruth explained that she had tried to protect him from painful encounters because she was afraid they would depress him. He managed to convince her it was no longer necessary and she agreed to stop running interference.

Being able to express the many resentments he had harbored over the years further released Ben from his passive role. His depression lifted in direct proportion to his feelings of mastery over his life.

THE USE OF QUESTIONNAIRES

We have found written questionnaires useful as an adjunct to our verbal discussions in helping us understand the belief systems of couples. The questionnaires consist of questions concerning the messages each spouse has received from family, peers, and the mass media that have shaped their expectations of themselves and their partner in relation to marriage, sex, independence, responsibility, power, and intimacy. The couple is asked to complete the questionnaires at home and bring them to the session for discussion. Their answers serve as a map for sorting out those beliefs and expectations that promote a positive sense of themselves as compared with those that lead to low self-esteem, conflict, and depression. The questionnaires stimulate couples to think about issues that do not automatically grow out of the session. They often open up many new and pertinent areas for discussion and provide each partner with a deeper understanding and empathy for what each is struggling with in their lives.

Recently we have begun to use intersession questionnaires (adapted from Fraenkel, 1992) in order to get immediate feedback from the couple on the impact of the session. The questions the questionnaires ask are:

What was the most important thing that happened or was said in today's session?
Which of your goals was addressed in this session?
What kind of change will this session make for your relationship as a whole?
How will the session today affect your or your partner's depression?

The questionnaires are given to the couple to fill out during a 10- or 15-minute break at the end of the session during which time the two cotherapists meet with the team to pool their ideas and formulate a message. The couple are then reconvened with the cotherapists and our message is given to them summarizing what we see as the salient aspects of the session and comparing our impressions with theirs.Since we view our therapy as collaborative, these questions give the couple an opportunity to play an active role in directing the course of the therapy. By reflecting on what happened in each session, they clarify their perceptions, define their goals, chart their progress, and develop an awareness of what is important to their partner. In addition, the questionnaires give the therapists immediate feedback as to whether or not they are on the right track.

SUMMARY

This chapter has described a multidimensional approach to treating depression within the context of couple therapy with a focus on gender differences. The approach attempts to integrate the biological, interpersonal, social, and cultural aspects of depression. Typically, treatments for depression have lumped men and women together as though there was no difference in the way they experience depression. In our work, we observed that men and women become depressed for very distinct reasons, cope with depressive symptoms differently, and are responded to differently by spouses. Women's depression is most often related to a disruption in a close personal relationship, while men's depression is most often related to a performance failure. These differences require a different therapeutic understanding and different methods of intervening. Case examples have been used to illustrate our multilevel approach.

We view our work as a beginning and hope our colleagues in the mental health profession will join us in developing new ways of understanding and treating this mysterious and devastating condition.

REFERENCES

Beach, S. R. H., Sandeen, E. E., & O'Leary, K. D. (1990). *Depression in marriage: A model for etiology and treatment.* New York: Guilford Press.

Beck, A. T., Rush, A. J., Shaw, B. F., Emery, G. (1979). *Cognitive therapy of depression.* New York: Guilford Press.

Braverman, L. (1986). The depressed woman in context: A feminist family therapist's analysis. In M. Ault-Riche (Ed.), *Women and family therapy* (pp. 90–101). Rockville, MD: Aspen Systems Corporation.

Coyne, J. C. (1995). Strategic marital therapy for depression. In N. S. Jacobson &

A. S. Gurman (Eds.), *Clinical handbook of couple therapy* (pp. 495–511). New York: Guilford Press.

Ferster, C. B. (1965). Classification of behavioral psychology. In I. Krasner & L. P. Ulmann (Eds.), *Research in behavior modification*. New York: Holt, Rinehart & Winston.

Fraenkel, P. (1992). *The therapy experiences scale.* Unpublished manuscript. Ackerman Institute for the Family, New York, NY.

Goldner, V. (1985, December). Warning: Family therapy may be dangerous to your health. *Family Therapy Networker,* 19–23.

Grinfeld, M. J. (1996). Mental illnesses to be among most prevalent by 2020, WHO study says. *Psychiatric Times, 13*(11), 1, 79.

Howard, B., & Weeks, G. R. (1995). A happy marriage: Pairing couples therapy and treatment of depression. In G. R. Weeks & L. Hillog (Eds.), *Integretive solutions: Treating common problems in couples therapy* (pp. 95–122). New York: Brunner/Mazel.

Jack, D. C. (1991). *Silencing the self.* Cambridge, MA: Harvard University Press.

Jacobson, N. S. (1984). Marital therapy and the cognitive–behavioral treatment of depression. *Behavior Therapist, 7,* 143–147.

Klerman, G. E., Weissman, M. M., Rounsaville, B. J., & Chevron, E. (1984). *Interpersonal psychotherapy of depression.* New York: Basic Books.

Kramer, P. D. (1993). *Listening to Prozac.* New York: Penguin Books.

Moltz, D. (1993). Bipolar disorder and the family: An integrative model. *Family Process, 32,* 409–424.

Papp, P. (1997). Listening to the system. *Family Therapy Networker, 21*(1), 52–58.

Real, T. (1997). *I don't want to talk about it: Overcoming the secret legacy of male depression.* New York: Simon & Schuster.

Strupp, H. H., & Binder, J. L. (1984). *Psychotherapy in a new key.* New York: Basic Books.

Taffel, R. (1991). The politics of mood: Depressive–caretaker relationships. *Journal of Feminist Therapy, 3,* 153–177.

Teichman, Y., & Teichman, M. (1990). Interpersonal view of depression: Review and integration. *Journal of Family Psychology, 3,* 349–367.

Yapko, M. D. (1999). *Hand-me-down blues.* New York: Golden Books.

CHAPTER 7

Embracing the Controversy

A Metasystemic Approach to the Treatment of Domestic Violence

Wendy Greenspun

"**S**tel-la! Stel-la!" That passionate, imploring wail of Stanley Kowalski in *A Streetcar Named Desire* provides a popular illustration of a couple in the throes of domestic violence. Shortly before, Stanley was beating Stella in a drunken rage; soon after, Stella rushes forgivingly into Stanley's arms for a fervent kiss. Illustrative of the cycle of abuse (Walker, 1979), where violence alternates with remorseful pleas for reconciliation, this prototypical interaction suggests that the bond of love may overpower the horror of violence that accompanies it.

At the same time, knowledge of the traumatic effects of battering are well documented (Herman, 1992; Walker, 1979). Approximately two million women are beaten by their husbands each year (Straus & Gelles, 1990), with over one million seeking medical assistance for injuries caused by battering (Stark & Flitcraft, 1982). These women often live in constant terror in the shadow of recurrent violence and intimidation, with consequent post-traumatic stress symptoms resulting (Browne, 1993; Herman, 1992; Walker, 1979).

How do we make sense of these contradictory images of violence within intimate relationships? And what form of intervention is best suited to address this complex, dangerous problem?

As couple therapists, we are particularly in need of information about how best to proceed. Holtzworth-Monroe, Beatty, and Anglin (1995) suggest that as many as one in two couples who come for treatment have experienced violence as part of their relationship. Since most couple therapists will therefore encounter this problem, we need to become educated regarding the facts, dilemmas, and treatment considerations in working with domestic violence.

This chapter will attempt to give an overview of the historical context of treatment within the domestic violence field, then outline the current controversy regarding how best to intervene. Finally, a comprehensive treatment approach will be described, one that takes into account the various complexities inherent in doing this work.

HISTORICAL CONTEXT

Public attitudes toward woman abuse have changed significantly in recent decades in the United States. Once considered a man's "inalienable right," physical assaults by men against their wives were outlawed in all states by the end of World War I (Ritmeester, 1993). But enforcement of such laws remained selective at best, since "domestic disputes" were often not taken seriously by police departments and the courts.

An outgrowth of the feminist movement, the first "safe houses" to shelter battered women were started in the early 1970s. Through the grassroots efforts of women who had been abused by their male intimates, the "battered women's movement" slowly evolved more fully, providing increasing numbers of shelters and advocating for changes in legislation (Schecter, 1982). As a result of their efforts, by 1986 more than half of the states had laws allowing women to take out orders of protection (i.e., restraining orders) against their violent mates (Ritmeester, 1993). More recently, newsworthy cases involving wife battering have focused media attention and public awareness on the problem of domestic violence.

A parallel change in attitude and awareness has occurred within the mental health profession. Earliest mentions of domestic violence in the literature were consistent with the prevailing epistemology of the time, focusing on individual psychopathology as its cause (see Ganley, 1989, and Herman, 1992, for further description). The female victim was regarded as masochistic, while the batterer was seen to have poor impulse control. Both victim and perpetrator were labeled "pathological."

The advent of family therapy brought a new perspective to problems within relationships. Instead of defining relational difficulties in terms of individual psychopathology, family systems theorists described circular processes and recursive sequences, suggesting that problems were created and/or maintained within the context of a relational system. Each member of a system was therefore believed to participate in a reciprocal manner in the difficulties. Domestic violence was handled similarly to other relationship problems, placing both victim and perpetrator in equal roles with regard to the violence (Mack, 1989; Weitzman & Dreen, 1982).

The feminist critique of both psychoanalytic theory and family therapy offered new perspectives that had significant implications for the treatment of family violence. Feminist theorists such as Nancy Chodorow (1978) and Carol Gilligan (1982) pointed to the differential developmental experiences of men and women in our society, challenging the notion that certain characteristic feminine traits such as dependency should be considered pathological. Now, within this gendered framework, a battered woman's choice to remain with her abusive partner could be seen in terms of her socialization toward "making relationships work," instead of regarded as a sign that she is overly dependent (Goldner, Sheinberg, Penn, & Walker, 1990).

In the family therapy field, feminist family therapists began to question the notion of reciprocity that was central to systems theory (Goldner, 1985; Hare-Mustin, 1978). By looking at the larger sociopolitical context, rather than just the family system, feminists argued that the gender inequities in our patriarchal society pointed to differential access to power within the family. Nowhere was this more clear than when applied to domestic violence, since abusing men obviously have more power than the women they abuse. To say that battered women are equally responsible for their abuse can be construed as victim blaming (Bograd, 1984; Dell, 1989; Goldner et al., 1990).

TREATMENT CONTROVERSY

As prevailing theoretical beliefs about domestic violence were challenged by feminist ideologies, a heated debate emerged related to its treatment (Bograd, 1992; Feldman & Ridley, 1995). Answers to the question of how best to intervene with couples when battering has occurred have tended to fall into two "camps," systemic and feminist, which will be briefly outlined below.

A family systems approach to battering views violence as symptomatic of underlying problematic dynamics in the couple (Cook & Frantz-Cook, 1984; Geffner, Mantooth, Franks, & Rao, 1989; Geller & Wasserstrom, 1984; Jennings & Jennings, 1991; Lane & Russell, 1989; Lipchik, Sirles, & Kubicki, 1997; Mack, 1989; Minuchin & Nichols, 1993; Weitzman & Dreen, 1982). From this perspective, addressing the dysfunctional patterns within the relationship should prevent further violence from occurring, helping to diffuse the "rising tide of emotion in the symmetrical feedback loop" (Mack, 1989, p. 202).

A distinction is made by most family systems thinkers between "expressive" and "instrumental" violence (Gelles & Straus, 1979; Neidig & Friedman, 1984). *Instrumental violence* is considered manipulative and purposeful, being used as a tool of power and control, and perpetrated most often by one member of the dyad against the other. Separation of the couple and gender-specific treatment groups are generally thought to be the best interventions in such cases. *Expressive violence,* on the other hand, is viewed mainly as an outgrowth of anger and conflict, with both members of the couple capable of violent acts. Systemic approaches generally recommend couple therapy in cases of expressive violence (Jennings & Jennings, 1991; Mack, 1989), since the escalation in conflict between members of the dyad can be addressed directly in such a format.

In terms of specific goals, couple therapy addresses the problematic communication patterns, conflict, and anger within the dyad that are believed to contribute to violence. Since both members of the couple are considered to play reciprocal roles in the mounting tensions, "if one or the other person can make a complimentary move during the escalating steps of the conflict, the process can be halted" (Mack, 1989, p. 196). Anger-management techniques, cognitive behavioral strategies to reduce emotional reactivity, and more traditional structural, strategic, and solution-focused interventions are utilized to address underlying systemic dysfunction (Cook & Frantz-Cook, 1984; Geffner et al., 1989; Geller & Wasserstrom, 1984; Jennings & Jennings, 1991; Lane & Russell, 1989; Lipchik et al., 1997; Mack, 1989; Weitzman & Dreen, 1982).

Another key feature of the couple therapy approach is the neutrality of the therapist (Lane & Russell, 1989). For instance, Mack (1989) asserts that clinicians treating spouse abuse need to maintain the "freedom from judgment" utilized in a systemic stance, rather than seeing separate victim and villain roles. Geller and Wasserstrom (1984) concur that this neutral position should be "no different with spouse abuse" (p. 39) than with other problems addressed in couple therapy.

Critics of family systems approaches to the treatment of domestic violence, mainly feminist thinkers, cite many dangers in working with the couple conjointly (Bograd, 1984; Dutton, 1992; Kaufman, 1993). The therapist who sees both members of the dyad together is defining the problem as relational, implicitly suggesting that the woman is equally responsible for her own victimization; this is a form of victim blaming. In addition, given the possibility of disagreement and anger emerging during couple therapy, the woman may be placed at greater risk as a result of what occurs during a session. Conversely, the woman may not be able to speak honestly in couple sessions for fear of later violent repercussions, rendering the therapy dishonest.

Feminist critics of the systemic approach to battering do not make the distinction between instrumental and expressive forms of violence (Adams, 1989; Bograd, 1984). Given the patriarchal society in which we live, the much higher incidence of violence and severity of injury from male violence toward women than female violence toward men (Berk, Berk, Loseke, & Rauma, 1983; Browne, 1993; Cantos, Neidig, & O'Leary, 1994; Kurz & Stark, 1988), and the disproportionate size of men and women, feminists view battering as a tactic of male power and control (Avis, 1992; Kaufman, 1993; Pence, 1989). From this perspective, battering occurs because traditionally there have been no repercussions for it (Ganley, 1989; Kaufman, 1993; Schecter, 1982). Feminists argue that social control is the most useful intervention: men should be arrested for the criminal act of assault against women. Therapy is more cautiously considered, since many feminists believe that "therapy has not been good for battered women" (Kaufman, 1993, p. 206).

From a feminist perspective, when therapy is contemplated as part of the intervention, it generally consists of separate treatments for batterer and victim. For the batterer, group therapy in which he can be helped to take responsibility for his behavior, and confronted for his denial and minimization of acts of intimidation and violence, is most often utilized (Adams, 1989; Holtzworth-Monroe et al., 1995; Kaufman, 1993; Pence, 1989; Pence & Paymar, 1993). The focus of treatment is on the resocialization of men, confronting patriarchal norms via feminist ideology. Feminist therapists, therefore, find it important *not* to remain neutral, but instead to take a clear moral stance against the domination of women by men. Therapy for the battered woman generally helps address her post-traumatic stress symptoms and maximize her safety, including assisting her to leave the relationship when possible (Dutton, 1992; Herman, 1992; Holtzworth-Monroe et al., 1995).

Critics of this feminist approach cite the lack of attention paid to the frequency with which women return to their abusive partners. While financial dependence and/or greater physical danger (from spousal retaliation) are often factors in women being unable to remain separate, many women return to their violent mates because of the power of the relational bond (Goldner et al., 1990). Often what they really want is to remain in the relationship, but without the violence. And a pure feminist approach seems to miss the underlying relational dynamics that may contribute to the cycle of violence (Cook & Frantz-Cook, 1984; Lipchik et al., 1997).

The controversy described above has resulted in polarization within the treatment field about how best to intervene. But both sides of the debate offer valuable knowledge, insights, and experience that can be utilized to help keep relationships safe. It was the embrace of this controversy that allowed for the development of the comprehensive treatment that will now be described.

A METASYSTEMIC APPROACH TO TREATMENT

In the mid-1980s, Virginia Goldner, Peggy Penn, Marcia Sheinberg, and Gillian Walker, therapists at the Ackerman Institute for the Family, decided to look more closely at how feminist ideas could inform systemic treatment. They chose to focus on battering in relationships, an area that clearly had implications in terms of both gender and relational factors. The theoretical underpinnings of this project are described in greater detail elsewhere (Goldner, 1992; Goldner et al., 1990; Walker & Goldner, 1995). This chapter will describe the treatment approach that emerged from the thinking and experience of this group, which has been codirected by Gillian Walker and Virginia Goldner for the past 10 years. I and several others joined Goldner and Walker later in the project's development.

Goldner (1992) and Goldner et al. (1990) discuss our utilization of a "both/and" rather than an "either/or" orientation in this treatment, referring to the capacity to incorporate seemingly contradictory viewpoints, rather than having to adopt a singular approach. Aspects from both sides of the treatment controversy are therefore used together in our project, for only in this meld of seemingly conflicting realities can the variety of factors relating to domestic violence be addressed. An overview of some of the assumptions that frame this treatment will help to illustrate:

1. We believe that violence is multiply determined. It is the outgrowth of both male abuse of power over women *and* the result of escalations within the dyad based on relational dynamics. In addition, individual factors, such as internalizations of early relationships, neurobiological predisposition and trauma history, further contribute to the use of violence and can become points of intervention.

2. We view violence by men against their intimate partners as both an instrumental *and* an expressive act, rather than one or the other. Men wield violence and threats in order to intimidate and control women, but they may also experience the moment of violence as a loss of control.

3. Social control, resocialization to egalitarian viewpoints, and psychological exploration can all serve as useful interventions in order to stop male violence. A comprehensive therapy must be able to utilize all these approaches when necessary in order to address the variety of factors that lead to violence.

4. Couple (conjoint) therapy can be employed as a treatment approach, but *only* when a clear moral framework is utilized that holds the man fully accountable for his use of violence. In this sense, the therapist cannot maintain the usual neutrality most often associated with couple therapy. Understanding the psychological and relational underpinnings should be used to deter the violence, but never to excuse it. *If the man will not take responsibility for his aggression, conjoint treatment should not be undertaken.*

The theoretical framework of this treatment consists of a complex tapestry of approaches woven together. From a feminist perspective, gender premises and power differentials are explored in order to address inequalities in the relationship and how they shape behavior and attitudes. From a systemic perspective, discovering the interactional sequences, complementarities, and symmetrical patterns that lead to affective escalations becomes an important tool to halt the cycle of violence. In addition, addressing problematic dyadic communication and improving conflict-resolution abilities provide necessary skills that can deter further violence. From a narrative perspective, utilizing the language of choice and personal agency helps to enlarge upon strengths and facilitate alternatives to violence. From a neurobiological perspective, the impact of possible attentional, learning, and impulse disorders on the ability to control aggression is assessed, with appropriate biological and behavioral interventions recommended when needed (Walker, 1999; Walker & Shimmerlik, 1994).

With this overview of the assumptions and theory that guide our approach in mind, a more detailed account of the treatment will now be presented.

DESCRIPTION OF TREATMENT

Our treatment project is still a work in progress, shaped collaboratively by the clinicians involved, along with the men and women who come to us for help. While specific ideas and interventions will be described, they represent a snapshot of an evolving process that will continue to be refined through ongoing research and clinical knowledge.

All treatment takes place within the Ackerman clinic setting. Clients are referred to our project after violence is identified as a problem during a brief telephone assessment. Most couples are self-referred, although a small percentage have been court-remanded to treatment. In this sense, the clients represent a self-selected group of couples who are seeking treatment together in order to address problems in the relationship. All the couples we have seen are heterosexual, since the focus of treatment has been on the impact of gender and power on relational dynamics. They span a wide range of socioeconomic, cultural, and racial groups, consistent with the fact that domestic violence is not discriminating in these areas (Feldman & Ridley, 1995; Holtzworth-Monroe, Smutzler, Bates, & Sandin, 1997). Therapy is provided by our team of clinicians, with one or two therapists interviewing the couples, and the rest of the team observing behind a one-way mirror.

As it is conceptualized at present, this treatment can be divided into three phases. The first phase involves a three-session evaluation of the viability of utilizing conjoint treatment. If deemed appropriate and safe to work with the couple together, we can move on to the second phase, short-term couple treatment. In the five sessions allotted for this brief dyadic work, we focus on stopping the violence and other abusive behaviors. In the third phase, eight sessions of group therapies are utilized to address ongoing couple dynamics and to create a community of peers who can provide support and confront abusive attitudes and actions.

Evaluation Phase

In the evaluation, we assess factors that are known to contribute to the use of violence and may therefore suggest alternate forms of treatment in addition to or instead of our program. With the men, given the high degree of substance abuse associated with battering (Feldman & Ridley, 1995; Kantor & Straus, 1987), we assess level of alcohol and drug use. Anyone with severe addictions would need to complete substance-abuse treatment prior to entering our project. We also evaluate the man's neurobiological predisposition and how it relates to his capacity for impulse control (Walker, 1999). For example, if a man suffered a severe head trauma that impairs his ability to control violence outside as well as inside the relationship, appropriate medical and behavioral interventions would be recommended to treat the problem. We have also seen a large number of other contributing neurobiological factors, for example, attention deficit disorder, which often require psychopharmacological intervention in addition to our treatment. A clear history of sociopathy may exclude a man from our program and require greater use of social control measures (e.g., recommendations for use of direct criminal proceedings). With the women, active substance abuse or severe eating disorders would again require separate intervention prior to beginning our project. In addition, when posttraumatic stress symptoms from a history of childhood trauma, coupled with the effects of battering, render a woman unable to think clearly or make adequate decisions, individual treatment would be suggested instead of our couple approach.

Suitability for Couple Work

One of the most important factors to assess during the evaluation phase is whether conjoint treatment is appropriate for the couple. The main criteria we utilize are the man's ability to take full responsibility for his use of violence, his capacity to tolerate hearing the woman's description of being victimized by him, and his willingness to work toward stopping his abusive behavior. While generally the men do not enter treatment believing that they are totally accountable, within the evaluation period they need to begin to accept responsibility for their choice of violence.

Consistent with recent findings that suggest a high frequency of bilateral violence within couples (Feldman & Ridley, 1995; Holtzworth-Monroe et al., 1995), we at times do see cases in which both the man and the woman have utilized violence in the relationship. We are clear to point out, however, that given the typical man's greater size and weight, his violence poses a greater threat and can cause far more severe injury than can the woman's use of force (Berk et al., 1983; Cantos et al., 1994;

Kurz & Stark, 1988). In addition, women frequently use violence in self defense after long periods of victimization (Browne, 1987; Holtzworth-Monroe et al., 1997). We consequently maintain the position that the man must take total responsibility for his abusive behavior, regardless of any provocation from the woman, and see his violence as at least partly a tactic of power and control. At the same time, we work with the woman to stop any violence she engages in as well.

In order to get the best representation of what happened, after explaining our program and talking briefly with both together, we meet separately with each member of the couple and ask about the violent incidents. It has been well documented (Adams, 1989; Kaufman, 1993) that men tend to minimize their utilization of violence. Our own experience confirms this view. For example, one batterer told us, "I just held her so that she wouldn't hit me." We then learned from his wife that his "holding" consisted of throwing her onto the ground and hitting her until she had a black eye and a broken nose. Hearing the woman's separate description of what occurred helps us ascertain the discrepancy between their perceptions and the degree to which the man denies the severity of his violence. In addition, in talking with the woman alone, we are able to assess whether she feels safe to meet conjointly with her partner, or if she was coerced into participation in this therapy.

Once we have determined that proceeding conjointly will not be detrimental, we continue the evaluation with both members of the couple together. However, we will meet with each person separately at any point in the treatment if we are concerned about safety. In meeting conjointly, we can address differences in their analyses of the violence, and see if the man is able to begin the process of acknowledging his responsibility for abusive behavior.

In the case of Clarissa and Gene, a couple who had been married for 8 years, Gene's initial description of his violent behavior was that Clarissa "forced" him to hold her back when she became "hysterical" during fights. His words reflected how little he felt responsible for his aggressive behavior, both minimizing his own violence and placing the blame on his partner. When Clarissa, listening to his depiction of events, became noticeably upset and described his brutality, Gene became increasingly defensive. The therapist worked with Gene to help him tolerate hearing Clarissa's report of her experience of events. Once Gene heard Clarissa's fear, which resulted from his violent behavior, he was finally able to look more objectively at his actions. He stated that if she had been scared as a result of his actions, he needed to acknowledge how violent he had been, even if it had not been his intent, or even if her account did not conform to his memory of events. The man's ability to accept his partner's account of events and utilize it as a "barometer" of having "gone too far" becomes an important indicator of whether the man can take responsibility for his violent actions.

If the man is not willing to take responsibility for the violence and/or if the woman does not feel safe or free to speak openly in conjoint sessions, traditional referrals can be made to a batterers group for him and a battered women's support group for her.

The Romantic Bond

One important dynamic we want to assess in the couple is the strength of the romantic bond between them. For couples where loving feelings have been completely eroded, there may be little motivation or reason to embark on the arduous path of couple treatment. For example, couples who merely remain together for economic reasons might be better helped to improve their financial resources in order to end the relationship rather than engage in conjoint therapy. At the other end of the continuum, we see numerous couples like Stella and Stanley in *A Streetcar Named Desire*, who describe passionate, ardent love for each other, which fuels their volatility and makes it hard to extricate themselves from their dangerous romance.

We have found it extremely useful to validate the strength of the bond between the couple when it exists, which is rarely done when batterer and abused woman are treated separately. Very often, the woman (especially) feels intense shame that she still loves someone who hurts her, and pathologizes the fact that she remains in the relationship. If they openly acknowledge their positive connection, their feelings of love do not have to go underground, and thus become more accessible to exploration. We utilize a feminist understanding of female development to point out that women are socialized to succeed in relationships at all costs. Consistent with the systemic approach, we also believe that the connection between them is a strength that can be built upon in treatment, while never losing sight of the fact that this bond also leaves them vulnerable to the cycle of violence.

Often we have heard couples say that they found in their partners a "soul mate" who understood their childhood pain firsthand, an important aspect of what drew them together. We can explore this aspect of the bond by constructing a thorough, problem-focused genogram. We inquire about patterns of violence in their families of origin, which often sheds light on the kind of pain they share. Consistent with re-search on batterers and battered women (Feldman & Ridley, 1995; Hotaling & Sugarman, 1986; van der Kolk, 1996), we find a high per-centage of these men and women were abused as children or witnessed violence between their parents. The internalization of childhood abuse experiences may predispose them to violence, for instance, through the man's identification with the aggressor or the woman's expectation of maltreatment. Furthermore, we need to assess the degree to which posttraumatic stress symptoms color the interactions between them and render them feeling powerless to change. If violent actions are se-verely dissociated, individual treatment may be warranted.

Brief Couple Therapy Phase

With much evaluative information gathered, and when deemed appro-priate to do so, we move into the second phase, that of brief couple therapy. In this phase, we can address the violence more directly and intervene to stop it. Here we utilize certain narrative therapy ideas, along with attempts to uncover the interior of the violent event. These will be briefly described below.

Unique Outcome

In terms of a narrative approach to the problem of violence, we borrow from the work of Michael White and David Epston (1990), utilizing a language of choice and the concept of unique outcome. We represent to the man that we think his violence is volitional, even if experienced by him as a helpless loss of control, and we clearly state that we do not believe the use of violence defines the whole of him. We are clear to talk about the times when he "chose" to be violent, emphasizing his control in the matter. We build on this idea by discussing "unique out-come" situations, occasions when he could have been violent, but chose not to be, suggesting that alternatives to violence exist for him and can be built upon. A case example follows.

Lynn and Harvey entered our program after the fourth time Harvey was violent to Lynn. The first tjree occasions consisted of Harvey grabbing and shaking Lynn; the fourth time occurred when Lynn told him to pick up his dirty socks from the floor, and Har-vey threw a chair at her. Although Harvey's violence was not long-standing or severe, he was quite verbally abusive, and Lynn was frightened that his aggression could escalate in a manner similar to what she had witnessed between her parents. Harvey expressed concern as well, stating that he did not want to use force, but that he had felt provoked.

When the therapist asked Harvey the unique outcome question—"Were there any times when you could have chosen to be violent with Lynn, but made a different choice?"—Harvey responded negatively. He believed that each time he had wanted to be violent, he had been violent. The therapist then posed a different form of the question, asking if there were other times or places in his life where Harvey may have wanted to be violent, but chose not to be. Harvey responded very quickly with "Sure!," then went on to describe his intense frustration and anger at certain bosses at work, whom he clearly knew he could not assault, although he often felt like doing so.

Once the fact that Harvey was able to make a nonviolent choice had been established, this could be explored in greater depth. Harvey was asked about how he was able to walk away when his boss was berating or demeaning him, and he described how he focused on "the matters at hand . . . the more important things," instead of his boss's behavior that seemed so unjust. Harvey acknowledged that, although initially it bothered him immensely, a day later whatever the boss had done seemed trivial, and he was glad he had not overreacted. He then spontaneously said that he could now view Lynn's asking him to pick up his socks in a similar manner, that it was not very significant, but that a "sense of injustice came up." The therapist framed this as the moment Harvey chose to focus on his sense of injustice instead of looking at the bigger picture. They were then able to talk about the meaning of unjust treatment for Harvey, as well as how to reinforce his capacity to attend to the most important matter, rather than to act on momentary anger.

Very often, addressing the unique outcome behaviors can also foster the development of a specific safety plan. Techniques that the man utilizes in order to refrain from violence can be built upon, since they are a logical outgrowth of a capacity he has already demonstrated. For instance, Harvey spoke about taking a deep breath and walking away from his boss, which translated into a safety plan of leaving the room if he felt provoked by Lynn, rather than becoming verbally or physically abusive. We find it helpful to be very specific in safety planning, including actions that both members of the couple can utilize in order to assure the woman's safety. Outlining and agreeing to such a plan during a session makes it more likely to be utilized, since it is mutually determined outside of the heat of an argument.

Internal Experience of the Batterer

Another way to directly intervene in the man's use of violence is to explore the interior of his experience surrounding the violent episodes. This has been referred to elsewhere as "deconstructing the violent moment" (Goldner et al., 1990) and involves detailed questioning about the specific thoughts and feelings the man experiences around his use of violence. This technique utilizes the psychodynamic premise that particular reactions in the present may often be fueled by unconscious, internalized experiences and relationships from the past. When these covert manifestations are brought into conscious awareness, the man is able to expand on his capacity to make choices other than violence.

In the case described above, Harvey was able to talk about how being "berated" by Lynn seemed to touch off a memory of his foster father's critical, demeaning treatment of him, an "injustice" that Harvey felt helpless to change. It was that helplessness that seemed to spark Harvey's disproportionate anger and left him vulnerable to acting out with Lynn what he could not do to his father.

At times deconstructing the violence can mean a connection to the man's own history of trauma, where he can gain awareness that he is now doing to another person what was once done to him. One man described superimposing the face of an abusive aunt onto his wife when he perceived her as "aggressive," then lashing out at that image. In addition to giving insight and other options for his behavior, this awareness may foster a greater capacity for the man to empathize with his partner's experience of victimization, another factor that may help deter his abuse. It may also shed light on the development of beliefs based on extreme sex-role stereotypes, which fuel the man's use of violence.

Trauma Work

Another important aspect of addressing the violence involves working with the woman's experience of trauma. Being able to acknowledge and validate her pain becomes a significant aid to her healing (Herman, 1995). Within the context of couple therapy, giving voice to her experience of abuse, and having the man understand it, can help empower the once-powerless woman and facilitate the man's empathic connection to her victimization. When Rita, a woman who was battered and intimidated by her husband Jack for 26 years, told Jack she just needed him to "listen to what it was like," she spewed out an eternity of

anger and suffering at his hands that she felt had completely under-
mined her sense of self. Jack was able to "bear witness" to her experience without defending himself, bringing them closer together and
helping Jack to stay aware of the repercussions of his behavior.

Addressing Safety Needs

The issue of safety is of paramount concern, and becomes an important topic to address. While we are clear that the man is responsible for
his use of violence, we believe that the woman can become responsible
for putting her safety needs first, to whatever extent is possible. This
does not mean that we think a woman has complete control over her
safety, since we know that repeated intimidation, coercion, threats, and
violence can undermine her self-esteem and decision-making abilities;
that financial and emotional dependence may preclude her developing
outside resources that could enable her to leave; and that unpredictable violence cannot be anticipated. Instead, we see that the woman
may not recognize points at which she does have input into her safety,
and that people outside the relationship may become mobilized to intervene on her behalf.

Therapists who work with domestic violence often feel an enormous responsibility to protect the woman. We have learned that when
the therapist or others express their concern for her, the battered
woman may feel less inclined to worry about the violence, and instead
be pulled more strongly by the intensity of love she feels for her partner, which places her in a potentially dangerous position. In *A Streetcar
Named Desire*, as Stella's sister and neighbor attempted to keep her
away from Stanley, Stella ignored their cautions and returned to Stanley once he appeared contrite, as if in letting others emphasize Stanley's aggression, Stella could attend to his goodness. To counteract this
tendency to split the good and the bad aspects of the batterer between
helper and battered woman, we actively investigate both sides of the
woman's ambivalent experience with the man, helping her to weigh out
those areas of the relationship that make her feel vulnerable to future
assault, and how best to think about keeping herself safe.

We attempt to work with decisions regarding safety within the context of treatment, actively exploring ways in which each member of the
couple can keep safety concerns at the forefront of the relationship.
The case that follows illustrates how we work therapeutically with this
issue.

Within their 5 years of marriage, Samuel had repeatedly battered his wife, Lavonne, during heated arguments, blackening her eye, bruising her arms, and cracking a rib at various times. Lavonne had taken out orders of protection, had kicked Samuel out of the house, and had sworn she would not see him again, but each time she gradually reengaged in the relationship after Samuel expressed remorse. They would generally return to a passionate, loving state, until the next big argument ensued.

In exploring the specifics of their altercations, we discovered a variety of dynamics that contributed to Samuel's violence and left Lavonne feeling she could not extricate herself from the danger. During arguments, Samuel's thinking seemed to become "muddy," and he then had difficulty tolerating Lavonne's superior verbal abilities. An assessment of his neurobiological functioning suggested that Samuel had considerable language-processing difficulties that had impeded his abilities in school and in conversing with others. When experiencing impediments to his thinking during an argument, Samuel viewed himself as a "failure," a feeling with which he had struggled throughout his life. As his anger and frustration mounted, Samuel began to withdraw. When able to take a "time out," he did not become physically aggressive, but when lacking an "escape," Samuel chose violence to express what he could not verbalize.

Lavonne, on the other hand, became furious when Samuel attempted to remove himself during a fight. She described feeling "cut off" and not heard, and said she needed to "talk out" problems until they got resolved. Even when Samuel stated that he needed to leave the house in order to "cool off," Lavonne would physically block the door in order to prevent his departure, a movement that often preceded his violent lashing out.

In exploring her experience during arguments, Lavonne was reminded of her past. She described feeling much as she did in childhood, when her violent stepfather berated and belittled her, and she was powerless to talk back to him. She said she had been determined since then to "have the last word" no matter what, even if it meant sacrificing her own well-being in the process. In addition, she had been abandoned at birth by her biological mother, and connected Samuel's wanting to leave in order to calm down as a potential sign of total abandonment.

We worked with both Samuel and Lavonne on separating their pasts from what occurred in their relationship. For Samuel, this meant addressing the ways he felt like a failure, and how to stop perpetuating this stance throughout his life. On a behavioral level, since he knew removing himself could help him choose to remain in control, we looked at ways he could separate himself mentally and physically regardless of what Lavonne said or did.

With Lavonne, we struggled to make the difficult distinction between helping her take responsibility for her own safety but not blaming her for the victimization. We acknowledged that Lavonne should be able to say whatever she needed to say to Samuel, without fearing for her safety if she used the voice she wasn't allowed to use as a child. At the same time, her wish to retaliate against her stepfather and prevent another loss seemed to cloud her judgment about valuing her own safety, and interfered with her capacity to let Samuel leave when he needed to. We helped come up with a "both/and" solution, where Lavonne could voice her thoughts and also value herself enough to know when she was in danger. We worked out a plan where they agreed to postpone discussions until it was safe for both to talk. This allowed Samuel time to calm down, but assured Lavonne that she would not be silenced again.

After addressing the violence and actively working on safety issues, our brief couple therapy focuses on consolidating the gains made up to this time. We continue to support nonviolent behavior, and seek to uncover all forms of emotional and verbal abuse as they exist. In addition, much work is done to intervene in the highly fused nature of the couple's interactions, including the large degree of reactivity that both members of the couple often display. For example, for many couples, helping them acknowledge and tolerate differences of opinion via a stance of "agreeing to disagree" becomes an important tool in preventing their dangerous escalations.

After the evaluation and brief couple therapy phases, a decision is made regarding further treatment needs. For some couples, more comprehensive couple therapy may be required, and we can refer out for further service. For most couples, however, we see the value of providing a group therapy experience to augment the changes that have already begun.

Group Therapy Phase

The value of group treatments for batterers and battered women is well documented (Adams, 1989; Almeida & Bograd, 1991; Feldman & Ridley, 1995; Herman, 1992; Kaufman, 1993; Pence, 1989; Pence & Paymar, 1993). Within our project, we believed that we could both serve more clients and provide an important resource for couples by offering group treatment following the couple work. We utilize both gender-specific and couples groups to serve the needs of this population, addressing certain related areas within each type of group, and alternating between the two formats as needed. In general, the groups provide support and confrontation by peers, reduce social isolation, increase the men's accountability, and reinforce gains made in the initial phases of treatment, especially maintaining nonviolence. We allow and even encourage contact outside of the groups, which fosters a self-help component that extends beyond the confines of our program.

The groups are run with two therapists in the room, with the rest of the team observing behind the one-way mirror. In the early sessions, therapists provide structure to facilitate trust and assist in the development of group process. For example, in the initial session participants might be asked to talk about both the romance of their relationships and what brought them to our treatment program. From this, they are able to extrapolate parallels in their experiences and start to broach previously shameful topics. Over the course of the groups, the structure generally entails one couple or individual at a time presenting relevant issues, with other group members adding comments and helping to problem solve. As sessions proceed, the therapists play a less central role (Yalom, 1985), with group members assisting each other as they develop the capacity to help themselves.

Although both exist within the group phase of treatment, the couple and gender-specific groups each provide certain unique therapeutic opportunities not always available in the other type of group. These will be described below.

Men's and Women's Groups

The use of gender-specific groups is the most common form of intervention in treating domestic violence (Feldman & Ridley, 1995; Holtzworth-Monroe et al., 1995). Separation by gender allows for the specific support and confrontation of peers with similar experiences. For the men, as in most groups for batterers, they are able to confront each other's sexist attitudes and abusive behaviors—often more effectively than a therapist can. For the women, they can understand each other's longing to remain in a relationship in spite of its dangers, yet also point out unnecessary risks, and bolster efforts to leave when necessary.

An example from a women's group can illustrate the therapeutic impact of sharing with others who can identify similar feelings. In this particular group session, Nora, a young lawyer who was still married to the man who abused her, spoke at length about how critical and mean she had been to her husband, Joe, during a recent evening out with friends. This friend was aware of Joe's abusive behavior toward Nora. Joe had not been violent since beginning our treatment program.

In talking about the events of that evening, she described Joe as acting quite silly, and noted that he "didn't know when to stop" behaving that way. One of the therapists asked whether Nora's sense of Joe "going too far" might connect to the experience of Joe being violent, which were times when he clearly went too far. Nora tearfully agreed with that interpretation, and went on to talk about how much she had been thinking about the abuse. She then described her ongoing anger at Joe for having battered her, as well as her tremendous anger at her neglectful mother and abusive father. She began to question when she would ever get over her rage at all of them, when she could forgive instead of always punishing those who hurt her.

As the group members listened and empathized, Nora spoke to another side of her emotions. She talked about her embarrassment in still loving someone who caused her harm. She described the feelings of shame involved in loving someone who had hurt her so much, especially when others knew it, and the lack of respect she felt for herself as a result. She questioned out loud whether anyone could understand this confusing experience.

In response, all the group members were able to elaborate on how they shared similar emotions, and went on to talk about their own ambivalent experiences of love. Lillian, another group member, responded that she hadn't previously been able to describe such feelings, even to her best friends, since she always hid from others the shame of her love. Only in the group did she feel she had a place to share these thoughts.

We also utilize men's and women's groups to explore gender premises and politics, thus fostering more egalitarian beliefs that can be supported by others of the same gender. In one technique used early on in the groups, we have participants describe what they were taught within their families of origin about being their particular gender. Within the group context, these internalized beliefs can be made conscious and new ideologies fostered through the support of peers.

In one men's group, the discussion of how they learned to become men highlighted many significant identifications that fostered the use of violence. Pete described how his father challenged him to a wrestling match when Pete was an adult. Pete stated his experience of his father this way: "So much of him is about machismo. There are so many ways he had failed. The only way he could show he was a man was to be violent." Even when a father's violence was less overt, intimidation and threat were often used to control women. John described how his father kept a belt hanging from the mantlepiece, a concrete symbol that he should never be crossed. Identifying their fathers' abusive tactics helped both Pete and John recognize how much they had internalized and played out similar attitudes within their own marriages.

In addition to the supportive and confrontational aspects of the gender-specific groups, the groups provide a format to foster an increased ability to differentiate from the couples' emotionally fused relationships. Very often there has been limited room within these dyads for each person to develop separate interests or relationships—frequently due to the batterer's need for complete control. The groups offer a safe context within which their separate identities can be nurtured by others who struggle with a similar dynamic.

Couples Group

Couples group therapy has been utilized for a variety of relational issues (Framo, 1982), but not often applied to the treatment of domestic violence. (For one example, see Heyman & Neidig, 1997.) We believe that the couples group format enlarges upon the benefits of both individual couple sessions and group therapies, providing a unique arena in which to address the complexities of violence within relationships. With both members of the couple present, each partner's perspective on events can be represented and addressed in a manner not possible in gender-specific groups.

Several key aspects of the couples group will now be described in greater detail. These include reducing social isolation, providing ongoing accountability, cross-coupling, and forming a community of nonviolence. The provision of these important aspects of treatment continues the therapeutic work dedicated to ensuring safety and preventing any further abuse.

The couples group offers an important format in which to counter the tendency toward social isolation, one key contributing factor in family violence (Adams, 1989; Dutton, 1988; van der Kolk, 1996). In joining a group of other couples, a dyad's generally closed boundaries are automatically opened to a community of peers, providing new input and possible resources. One couple described how they had "lived in a cocoon" prior to joining the group, sharing very little about their interpersonal dynamics with anyone. In the process, the intensity and fusion often characteristic of these relationships can be diffused by the inclusion of people outside of the twosome.

There are a variety of reasons that these couples become isolated, including the batterer's need to limit and control the woman's access to others (Adams, 1989). Once violence occurs, the need to keep the shameful truths of the relationship secret further contributes to the couple's seclusion. In joining the group, couples find others with similar experiences, and often for the first time can speak honestly about what occurs in their relationships. The confusing array of feelings—of love, anger, fear, remorse, insecurity, shame, and courage—can be validated by those who understand firsthand. This confirmation can deepen the therapeutic work needed for healing, by sharing, identifying, and learning through the experiences of others.

The group also provides a needed arena for ongoing accountability. Group members come to hold each other responsible for their behavior, especially any use of physical, verbal, or emotional abuse. A number of men said they were able to choose nonabusive behaviors by remembering their accountability to the group. In many ways, the couples group serves the function of social control as well as the function of therapy. With both members of the couple present, any violations can be openly discussed, greatly reducing the possibility of denial and minimization on the part of the batterer. In this sense, a couples group format addresses the criticism launched against batterers' groups that do not utilize input from the battered women to validate the men's perceptions (Adams, 1989; Kaufman, 1993). A case example follows.

In one couples group, when asked how they were doing, Bob sheepishly acknowledged that he and his wife, Cindy, had had "a pretty bad fight" that week. He described how Cindy had introduced "the black cloud of the moment" after having a pleasant evening out, which disappointed him. He spoke of how he got very angry at her, and ended up pushing her arm away from him, then how she started to also complain about the way he pushed her arm. Bob added that Cindy remained angry at him even after he apologized, something he didn't fully understand. Because she was also present, Cindy was able to describe more fully her experience of this push. She spoke about how it felt like he wasn't just trying to push her away in order to have distance, but was intentionally trying to hurt her. She then cried as she recalled her belief that he was being abusive once again. With Cindy's added input, group members got a fuller picture of what had occurred, which they then could confront.

One very unique aspect of couples groups is the capacity for what I call "cross-coupling." This refers to the ability of a member of one couple to confront the opposite-gendered member of another couple in a meaningful way. When receiving input from someone other than the spouse, an individual seems to have a less volatile emotional reaction, and a concomitant increased ability to hear the perspective and suggestions of someone parallel to the partner.

An example of cross-coupling occurred in the group cited above, when Bob's behavior was confronted. As Bob described the experience of feeling the "rage building up inside" prior to pushing Cindy's arm, Eleanor (another woman in the group) responded to him. She began to suggest that he catch himself before he acted on his anger, just when the rage was "starting to come up." She then went on to give Bob feedback, stating that as a woman who was not his wife, but who similarly had been abused by the man she loved, she could let him know how it felt. She described that once a woman has been battered, even the smallest aggressive word or action could feel the same as a severe assault. Bob then acknowledged that he was aware that Cindy had been scared, which helped him to walk out of the room at the time. Eleanor again confronted his behavior, stating that he needed to be able to leave *before* the push occurred. She spoke of how his push would set back Cindy's trust in him for a long time, and that he must learn to recognize the rage before acting on it. She forcefully stated that no matter what Cindy might have done that was provocative, it was his responsibility to stop any abusive impulse.

Another significant aspect of couples group treatment is the development of a community dedicated to nonviolence. Given the high potential for recidivism (Holtzworth-Monroe et al., 1995; Rosenfeld, 1992), we believe that the potential for violence may always be present once someone has utilized it previously. Consequently, we borrow certain concepts from the addiction literature, where ongoing acknowledgment of the problem and a community of peers who can support positive change become essential components of remaining symptom-free (Chappel, 1992). In terms of our couples groups, a community of others who have embraced egalitarian ideals for their relationships and will not condone any form of abuse helps the men choose alternatives to violence in an ongoing manner.

Much of the work of the community extends beyond the confines of our group sessions. Since group members are encouraged to have contact outside, they frequently turn to each other whenever they need help. For example, when Bob and Cindy started to argue with more frequency, Bob would call male (and sometimes female) group members for input on how to "stay cool," even going out for coffee with the men in order to "talk out" his feelings rather than overreacting to Cindy. One group we ran decided to meet on their own when our clinic was closed for vacation, ensuring that they had ongoing contact with each other and a place to process their relationships.

As we have continued to grow, we have added another way to extend group members' participation in the nonviolent community. Similar to the work of Rhea Almeida (Almeida & Bograd, 1991), we have asked group members who have "graduated" to become mentors of sorts for newcomers to our program, reaching out as needed and even cofacilitating groups with the therapists. This benefits both the neophytes, who gain the wisdom of experience from senior group members, and allows the "graduates" the ongoing reminder of their dedication to nonabusive behavior and attitudes. In this way, the group can transmit nonviolence between "generations" of members, helping combat the internalized abusive attitudes that pervaded prior to treatment.

CONCLUSION

This chapter presented a metasystemic approach to the treatment of domestic violence, incorporating the feminist and systemic ideas from both sides of the treatment controversy. We recognize that this treatment serves a somewhat limited population: those couples who are choosing to remain together and men who are willing to take responsibility for their violence. Still, we believe that many of the ideas inherent in this approach can be utilized to facilitate more comprehensive ways to address this problem. We have begun outcome research in order to produce more empirical data regarding this approach, and hope to continue to embrace various aspects of the treatment controversy to bridge the polarities present in the field.

ACKNOWLEDGMENTS

I wish to thank Virginia Goldner and Gillian Walker for their ideas, mentoring, and support throughout the project. Thanks also to Thomas Moore, my coteam member, for assistance in researching this field of study.

REFERENCES

Adams, D. (1989). Feminist-based interventions for battering men. In P. L. Caesar & L. K. Hamberger (Eds.), *Treating men who batter: Theory, practice, and programs* (pp. 3–23). New York: Springer.
Almeida, R., & Bograd, M. (1991). Sponsorship: Men holding men accountable

for domestic violence. In M. Bograd (Ed.), *Feminist approaches for treating men in family therapy* (pp. 243–259). New York: Haworth Press.

Avis, J. M. (1992). Where are all the family therapists? Abuse and violence within families and family therapy's response. *Journal of Marital and Family Therapy, 18*, 225–232.

Berk, R. A., Berk, S. F., Loseke, D. R., & Rauma, D. (1983). Mutual combat and other family violence myths. In D. Finkelhor & M. A. Straus (Eds.), *The dark side of families: Current family violence research* (pp. 179–212). Beverly Hills, CA: Sage.

Bograd, M. (1984). Family systems approaches to wife battering: A feminist critique. *American Journal of Orthopsychiatry, 54*, 558–568.

Bograd, M. (1992). Values in conflict: Challenges to family therapists' thinking. *Journal of Marital and Family Therapy, 18*, 245–256.

Browne, A. (1987). *When battered women kill.* New York: Free Press.

Browne, A. (1993). Violence against women by male partners: Prevalence, outcomes, and policy implications. *American Psychologist, 48*, 1077–1087.

Cantos, A. L., Neidig, P. H., & O'Leary, K. D. (1994). Injuries of women and men in a treatment program for domestic violence. *Journal of Family Violence, 9*, 113–125.

Chappel, J. N. (1992) Effective use of Alcoholics Anonymous and Narcotics Anonymous in treating patients. *Psychiatric Annals, 22*, 409–418.

Chodorow, N. (1978). *The reproduction of mothering.* Berkeley and Los Angeles: University of California Press.

Cook, D. R., & Frantz-Cook, A. (1984). A systemic approach to wife battering. *Journal of Marital and Family Therapy, 10*, 83–93.

Dell, P. (1989). Violence and the systemic view: The problem of power. *Family Process, 28*, 1–14.

Dutton, D. G. (1988). Profiling of wife assaulters: Preliminary evidence for a trimodal analysis. *Violence and Victims, 3*, 5–30.

Dutton, M. A. (1992). *Empowering and healing the battered woman.* New York: Springer.

Feldman, C., & Ridley, C. (1995). The etiology and treatment of domestic violence between adult partners. *Clinical Psychology: Science and Practice, 2*, 317–348.

Framo, J. (1982). *Explorations in marital and family therapy.* New York: Springer.

Ganley, A. L. (1989). Integrating feminist and social learning analyses of aggression: Creating multiple models for intervention with men who batter. In P. L. Caesar & L. K. Hamberger (Eds.), *Treating men who batter: Theory, practice, and programs* (pp. 196–235). New York: Springer.

Geffner, R., Mantooth, C., Franks, D., & Rao, L. (1989). A psychoeducational, conjoint therapy approach to reducing family violence. In P. L. Caesar & L. K. Hamberger (Eds.), *Treating men who batter: Theory, practice, and programs* (pp. 103–133). New York: Springer.

Geller, J. A., & Wasserstrom, J. (1984). Conjoint therapy for the treatment of domestic violence. In A. R. Roberts (Ed.), *Battered women and their families: Intervention strategies and treatment programs* (pp. 33–48). New York: Springer.

Gelles, R., & Straus, M. A. (1979). Determinants of violence in the family: Toward a theoretical integration. In W. R. Nye & I. L. Reiss (Eds.), *Contemporary theories about the family* (pp. 549–581). New York: Free Press.

Gilligan, C. (1982). *In a different voice.* Cambridge, MA: Harvard University Press.

Goldner, V. (1985). Feminism and family therapy. *Family Process, 24,* 31–47.

Goldner, V. (1992). Making room for both/and. *Family Therapy Networker, 16,* 54–62.

Goldner, V., Sheinberg, M., Penn, P., & Walker, G. (1990). Love and violence: Gender paradoxes in volatile attachments. *Family Process, 29,* 343–364.

Hare-Mustin, R. (1978). A feminist approach to family therapy. *Family Process, 17,* 181–194.

Herman, J. (1992). *Trauma and recovery.* New York: Basic Books.

Herman, J. (1995). Crime and memory. *Bulletin of the American Academy of Psychiatry and Law, 23,* 75–87.

Heyman, R. E., & Neidig, P. H. (1997) Physical aggression couples treatment. In W. K. Halford & H. J. Markman (Eds.), *Clinical handbook of marriage and couples interventions* (pp. 589–617). New York: Wiley.

Holtzworth-Munroe, A., Beatty, S. B., & Anglin, K. (1995). The assessment and treatment of marital violence: An introduction for the marital therapist. In N. S. Jacobson & A. S. Gurman (Eds.), *Clinical handbook of couple therapy* (pp. 317–339). New York: Guilford Press.

Holtzworth-Munroe, A., Smutzler, N., Bates, L., & Sandin, E. (1997). Husband violence: Basic facts and clinical implications. In W. K. Halford & H. J. Markman (Eds.), *Clinical handbook of marriage and couples interventions* (pp. 129–155). New York: Wiley.

Hotaling, G. T., & Sugarman, D. B. (1986). An analysis of risk markers in husband to wife violence: The current state of knowledge. *Violence and Victims, 1,* 101–124.

Jennings, S. P., & Jennings, J. L. (1991). Multiple approaches to the treatment of violent couples. *American Journal of Family Therapy, 19,* 351–362.

Kantor, G. K., & Straus, M. A. (1987). The "drunken bum" theory of wife beating. *Social Problems, 34,* 213–229.

Kaufman, G. Jr. (1993). The mysterious disappearance of battered women in family therapists' offices: Male privelege colluding with male violence. In E. Imber-Black (Ed.), *Secrets in families and family therapy* (pp. 196–212). New York: Norton.

Kurz, C., & Stark, E. (1988). Not so benign neglect: The medical response to battering. In K. Yllo & M. Bograd (Eds.), *Feminist perspectives on wife abuse* (pp. 249–266). Beverly Hills, CA: Sage.

Lane, G., & Russell, T. (1989). Second-order systemic work with violent couples. In P. L Caesar & L. K. Hamberger (Eds.), *Treating men who batter: Theory, practice, and programs (pp. 134–162).* New York: Springer.

Lipchik, E., Sirles, E. A., & Kubicki, A. D. (1997). Multifaceted approaches in spouse abuse treatment. *Journal of Aggression, Maltreatment and Trauma, 1,* 131–148.

Mack, R. N. (1989). Spouse abuse: A dyadic approach. In G. Weeks (Ed.), *Treating couples: The intersystem model of the Marriage Council of Philadelphia* (pp. 191–214). New York: Brunner/Mazel.

Minuchin, S., & Nichols, M. (1993). *Family Healing.* New York: Free Press.

Neidig, P. H., & Friedman, D. H. (1984). *Spouse abuse: A treatment program for couples.* Champagne, IL: Research Press.

Pence, E. (1989). Batterer programs: Shifting from community collusion to community confrontation. In P. L. Caesar & L. K. Hamberger (Eds.), *Treating men who batter: Theory, practice, and programs* (pp. 24–50). New York: Springer.

Pence, E., & Paymar, M. (1993). *Education groups for men who batter: The Duluth model.* New York: Springer.

Ritmeester, T. (1993). Batterers' programs, battered women's movement, and issues of accountability. In E. Pence & M. Paymar, *Education groups for men who batter: The Duluth model* (pp. 169–178). New York: Springer.

Rosenfeld, B. D. (1992). Court-ordered treatment of spouse abuse. *Clinical Psychology Review, 12,* 205–226.

Schecter, S. (1982). *Women and male violence: Visions and struggles of the battered women's movement.* Boston: South End Press.

Stark, E., & Flitcraft, A. (1982). Medical therapy as repression: The case of battered women. *Health and Medicine, Summer–Fall,* 29–32.

Straus, M., & Gelles, R. (Eds.). (1990). *Physical violence in American families: Risk factors and adaptations to violence in 8,145 families.* New Brunswick, NJ: Transaction Press.

van der Kolk, B. A. (1996). The complexity of adaptation to trauma: Self- regulation, stimulus discrimination, and characterological development. In B. A. van der Kolk, A. C. McFarland, & L. Weisaeth (Eds.), *Traumatic stress: The effects of overwhelming experience on mind, body, and society* (pp. 182–213). New York: Guilford Press.

Walker, G. (1999). The initial assessment in therapy with couples where battering is an issue. Unpublished manuscript. Ackerman Institue, New York, NY.

Walker, G., & Goldner, V. (1995). The wounded prince and the women who love him. In C. Burck & B. Speed (Eds.), *Gender, power, and relationships* (pp. 24–45). London: Routledge & Kegan Paul.

Walker, G., & Shimmerlik, S. (1994). The invisible battlefield. *Family Therapy Networker,* May–June, 50–60.

Walker, L. E. (1979). *The battered woman.* New York: Harper & Row.

Weitzman, J., & Dreen, K. (1982). Wife beating: A view of the marital dyad. *Social Casework, 63,* 259–265.

White, M., & Epston, D. (1990). *Narriative means to therapeutic ends.* New York: Norton.

Yalom, I. (1985). *The theory and practice of group psychotherapy, third edition.* New York: Basic Books.

CHAPTER 8

A Tourist's View of Marriage

Cross-Cultural Couples—
Challenges, Choices, and Implications
for Therapy

Esther Perel

We can no longer afford to ignore the rapidly increasing heterogeneity of the world—a potent cultural mix that is no longer limited to major cities, but wired into our lives via cable television and the Internet, faxed onto our desks in the workplace, and appearing in our homes in the increasingly frequent romantic choices people make of partners from different cultural backgrounds.

So far cross-cultural relationships haven't received adequate attention, in part because the phenomenon is so new—largely a product of the last 50 years. Increased mobility, advances in travel and education, military and political incentives, the introduction and effects of broader civil rights, and the easing of U.S. immigration restrictions during this period have all contributed to the increase of marriage between people of different faiths, cultures, nationalities, and races.

The study of mixed couples yields a number of compelling insights and helps us understand how people adapt to cultural conflict and how they react to the very contemporary phenomena of marginality and cultural change. Of particular relevance to the field of family therapy, it sheds light on new family and personality types that reflect and are particularly suited for life in a mobile modern world.

All marriages encompass the discovery of and subsequent discussion about differences. Dealing with differences in intermarriage also requires a reconciliation of the conflicting Claims and Pulls of the two worlds.

One world is the world of "Marriage." In the West, the modern concept of marriage is based on the centrality of love. In this formulation, marriage is a result of a free choice. It is a private decision made by the couple, and it aims to promote their happiness, intimacy, and mutual self-fulfillment. In this world, each partner connecting to the other often requires a separation from or a weakening of the attachments to family or tradition.

The other world is the world of origins—race, religion, culture, and/or nationality—which brings with it assorted collective responsibilities and loyalties. Let's call this "Inter." This world strongly pulls against the individual character of the modern ideology of love. Inter is governed by the notion of a larger web of connections in which the person is part of a national and family history and tradition, and feels communal allegiance. Marriage is not simply between two individuals but two families. In this world, the needs of the community supersede the needs of the individual.

If "Marriage" describes Romeo and Juliet, "Inter" describes the Capulets and Montagues.

Consider Manuel, a Colombian man, married to Mary, who was born in New England. "For me," he says, "marriage is between two families. Who am I without my family? For Mary it's between the two of us. I guess our basic view of who is involved in our marriage is different. Our views of boundaries diverge, and you can imagine just how polar are our expectations of how much our families should be involved with us and our children." Marriage as an enterprise of free choice is rejected in Manuel's culture. Mary's American emphasis on individual choice both attracts Manuel and prompts a sense of guilt in him for violating his own entrenched cultural expectations of what a marriage is "supposed" to be. This division allows us to see, in simple fashion, some of the main causes of tension in cross-cultural marriages.

These tensions can sometimes seem overwhelming. There are usually many facts to be learned about each other, terms and assumptions to be defined, from the simplest words to the most fundamental concepts of birth, marriage, child rearing, gender roles, work, family, tradition, even death. Very little can be taken for granted.

In fact, cross-cultural partners are like immigrants or tourists. Sometimes they actually cross borders, sometimes they undergo the transition in their own living room. Plunged into an unfamiliar world, each "tourist"-partner wonders, "How can I feel comfortable here?" The "tourist" notices all kinds of things the indigenous local misses or takes for granted—"Why is this building here? What does that sign mean?"—often reawakening the local's own curiosity about his or her own surroundings, and his or her place in those surroundings, affording a fresh look at customs or landmarks or traditions that the local formerly hadn't noticed for years—if at all.

In one type of cultural adjustment, the newcomer slowly takes hold of this new world by imitating, identifying, and internalizing its key aspects and familiarizing himself or herself with its landmarks. However, the "tourist"-partner must continually adjust to this newfound home because there he or she is always confronting new or unfamiliar cultural aspects as new events, decisions, crises, and life-cycle transitions occur. In capsule, this describes the experience of a partner in a cross-cultural couple who lives in the "home" country or culture of the other.

Safia was born in Pakistan, married an American, and now lives in the northeastern United States. "In my adjusting here I go for a few years with a comfortable sense that I have found ways to maneuver through this place, but when my kids go to school I acutely feel my foreignness again. When they come home they bring the outside culture through the front door and I am confronted with the fact that I didn't grow up here. I don't know the system. I don't know the rhymes. So every time I confront a new institution, I again experience my foreignness. The transition is never-ending."

Certainly the therapist who works with "mixed" or cross-cultural couples needs to be as alive to the couple's differences and what they mean to the couple themselves, and to develop a tourist's sense of landmarks in unfamiliar territory, learning to ask the right questions about what things mean and how things work. This quality of attention is more and more urgently required.

REACTIONS TO CROSS-CULTURAL MARRIAGES
IN THE UNITED STATES

Reactions to cross-cultural marriage in the United States during the past half-century or so have tended to gravitate to one of two poles:

welcome and tolerance or xenophobia. At one pole is the view that these unions are a testament to the power of love to transcend traditional boundaries. On the other is an alarmist view that sees such unions as a threat to the prevailing national identity, a doomed endeavor inevitably leading to divorce. Literature written after the first wave of mixed marriages involving Asian war brides and American servicemen, tended to reflect this latter view.

Until the 1960s, the lines transcended were primarily ethnic, say, between Irish and Italians. When the religious Rubicons were crossed, they generally implied Catholic and Protestant unions. Interracial relationships remained criminal until groundbreaking federal civil rights legislation was passed in 1967.

A dramatic indication of the recent cultural change has been the rate of increase of Jews marrying non-Jews over the past 30 years—rising from 5% in 1964 to 52% in 1997.

In general the history of cross-cultural marriage in the United States indicates a mutation in two directions: on one side, a pull toward assimilation, diminishing cultural distinctions in the public and private domains founded on ideas of equality, a premise that gives primary allegiance to the national (and mythical) identity of the United States as a "melting pot." On the other side has been an increasing recognition of the enduring nature of ethnic and religious values, and identification of the role they play in family life and personal development throughout the life cycle.

REACTIONS TO CROSS-CULTURAL MARRIAGES IN THE LITERATURE

Most studies done in the field of cross-cultural marriages have been of limited use partly because of the narrow focus of the various sociological, anthropological, religious, national, and psychotherapeutic factions conducting them. Their researches are often constrained by whatever investment the particular faction has in the topic—an investment that typically does not invite, much less examine, the findings and approaches of any other faction. In addition, focused research presumed that deviation equals difficulty (Cotrell, 1990). As a result, research on interracial marriages doesn't look at the effects of religion or language, research on interfaith marriages doesn't address any issues but the religious ones, and so on.

However, some of the more recent literature is helpful in its acknowledgment of the confluence of many factors and offers more in-sightful clinical information and therapeutic skills. (See the work of Ibrahim, 1984, 1990; Soncini, 1997; Perel, 1990, 1991; Romano, 1996; Tseng, McDermott, & Maretzki, 1977; Tseng & Hsu, 1991; McGoldrick & Preto, 1984; McGoldrick, Pearce, & Giordano, 1996; and Ho, 1984, 1990.) Also of particular interest are the writings of Kluckhohn (1951) and Kluckhohn and Strodtbeck (1961) and the cultural variables devel-oped in the business anthropological literature by Hall and Hall (1980), Hall (1990), Hofstrede (1980), Trompenaars and Hampden-Turner (1998), and Stewart and Bennett (1991), and which offer generative models outlining a cultural map.

The following model is designed to clarify the underlying assump-tions guiding what otherwise appear to be unrelated daily occurrences. It involves a macrolevel analysis of cultures to help illuminate the interper-sonal reality of couples who come for treatment. Edward T. Hall (1990) provides the useful concepts of "high-context" and "low-context" societ-ies. Although they were originally applied specifically to communication, I will employ them in a broader sense. Most cultures tend to gravitate to-ward one pole or the other in this spectrum. Another way to conceive of the spectrum is individualism versus collectivism. In low context societies such as Germany, the Scandinavian countries, the Netherlands, England, Australia, and the United States (often countries rooted in Protestant Calvinism; see Weber,), people compartmentalize personal relation-ships and work, and focus on short-term relationships. Factual informa-tion is stressed, as is explicit verbal expression. The high-context societies are more rural and less industrialized than the low-context societies. In Latin America, Africa, the Mediterranean countries, the Arab world, In-dia, China, and Indonesia extensive information networks exist among family, friends, and colleagues. This shared experience allows for a greater degree of tacit understanding. People are often involved in close and lasting personal relationships.

These two categories can function as receptacles for a multitude of other cultural dimensions (see Table 8.1).

The situation of one couple offers a quick illustration of how these polarities influence everyday life. Indira comes from a large family who live near Bombay in India, and Peter is a white Protestant from Phila-delphia. They fell in love with each other while in graduate school in Boston. Their differences since marrying had become so acute that they sought therapy, mostly at Peter's insistence. Peter first complained about Indira's family coming for a 2-month stay, and expressed puzzle-ment at why Indira could ever have let her family intrude upon them

TABLE 8.1. Low Context versus High Context

Low context	High context
Individualism	
Individualistic; "I" predominates over "We"; independence and self-reliance highly valued ("It's everyone for himself"); few obligations between people (except for very close family); social control based on individual guilt and fear of losing self-respect; universalistic, strive for generalizable laws, rules, widely applicable models and prescriptions.	Collectivistic, value group interest and group identity over individual needs, personal identity inscribed in a larger social network; social control is based on fear of losing face and being shamed; harmony more important than speaking one's mind; particularistic, emphasizes difference, uniqueness, and exceptions, relationships more important than rules and laws. ("For a friend, I can change all the rules if needed").
Time	
Monochronic; felt to be linear; one thing is done at a time; deadlines set and adhered to; time is to be managed; time is referred to as being "spent," "saved," "wasted," or "lost"; youth-oriented society; change is a virtue.	Polychronic: involved in many things at once; distractible, subject to interruptions; time is to be enjoyed; emphasis is on quality of life; age is respected; constancy is a virtue; people are more important that schedules.
Nature of the universe and attitude toward life	
Pragmatic, task-driven, focus is on measurable accomplishments, doing not being ("If at first you don't succeed, try, try again"); work to live; work and relationships are separate; acquiring goods; privacy is valued; emphasis on personal achievement; belief that individuals control their own destiny and environment ("Life is what you make of it"); seek to control nature to meet the needs of people.	Emphasis on affiliation, character, and personal qualities; traditional; focus on ascription not achievement ("It's who you are, not what you do"); focus on relationships, experience, and quality of life; work to live; events are determined by chance, luck, destiny, or a supernatural force; circumstances just happen ("What can you do about fate?"; "It's God's will"); fatalistic; people are subject to the forces of nature.
Family structure	
Couple is the main deciding unit; marriage is between two individuals; individual needs are separate from family needs ("You should do what's right for you"); family obligations minimized; child rearing focuses on fostering a strong sense of self, autonomy, self-reliance, independence.	Extended family are important; marriage is between two families; family needs are intertwined with individual needs; respect for ancestry ("Your grandmother would turn over in her grave . . . !"); child rearing focuses on fostering a strong sense of connection and loyalty; family cohesiveness.

(*continued*)

TABLE 8.1. (*continued*)

Low context	High context
Emotional expressiveness and communication	
Utilitarian, instrumental, pragmatic, impersonal, goal-oriented, direct ("Say what you mean"); informal ("Let's just be ourselves"); meets conflict head-on; explicit communication; seeks high degree of objectivity; goal is to exchange information, facts and opinions; what is said is more important than how ("Get to the point"); emotionalism is irrational and embarrassing.	Communication is more than words; meaning implicitly derives from group understanding, voice, tone, body language, use of silence; indirect, face-saving ("I don't know"; "If you say so"); avoiding conflict takes precedence over open confrontation; formal and respectful; expressive, strong display of emotions; high degree of subjectivity; those who hide their feelings may be perceived as "cold fish" or even deceitful.
Thinking	
Inductive thinking, derives principles and theories from empirical observation and experimentation; linear orientation, break problems apart to reach manageable, precise, pragmatic results.	Deductive reasoning, priority is given to the reality of ideas, moral values, theories, emphasis on the conceptual world, on abstract and symbolic thinking; why rather than what and how; systematic orientation, stress integrated, "holistic" approach to problem solving; use of analogy, metaphor, simile for explanation.
Power and gender roles	
Man and woman experience greater role flexibility and the concomitant confusions; emphasis on equality and more even power; women more economically independent, more openly critical, more sure of their rights.	Fixed roles, high degree of differentiation between the sexes and a clear demarcation of power distribution; women more defined by their alliance to a man than by any independent accomplishments.

for so long. He was also upset about Indira's passive reaction to a recent miscarriage. To her it had been "fate," something over which she had no control, but he believed that if she'd taken better care of herself, she might have avoided the miscarriage. Moreover, he was annoyed at her family's offer to take care of the child Indira was now expecting (she had recently become pregnant again) for several months or even a year in India. Peter saw this as completely inappropriate—akin to wanting to kidnap the child. This wariness was connected to his feeling that he had no privacy when Indira's family visited. His decision to seek therapeutic help grew out of his conviction that "these things need to be talked about," a conviction at odds with Indira's view that they were best left unsaid and that they would eventually sort themselves out.

Clearly, numerous culturally determined assumptions are at war here: Indira's (collectivist, constrained-orientation) sense of fatalism versus Peter's (individualistic, control-orientation) instinct to act and his belief that circumstances are the result of personal choice; Indira's sense of family identity versus Peter's sense of autonomy; her feeling that her family is as important as her connection to Peter versus Peter's craving for privacy and belief that they (as a couple) are the most powerful family unit; Indira's fear that "spelling things out" leads to conflict (not to solutions) versus Peter's belief that it is only by talking about conflict head-on that it can be resolved. While not all people fall so neatly into these cultural categories, most people do feel consistently drawn to one pole or the other.

Cultural maps exist to serve as frameworks. In our work with cross-cultural couples, we will often be able to ascribe the experience of partners at various points on the continuum between the high- and low-context poles. As demonstrated through Indira and Peter, each of their cultural orientations function as a cluster of interrelated values. Knowing these categories will help the therapist understand individuals in cross-cultural relationships. Even though no single individual (or culture) will completely embody every aspect of any one model, doing so can clarify the underlying assumptions guiding what otherwise appear to be unrelated daily occurrences.

THE MANY FACETS OF COMPLEMENTARITY

Why do some people cross cultures to marry, while others stay with partners in their own culture?

A significant dividend of embarking on and sustaining a cross-cultural relationship is the widening of experience and perspective it provides the couple. Such a relationship offers new options for thought and behavior, as well as holds up a mirror each partner would not have had the opportunity to look into otherwise: in the Other, we discover ourselves. As John Locke said, "The self, once expanded, cannot contract to its former dimensions."

Many cross-cultural couples possess a general longing for this broadening change in outlook. Those who enter into an intercultural relationship are referred to alternately as escapists, rebellious, detached, adventurous, and embracers (Tseng et al., 1977; Romano, 1996; Soncini, 1998).

Man Keung Ho (1990), for example, says that a common motive is to escape one's background. This desire to escape may be induced by political, religious, familial, or other conditions the partner finds repressive, but the yearning often has other personal components as well. Edwin Friedman (1982) points out that most partners who marry outside their culture are firstborns. The irony is that firstborn children typically display the greatest loyalty to family and are most involved in their parents' relationship. In families where there is a high degree of emotional intensity, a person is likely to confuse feelings about his family with feelings about his culture; he attributes the undesirable traits in his family to the culture. Thus, a person may seek to distance himself from his relatives by distancing himself from his culture. Yet if intermarriage disrupts a family, it can also enrich it: new doors are opened for diversity, behavior, and connections.

For some, intermarriage presents an opportunity to readjust the undesirable characteristics that they attribute to their background (McGoldrick & Preto, 1984). In this way, intermarriage may be seen as an attempt to establish complementarity through culture. For example, one partner is often attracted to cultural traits from which the other partner is trying to distance himself or herself. When a person from a culture that tolerates higher emotional expressiveness is attracted to someone from, say, a white Anglo-Saxon Protestant (WASP) background, with its emphasis on self-contained autonomy and respect for boundaries and privacy, the WASP partner often simultaneously wants to move away from those qualities and toward more emotional expressiveness.

No matter what motives someone may have for a cross-cultural relationship, the initial complementarity sought by one partner in the other often turns out to be at the root of later problems: what one is attracted to initially because of its foreignness often becomes the source of conflict later. For example, the initial attraction of a WASP to a Mediterranean spouse's family cohesiveness and expressivity can later be felt as overwhelming and intrusive; the Mediterranean's attraction to the WASP's attitudes toward privacy and independence can be felt as disengagement or distance—a lack of caring and involvement. Crisis exacerbates those differences. And during crises couples often lack shared rituals and assumptions that could help them manage these events.

Another challenge is the fact that traits perceived to be positive or attractive in the partner are always attached to a whole network of other habits, characteristics, and behaviors that are not as pleasing as the "attractive" traits; indeed, some of them may turn out to be decidedly unattractive or even intolerable. Studies of marriages between American servicemen and Japanese women, for example, have found that many husbands were initially attracted by their wives' submissiveness. However, that submissiveness often carried with it a passivity and a lack of initiative that later clashed with the husband's desire for assertiveness, action, and hard work—known as effort optimism—that Americans in particular tend to value.

By the same token, the Japanese wife idealized her husband's take-charge attitude and his ability to free her from the restrictions imposed on her by her native Japanese culture. Yet these positive traits were often attacked to characteristics that were far less appealing: materialism, self-absorption, lack of concern with tradition, and little sense of responsibility to the family.

What needs to be done when a couple reaches this impasse is to remind them why they were attracted to each other in the first place—to move from polarity back to complementarity. You remind the Mediterranean woman that she once loved her American WASP husband for his cool-headedness and the WASP that he loved his Mediterranean spouse for her passion; you remind the American husband that he once treasured his Japanese wife's supportiveness and his wife that she cherished her husband's assertiveness. This can help them reclaim their choice.

Cross-cultural couples come up with their own strategies to ward off conflicts. But the drawbacks of these makeshift tactics may not be apparent for quite some time, particularly if (like most couples) one partner or both have an investment in denying difference or blocking out awareness of it. With premarital couples, in particular, one can see such concealment at work. Often they feel caught between remaining silent to ensure togetherness, yet at the same time desiring greater self-revelation, which will inevitably lead to the uncovering of tribal affinities or spiritual feelings. This results in a paradox: the very efforts to maintain the relationship could in the long run injure it. The couple creates a conspiracy of silence in order to keep out those issues and beliefs that could topple their relationship. It may only be when a major life event, experience, or rite of passage (like death, birth, or marriage) occurs that these denied or buried differences reappear—usually with unanticipated intensity. Consider Ethan, a Jew, and Linda, a Catholic.

They initially vowed to bring up their child with elements of both religious traditions, but without ever spelling out precisely what they meant by this compromise. When she gave birth to their first child, a boy, Ethan assumed the boy would have a ritual circumcision while Linda assumed the baby would be baptized.

Thus, intermarriage is the crossroads of the wish to assimilate and the wish to retain one's cultural, racial, or religious identity. Now let's look at three particular flashpoints: religion, child rearing, and gender.

INTERMARRIAGE FLASHPOINTS

Religion

With interfaith marriages, it is often more difficult to navigate differences because it is harder to accept religious certainties as "relative."

Because religious beliefs are inculcated in childhood, the strength of these traditions may be felt but still be hard to articulate, as hard to describe as they would have been at the time they were first acquired. This explains why people who are otherwise capable of sophisticated abstract thinking, open-minded listening, and compromising in other areas of life, revert to simple, concrete childlike language when they try to speak about religion. Freud concurred in his assertion (about himself) that the more powerful the religious feeling or identification, the harder it was to articulate it.

Let's examine another Jewish and Christian intermarriage.

Sam, who comes from an assimilated American Jewish family but who identifies himself strongly as Jewish, and his partner, Grace, who comes from a Roman Catholic family, are similar to Linda and Ethan in that they suddenly experienced their religious beliefs and traditions more powerfully when they decided to get married. Sam and Grace stayed together in relative harmony for 4 years before these issues became urgent.

"For four years this has never been an issue," Grace said, "but now, when marriage comes up, we suddenly become fierce representatives of our religions, which we both thought we'd long abandoned."

It turns out that Sam hadn't "abandoned" his Jewishness as Grace thought he had: "I feel very strongly about being Jewish. I can't explain it. I am not religious but I do want to raise my children Jewish."

Grace expressed her resentments about this: "Why should I give up my beliefs and practices when you don't follow your religion? I have a feeling that Judaism is being forced upon me with no respect for my own cultural beliefs and how important my own heritage is to me. In your desire to have a Jewish home, you are not ready to accept any other influence. Why is the non-Jewish partner supposed to bend completely?"

Sam acknowledged that he knew it didn't make sense to Grace, and that he didn't understand why his own reaction was so strong. "I don't even believe in God, but I feel very strongly about the history of my people and there is a part of me that feels that I would be abandoning the dead."

When Grace asked him if he were simply parroting his parents' beliefs, Sam replied, "The fact that my parents think like me doesn't make what we agree on any less my thoughts. Actually I disagree with them that you should have to convert, but I do want a commitment on having a Jewish family."

Grace countered: "How much Jewish commitment will ever be enough for them? They will never accept me as one of them. You, on the other hand, are totally welcome in my family." Sam replied that his parents liked her very much. Grace responded, "Yes, but they would like me *more* if I came in a *Jewish* form."

In these situations, partners are likely to return to the familiar territory of their culture or religion as frames of reference to guide them through the changes. Long-dormant ethnic and religious feelings may explode at these critical moments when one or both partners experience a reawakening of their cultural allegiances.

Sam and Grace provide a good example of how religion can be powerfully felt but only dimly understood. Sam is a Jew for whom Jewishness involves a powerful sentimental attachment to the past. He has a strong but unintegrated feeling of being a Jew, and often feels that his Jewishness, precisely because it is so unintegrated, could easily be taken away from him. It lacks any active expression in his life, and thus tends to express itself as a deep sense of vulnerability. His Jewish identity is a strong but passive and mostly unarticulated group loyalty that Grace's mere presence threatens. Her "otherness" stirs the specter of betrayal in Sam, a betrayal of group and history, which provokes a fear of loss.

Not yet known is whether his reaction stems more from his fear of being overwhelmed by Grace's foreignness or from his attachment to Judaism and the role Judaism plays in his life. This must become clear if Sam is to broach any of the critical topics of religious and marital pursuits. Right now his participation in Judaism is not expressed in any activity; he says he's waiting to have children to become proactive again.

Sam finished his Jewish education at 13, on the day of his bar mitzvah. Grace attended parochial school for some time in her girlhood and was confirmed at age 11. Neither demonstrates a vocabulary adequate to translate their childhood religious feelings and identities into adult terms. Sam tends to revert to a limited leitmotif ("I'm not religious . . . but I want my children to be raised as Jews") when he speaks of his commitment to Judaism, but this leaves little entry for Grace, or much inducement for her even to try to enter. All he offers her of Judaism now is a simplistic historical legacy of persecution, stripped of most of the content and meaning of living Judaism.

In my experience, generally Jews and Christians use a different language when they talk about their cultural and religious ties. When asked what is essential about his Jewish identity, a secular cultural Jew will usually stress the feeling of belonging to a community, a historical consciousness, an attachment to a collective past. He may say that he feels guilty for having betrayed his people by marrying out of the religion. But the important point here is that a "peoplehood" notion of Jewishness supersedes the religious one. God, belief, spirituality, and faith are underrepresented in this Jewish discourse, of which Sam's words to Grace are clearly a part.

Grace, like many Christians, talks about individual faith, a personal relation to God, the soothing comfort of church, and the spiritual and family feelings of Christmas. She may disagree with the values of the Roman Catholic Church pertaining to sex, abortion rights, and women's rights, but not about Jesus, whom she thinks about much as she did at age 11. When feelings of betraying the Catholic Church arise for someone like Grace, they are usually connected to very personal experiences: not being completely honest at confession, failing to baptize a child, and other sins that jeopardize her individual soul. This is a far cry from threatening the collective Jewish soul that Sam thinks of when he hears that word.

These differences lead both partners to examine themselves more intensely. In the presence of the Other, we are forced to define ourselves. This is why Sam and Grace need to understand the meaning and importance of their respective traditions. At stake in any discussion of their cultural and religious differences is a meaningful resolution that will affect their marital life, their ethnic and religious identity as a family and as individuals, and the future identity of their child.

Clearly, mixed marriages require greater than normal adjustments. If Grace chooses to accommodate Sam, they both need to recognize that she was able to make that accommodation because she has more latitude—that is, she is less connected to her religion or to her family's wishes, she has a more flexible personality, she sees it as the woman's role. In such couples, one partner ends up compromising because the other was unable to.

Note that by accommodating, the compromiser is invested with enormous power since she (or he) is the one who sustained the relationship. The person whose religion (or country or culture) is observed must acknowledge and appreciate the loss and the adjustment that the partner is experiencing throughout their entire union.

The "Time Bomb" Issue of Children

The dilemma of children for the cross-cultural couple is usually complicated and emotionally volatile. The couple wonders how they can synthesize two backgrounds into one that their child will grow up in. Children symbolize the continuity of family, values, and traditions. They bring to focus the differences in partners' backgrounds in dramatic ways. As we saw with Sam and Grace, the prospect of having children and the decisions a cross-cultural couple faces about their upbringing can constitute a time bomb. Accommodations made or promised at the beginning of the relationship—for example, one partner's agreement that the children will be brought up in the other partner's faith or country—may suddenly feel impossible to carry out when the baby is actually conceived or born.

For mixed couples especially, a child is sometimes seen as a blank screen onto which the parents can project feelings they may be loath to confront within themselves. A constellation of concerns often includes the fear of alienation from the child if he is raised in a different religion or culture from the parent's own. A parent must figure out how to transmit an alien heritage, for example. The intent may be to divide the influence equally, but carrying out a 50–50 split poses more questions than it answers. How do you do it? The idea that "the child will choose" is impossible: a child of 3 or 6 isn't equipped to choose something as complex and overwhelming as religious faith and tradition. Nor does exposure to both parents' traditions and faiths foster an "equal identity." Children need consistent socialization in which religion and culture are incorporated into the building of self. From the place of the child within the family to attitudes about parental authority, couples must grapple with a wide range of issues dealing with child rearing.

One couple, Sally and Nigel, illustrate the problem. Nigel, from England, and Sally, an American, are married with two children, ages 3 and 5. Their conflicts typically arise around the issue of discipline. On a recent Sunday morning, when they had planned a family outing to the zoo, the kids woke up and decided they didn't want to go. Sally's instinct was to say "OK, we don't have to go through with this if the kids don't want to go. After all, we're doing it for them." But Nigel would have none of that. "They're going to go because we decided on it!" As far as he was concerned, the children were too young to enforce their wishes on the family. Where Nigel believes that what Mom and Dad say goes, Sally subscribes to a more collateral model, whereby you listen to your children's wishes and, to the extent possible, try to fulfill them.

When Nigel got his way and they began to drive to the zoo, the children asked to hear "Hercules" on the audiotape deck. Nigel said it was fine to listen to music, but that they should pick something everyone wanted to listen to (and he'd had it up to here with "Hercules," which his kids played at home nonstop—at least until Nigel made them turn it off). Again Sally's instinct was to grant the kids their wish. Back home after the zoo, at the dinner table, their children wanted to leave the table when they were done eating, and once again Nigel wouldn't hear of it: "Kids should stay at the table until they're finished, just like I had to!" Once again, this caused friction with Sally, who didn't see why it was such a big deal to allow the children to leave.

Nigel's assumption that children should adapt to the world of adults, versus Sally's assumption that the child's individuality should be fostered whenever possible, did not at first strike either of them as culturally determined. Because language was not an obstacle, and because they shared many other approaches to life, this realm of dissension had always struck them as far more personality-based than a product of cultural indoctrination. However, when each was asked to talk about his or her own experience of growing up, the cultural divisions became clear: Nigel grew up in a lower income family in northern England where children were to be "seen and not heard." Neither he nor his siblings would ever have dreamed of rebelling against their father and mother's wishes. Sally was allowed, from about age 2, to express herself and to choose what she wanted to do far more freely. She was asked what she wanted, and generally permitted to have or to do whatever that was. The underlying cultural notion in Sally's case is that by knowing what you want, you cultivate a sense of self (even at the age of 2). The underlying cultural notion in Nigel's case is that small children aren't equipped to make reasonable choices by themselves and need firm guidance until they are older. Think back to the cultural map described earlier: In a society where individual independence is central, one is likely to encounter an approach to child rearing that encourages self-expression. In a society where the family takes precedence over the individual, a parent is more likely to enforce communal values.

Once Sally and Nigel could acknowledge the assumptions that their respective cultures had transmitted, they entertained the possibility that they might not have to choose one style of parenting over the other, but could decide whose style to follow on a case-by-case basis. The question they began to ask themselves before making a decision about their children began to shift from choosing between "the right way" and "the wrong way" to choosing between "your style" or "my style." Now they can use humor to arrive at a flexible approach that balances their respective values and enables them to negotiate conflict (Falicov, 1986). This can ultimately create a new code that integrates parts of both cultures.

Gender

Expectations about gender roles are another potential flashpoint, although these conflicts may be masked as personality differences or communication problems.

Consider the case of Ahmed and Irene. Ahmed, who escaped Yemen, his country of birth, for political reasons as a young man in his 20s and his wife, Irene, who had a fairly typical U.S. middle-class family background (she grew up in a suburb of Philadelphia), came to therapy to talk about their frequent fighting, not their cultural conflict. They just said that they frequently couldn't "get along" and that their differences led to terrible, sometimes even physically violent, fights. To them, the fights seemed to be based on warring personalities. When Ahmed did bring up cultural reasons for his behavior, Irene felt that it was a cop-out. "I'm not here to talk about your culture," she once said when he offered a cultural rationale for why he sometimes ignored her when they visited his Yemeni friends in Queens. (He said that it was inappropriate for a Yemeni man in male company to be openly demonstrative to or to pay too much attention to his wife.) "We're here to talk about why you won't listen to me!" she said.

Irene was also not aware of the assumptions on which her own distress was based (i.e., a belief in sexual parity, the idea that men and women are "equal"): Ahmed's behavior simply seemed wrong to her. Whether received from culture or family, values perceived to be "basic" are always characterized by their feeling of rightness (much like religious values, which may carry an even stronger sense of immutable truth). Such values appear to their adherents as self-evident and inarguable. It is therefore difficult to communicate them to a partner who not only does not share them, but who may dismiss them, or even be appalled by them.

Part of what enabled Irene and Ahmed to understand why it feels so threatening when one challenges the basic values of the other was to use the metaphor of the immigrant or tourist when they visited certain of each other's friends and family. Although they were still physically in New York City when they took the subway to visit Ahmed's friends in Queens, it nonetheless felt as if they had crossed the actual geographical border into Yemen when they got there. Ahmed had lived with Irene in the United States for years, and he liked many of the liberating aspects of U.S. culture. He liked the fact that she held a job, that they could be openly affectionate on the street, that she was outspoken and independent. But visiting his Yemeni friends was like visiting his homeland, with its own culture and codes of behavior. There, he felt her demands were inappropriate and out of context, that she was failing to acclimate, even briefly, to his culture. Similarly, Ahmed told Irene that when they fought and he yelled at her, she should "make yourself not hear," be silent. He wanted her to respond as a Yemeni woman would in this particular instance, despite his appreciation for her outspokenness in other contexts.

At one point in couple therapy when the therapist said of Irene (who had just berated Ahmed for not treating her as an equal in their social life) that "she is angry," Ahmed stopped for a moment, looked at her, and replied, "Yes. You can see it in her eyes." In that moment the therapist realized that Ahmed was, as a consequence of growing up in a Muslim culture where women covered the bottom halves of their faces with veils, extraordinarily sensitive to the messages in eyes: while growing up, when interacting with women, they were the only facial characteristics he could see.

Each partner has fleeting moments when he or she feels like a "tourist" in another culture. Learning to be sensitive to those moments not only reinforces just how ever-present cultural influences are, but can enrich the observing partner's appreciation of just how one spouse perceives a world in many ways essentially alien to the way of the other. However, as we'll see in the next section, on therapy, partners can create what I call a "third reality," a place where they can meet as fellow travelers. For example, now when Ahmed and Irene go to visit Ahmed's friends in Queens, Ahmed asks her: "Have you got your passport?" and Irene winks back, "Yes, and my veil too." They acknowledge—importantly, with humor—that they are going on a "trip" to another culture, preparing themselves for it by giving a quick nod to their differences, thereby to some degree integrating their two cultures.

Cross-cultural partners are sometimes tourists even when they haven't left their living rooms. Evoking what it means to be a tourist or an immigrant reminds them of the natural awkwardness and confusion felt by anyone visiting an unfamiliar culture or country ("I'm a tourist here—how could I be expected to know what to say, eat, wear?").

It's harder to play tourist at some times than at others, of course, especially when the issue of appropriate gender behavior and identity arises. A trip Ahmed and Irene took on the subway together from Queens to Manhattan provided the frame for another recent argument. It was late and they were in a subway car with a gang of teenagers who looked dangerous. Adding to their insecurity was the fact that they were lost: they'd gotten on the wrong train and didn't know how to connect back to the right one. Irene finally sought and found a police officer and asked him for directions, a decision and an action she felt was appropriate and effective, and also one that provided them with some measure of protection. However, Ahmed felt dismissed and emasculated by her taking charge; he felt it was his responsibility as "the man" to take care of her, not the other way round, and that she ought to have waited for him to do so.

Ahmed felt emasculated by his wife taking control, particularly at a time of danger when it especially appeared to him that it was his responsibility to protect his wife. Irene, meanwhile, felt that by taking charge she was not threatening his role as a man. Understanding those positions is an especially difficult challenge for both of them. Cultural influences intensify feelings about gender roles. In the "Therapy" section we'll see how various couples, including Ahmed and Irene, managed to look at those assumptions more dispassionately and work out "asymmetrical compromises," the very notion of which first struck Irene a priori as wrong, but which she's come to accept as she understands more about what they mean and how they can work.

An essential in working with cross-cultural couples that is often overlooked is language. In a session with a visiting therapist from Israel, Ahmed had difficulty understanding certain words. The therapist used the word "authoritative," for example. "Physical force—pushing?" Ahmed asked. "No, a different kind of power—taking charge," the therapist answered. Ahmed now understood: he demonstrated his understanding of the word by saying, "In my house, I am the king, and Irene is the queen." At another point, the Israeli therapist apologized for his funny Israeli accent. "I like it!" Ahmed quickly announced, forming an instant bond with someone who, like himself, faced the challenge of using a foreign language.

An interesting paradox occurs when a person breaks one of the strongest intimacies anyone can know, that of one's mother tongue, to establish closeness with someone in a secondary or foreign language. How do we express intimacy in a language we're not intimate with, when so much is "lost in translation"? Culture shapes language and language shapes culture. In this symbiotic relationship the way people use language speaks volumes about the effects on them of their environment. (One of the oldest recorded European aphorisms relates to language: Charles V, the Holy Roman Emperor, is supposed to have said: "I speak Spanish to God, Italian to women, French to men, and German to my horse!")

THERAPY

The reasons cross-cultural couples come to therapy include those explicitly connected to cultural difference: conflicts about religion, child rearing, marriage, and the comparative priorities of career and personal/family relationships. They may also complain about lack of family support and/or other external social pressures that can be seen to be "cultural." But many couples' complaints aren't manifestly the product of culture at all—they may be expressed simply as not being able to "get along," frictions that may strike the couple as having more to do with personality than cultural influences. These conflicts often turn out to be more connected to culture than couples realize—although naturally intrapsychic sources of conflict are generally simultaneously at work. Other couples, on the other hand, often err by focusing exclusively on their cultural differences as the source of all pain, thereby eschewing taking responsibility for their actions.

As I've suggested, the metaphor of immigration isn't only a generative one for the cross-cultural couple: it's equally helpful for the therapist to whom they go for counsel. Just as each partner in the couple needs to examine his or her own assumptions and expectations, so does the therapist need to examine his or hers. One couple—the man came from Mexico, the woman grew up in the midwestern United States—illustrates the importance of this. My name had been recommended to the woman by a mutual acquaintance. A cursory rundown of my qualifications was all she needed to hear to trust my expertise.

However, the man had no interest in my curriculum vitae. He wanted to know: Was I married? Did I have children? Had I encountered problems like the ones they were facing myself? He had completely different criteria he wanted me to meet—none of which had to do with academic training at all.

In addition to developing a sensitivity to the couple's expectations not only concerning each other but concerning therapy and their therapist, the therapist's task is furthermore to see, and help the couple to see, how much of the problem the couple brings to therapy is its "content"—misunderstandings about cultural meanings, a product of their manifest differences—and how much is the product of "process," underlying interpersonal and family dynamics that "content" (especially when it is as packed as it can be in cross-cultural couples) often quite effectively screens.

Luckily, partners in cross-cultural couples tend to begin the relationship at a higher developmental state than many others. In fact, Gabrielle Varro, in *The Transplanted Woman* (1988), has identified a series of traits common to women who marry outside their cultural and/or national boundaries that bear this out. Such women, Varro says, tend to be better prepared for the demands of marriage, and evince a higher degree of commitment, self/other differentiation, tolerance and respect. The children they raise tend to be more "cultured"—more flexible, more able to deal with different cultural claims and demands. In all, their commitment and flexibility seems to add significantly to the vitality of their families' lives.

The main point is that cross-cultural couples often have to confront hard questions involving what religious traditions to follow, how to raise the children, and the like. much sooner than couples who share the same background. This means that they often come to therapy more capable of acknowledging and addressing questions about their assumptions than other couples who haven't been similarly forced to confront them on a regular basis. The tourist/immigrant metaphor works so well for cross-cultural couples because it is so recognizably apt and ubiquitous: "That's exactly how I feel when I go to 'Yemen' in Queens!" Irene said when she was introduced to the idea.

The basic goals of therapy for the cross-cultural couple are these:

1. To help them acknowledge their differences, their complementarity
2. To validate the choices they made based on that complementarity, and to normalize each other's approaches and beliefs

3. To create a "third reality"—a transcultural reality—that connects them even at moments of crisis or transition, and even if it involves implementing asymmetric compromises (i.e., compromises that are not based on a strict 50–50 split of responsibility or reward). This presents the couple with the challenge of establishing in each situation who is more able to make the sacrifice that will lead to a compromise and acknowledging that the partner who made the accommodation is the only one who could have made it.

First Step: Acknowledging Complementarity

Identifying the source of the partners' differences can be accomplished by asking questions designed to clarify the different family (and cultural) styles they learned. Table 8.2 presents two series of statements it can be helpful to ask the partners to examine, checking each statement that applies to him or her. At the end, partners will have much clearer ideas about their own and each other's assumptions.

Second Step: Validating and Normalizing Choices

Malika, who comes from Morocco, is married to Giancarlo, who comes from Italy. Each departed in significant ways from their families' expectations in choosing the other: Giancarlo because he married out of the Roman Catholic faith; Malika not only because she married outside the Muslim faith but because she was highly educated, with degrees both from European and American universities, which is highly unusual for a woman of her background.

Malika is aware that some of her motives are contradictory: "Giancarlo wants me to be Moroccan, but I wanted to get away from Morocco. And yet every time he encourages me to learn Italian so that I can speak to his family and feel more at home when we go to Italy, I resist. Learning Italian feels like it would be giving up my identity."

Giancarlo was exasperated by something he regarded as far more urgent. Malika was pregnant by the time they decided to marry, and he couldn't understand why she wouldn't pick up the phone and tell her family, and introduce her family to him. "I knew she wanted them at the wedding, and the wedding obviously had to be soon. Why was she waiting, and what was she afraid of?"

Malika did not like confrontations, and she was afraid her family would turn against her both for marrying a non-Muslim and for being

TABLE 8.2. Exercise to Identify and Clarify Family Styles

Number a piece of paper from 1 to 22. Respond to each number by recording which column (A or B) best describes the message you received from your family. In your discussion with your partner, you will contrast these statements with your current beliefs.

Column A	Column B
1. Money is to be spent only when necessary.	1. Money is to be enjoyed.
2. Success is to be pursued by all legitimate means.	2. Success should not be pursued at the expense of family ties.
3. Women have a right to achieve as much as men.	3. Women's primary role is in the home.
4. Modesty is noble; being boastful is crude.	4. A person has a right to be openly proud of his/her achievements.
5. Problems can only be solved through action.	5. Problems are best solved by talking them through.
6. Words can be used for effect. Exaggeration is a way to make a point.	6. Words are to be used carefully, not wasted.
7. Marriage is between two families.	7. Marriage is between two individuals.
8. Anger is expressed by fighting and debate.	8. Anger is shown by distancing and silencing.
9. The authority of the parent is nondebatable.	9. Family rules can be negotiated by everyone.
10. Your problem is my problem.	10. Don't interfere in others' affairs unless solicited.
11. Food is an expression of giving and love.	11. Food is sustenance. Eat in moderation.
12. A little clutter makes the house look lived in.	12. Cleanliness is next to godliness.
13. Care for the elderly is the primary responsibility of the family and takes place at home.	13. Care for the elderly is the primary responsibility of professional health care providers.
14. Relatives play a central role in child rearing.	14. Child rearing is the exclusive province of parents.
15. It is important to sacrifice today for a better tomorrow.	15. It is important to live for today and to appreciate every moment.
16. Children have as much say as adults.	16. Children should be seen and not heard.
17. Showing feelings and vulnerability is a sign of maturity.	17. Being strong and showing self-control is highly valued.
18. The world outside the family is dangerous and not to be trusted.	18. The world outside the family is safe and hospitable.
19. Suffering is to be borne silently.	19. Everyone feels everyone's pain.
20. Feelings should be contained.	20. Feelings should be expressed.
21. People are basically selfish and can't be trusted.	21. People are inherently good; if you treat them well, they will treat you well.
22. Men are impulsive creatures. You can't expect them to be totally monogamous.	22. If either partner has sex outside the relationship, it seriously jeopardizes its survival.

pregnant before marriage. When she finally spoke to them, they were more supportive than she had dared to hope, although her mother did urge her not to tell any relatives that she was pregnant when she got married—a difficult secret to keep since she was 5 months into her term when she walked down the aisle. Giancarlo thought this was hypocritical; he had wanted Malika to be upfront about him and about her pregnancy. At the wedding, when Malika's relatives greeted her, they tactfully let on that they knew: "Please come to visit us with your family," they said. Malika understood this as a gracious indirect communication, but Giancarlo heard it as a kind of underhanded jab or insult.

Giancarlo's more Western "bring it all out in the open" style was part of what attracted Malika to him; Malika's greater reticence was part of what attracted him to her. However, the larger assumptions to which each style was attached were very foreign and a good deal less appealing to both of them. Once they identified their family/cultural styles, and were encouraged to see that each approach had its merit, they began to accept that they could coexist as a couple despite their differences. More comfortable now that she had attained some degree of acceptance both from her family in Morocco and from Giancarlo, Malika even signed up to take lessons in Italian. Giancarlo is able to see Malika's family's "nonconfrontational" tactics not as hypocrisy or passive aggression but as evidence of subtlety and graciousness: each's view of the world and each other has widened, first by recognizing and validating each other's approach, then by normalizing it—that is, conceding its logic and effectiveness. This has freed them to remember and revel in what they first found attractive in each other, to reclaim the romantic feelings that first brought them together. They exist now in a "third reality" which is not so much a mixture of their styles as it is a kind of alternating current between their two styles: like Nigel and Sally, they ask, "Whose style do we follow today?"

Third Step: Creating a Third Reality

Philippe, originally from Lyons, France, and Margaret, a third-generation Polish American, have similarly created a "third reality" that can encompass their considerable differences. Philippe's father and grandfather ran an inn in Lyons and he grew up with family, friends, and crowds of guests of the inn at the dinner table—every night was a party. Margaret's grandparents, who grew up in Soviet-dominated Poland, had, predictably, a much harder existence, and passed on, through Margaret's mother, a stern sense of thrift and wariness: food was not something you indulged in to excess; physical pleasure was something you were well advised to be wary of. When Philippe began inviting friends over for Sunday dinner—Margaret complained that they came at 11:00 in the morning and rarely left until after 11:00 at night—Margaret was appalled at the expense and the mess of preparing the "feasts" Philippe felt he had to prepare to entertain them. "Why can't we have a weekend alone once in a while? And why do you have to spend so much on food?" Philippe, originally attracted to Margaret's good sense and clear sense of purpose in life, now began to see her as a killjoy; Margaret had long since forgotten that it was precisely Phillipe's joie de vivre that had first attracted her to him.

In therapy, however, when Phillipe began to paint a picture of his childhood and how much the family business meant to him, Margaret was able slowly to reconnect to her earlier feelings of love for Phillipe—and to understand that Phillipe was as much a product of French culture, which revered the arts of eating, drinking, and taking pleasure in other people's company, as she, in a slightly more removed way, was a product of her own family's tradition of austerity. Further, when Margaret consented to allow Phillipe to continue his Sunday parties, Phillipe understood the nature of the "assymetric" compromise she had agreed to, and he was genuinely grateful to her for what he knew was the significant concession she was making. He now was more disposed to carve out time at other times during the week when he could be alone with her as she had wished.

Margaret understood something Irene also appreciated about Ahmed—the nature of what Man Keung Ho (1990) refers to as "healing webs," the networks of friendships that "displaced" partners—partners not living in their home countries—benefit from seeking out. "I need one time during the week," Phillipe said, "where I can speak my language and not worry about whether I am doing the appropriate 'American' thing. I need some place to relax completely and be myself."

The "third reality" that Phillipe and Margaret have created is not some undifferentiated "mix" of their styles and personalities, but rather a stage upon which they can each be their separate and idiosyncratic selves—while still maintaining sensitivity to each other's reactions. They now have a 4-year-old boy, Alain, who has been back and forth between Europe and America three times already and is fluent in both French and English. "He astonishes our friends," Margaret says. "He's the quintessential American kid with me—and a born Lyonnais with his papa. It doesn't seem to confuse him at all. Which makes me think that Alain could teach us all a bit about what living cross-culturally really means."

CONCLUSION

The "third reality," the world of the tourist, is to me the best kind of compromise to diffuse conflict and polarization. It is a respectful stance that incorporates elements of both partners, transcending the limits of each's ethnocentrism. In this realm the couple can now tolerate confusion and exercise flexibility to alter their views or opinions: "Maybe my way *isn't* the only way." They often feel an enhanced curiosity about and interest in each other's points of view. In the "third reality," each partner can achieve a balance between loyalty to his or her background and differentiation from it, a balance between sameness and difference.

REFERENCES

Alba, R. (1986). Patterns of interethnic marriage among American Catholics. *Social Forces, 65*, 202–223.

Bizman, A. (1987). Perceived causes and compatibility of interethnic marriage: An attributional analysis. *International Journal of Intercultural Relations, 11*(4) 387–399.

Brake, T., & Walker, D. M., & Walker, T. (1995). *Doing business internationally: The guide to cross-cultural success*. Burr Ridge, IL: Irwin.

Brislin, R. V. (Ed). (1990). *Applied cross cultural psychology*. Newbury Park, CA: Sage.

Cottrell, A. (1990). Cross-national marriages: A review of the literature. *Journal of Comparative Family, 21*(1), 151–168.

Crohn, J. (1995) *Mixed matches: How to create successful interracial, interethnic, and interfaith relationships*. New York: Fawcett Columbine.

Falicov, C. J. (1986). Cross-cultural marriages. In N. S. Jacobson & A. S. Gurman (Eds.), *Clinical handbook of marital therapy* (pp. 429–451). New York: Guilford Press.

Fay, M. (1993). *Children* and *religion: Making choices in a secular age*. New York: Simon & Schuster.

Friedman, E. (1982). The myth of the Shiksa. In M. McGoldrick, J. K. Pearce, & J. Giordano (Eds.), *Ethnicity and family therapy* (pp. 499–526). New York: Guilford Press.

Geertz, C. (1973). *The interpretation of culture*. New York: Basic Books.

Giladi-McKelvie, D. (1986). Intercultural marriage: A phenomenological study of couples who succeed. *Dissertation Abstracts International*, 8713036.

Gordon, A. (1964). *Intermarriage: Interfaith, interracial, interethnic*. Boston: Beacon Press.

Hall, E. T. (1990). *The silent language*. New York: Doubleday.

Hall, E. T., & Hall, M. R. (1980). *Understanding cultural differences*. Yarmouth, MA: Intercultural Press.

Ho, M. K. (1984). *Building a successful intermarriage between religions, social classes, ethnic groups, or races.* St. Meinrad, IA: St. Meinrad Archabbey.

Ho, M. K. (1990). *Intermarried couples in therapy.* Springfield, IL: Thomas.

Hofstrede, G. (1980). *Culture's consequences: International differences in work-related values.* Newbury Park, CA: Sage.

Ibrahim, F. (1984). Cross-cultural counseling and psychotherapy: An existential psychological approach. *International Journal for the Advancement of Counseling, 7,* 159–169.

Ibrahim, F. (1990). Cross-cultural couples counseling: A developmental, psycho-educational intervention. *Journal of Comparative Family Studies, 21*(2), 193–205.

Johnson, W., & Warren, D. (Eds.). (1984). *Inside the mixed marriage: Accounts of changing attitudes, patterns, and perceptions of cross-cultural and interracial marriages.* Lanham, ND: University Press of America.

Kluckhohn, C. (1951). Values and value-orientations in the theory of action. In T. Parsons & E. A. Shields (Eds.), *Toward a general theory of action* (pp. 388–433). Cambridge, MA: Harvard University Press.

Kluckhohn, F. R., & Strodtbeck, F. L. (1961). *Variations in value orientations.* Evanston, IL: Row, Petersen.

McDermott, J., & Fukunaga, C. (1977). Intercultural family interaction patterns. In W. S. Tseng, J. McDermott, & T. Maretzki (Eds.), *Adjustment in intercultural marriage* (pp. 81–92). Department of Psychiatry, University of Hawaii.

McGoldrick, M., Giordano, J., & Pearce, J. (Eds.). (1996). *Ethnicity and family therapy* (2nd ed.). New York: Guilford Press.

McGoldrick, M., & Preto, N. G. (1984). Ethnic intermarriage: Implications for therapy. *Family Process, 37*(3), 347–364.

Perel, E., & Cowan, R. (1992, May–June). A more perfect union: Intermarriage and the Jewish world. *Tikkun,* pp. 53–64.

Perel, E. (1990). Ethnocultural factors in marital communication among intermarried couples. *Journal of Jewish Communal Services, 66,* 244–253.

Perel, E. (1991). Communication in and about intermarriage: Exploring content and process. *Proceedings of the Paul Cowan Conference.* City University of New York Graduate School, Jewish Outreach Institute.

Rohlich, B. (1988). Dual-culture marriage and communication. *International Journal of Intercultural Relations, 12,* 35–44.

Roland, A. (1996). The influence of culture on the self and self–object relationships: An Asian–North American comparison. *Psychoanalytic Dialogue, 6*(4), 461–475.

Romano, K. (1996). *Intercultural marriage: Promises and pitfalls.* Yarmouth, ME: Intercultural Press.

Soncini, J. T. (1997). *Intercultural couples: Cultural differences, styles of adjustment and conflict resolution techniques which contribute to marital harmony versus conflict.* Doctoral dissertation, New York University, New York, NY.

Stewart, E., & Bennett, M. (1991). *American cultural patterns: A cross-cultural perspective.* Yarmouth, ME: Intercultural Press.

Trompenaars, F., & Hampden-Turner, C. (1998). *Riding the waves of culture.* London: Brealey.

Tseng, W., & Hsu, J. (1991). *Culture and family: Problems and therapy.* New York: Haworth Press.

Tseng, W., McDermott, J., & Maretzki, T. (Eds.). (1977). *Adjustment in intercultural marriage.* Honolulu: University of Hawaii Press.

Varro, G. (1988). The transplanted woman: A study of French-American marriages in France. New York: Greenwood.

Vinsonneau, G. (1985). Le couple-mixte en situation psycho-sociale particuliere. *Journal des cahiers de sociologie economique et culturelle, 3,* 93–117.

CHAPTER 9

Therapy with African American Couples

Lascelles W. Black

Being a marital and family therapist is a lot like being a jug-
gler: you often have a lot of balls in the air and need to concentrate on
more than one simultaneously. A couple comes to the therapist for assistance in dealing with a specific problem, but while working on the
identified problem the therapist also discovers the many concrete, real-
life issues that contribute to the difficulties surrounding the problem.
African American individuals and couples face the acute pressures of
coping with racism in addition to the many other difficulties that individuals and couples face in modern life. People of African descent experience a form of discrimination quite unlike that encountered by
other immigrants to our country (Hacker, 1992). Therefore, therapists
working with them should have some knowledge of their history in
America, their culture, and the conditions they encounter in our country today. As therapists we are not only working with the couple, we are
also working with the culture from which they came, because this culture contributes to the couple's strengths and shapes their values, their
beliefs, their views of marriage and the family.

But how many "isms" can we therapists work on and how many
layers of complexity can we uncover without our work overwhelming
us? As a therapist of color, it has become abundantly clear to me that
all therapists need to assist their clients in dealing with racism, sexism,

205

classism, and ageism because these forms of prejudice affect the way they experience their daily lives. A late-middle-age African American man may be facing both racism and ageism on the job. These prejudices could generate feelings of humiliation that may be the cause of his noncommunicative behavior at home. An African American woman may be trying to cope with issues of racism and sexual harassment at work, and so does not feel sexually responsive to her husband. At the same time, she may hide her work problems from him because she believes he has enough to cope with already. She may think she is protecting him the way her upbringing taught her to protect "her man," but the stress of keeping her secret may be pulling their marriage apart. The therapist working with these couples needs to discuss the relevant presenting issues in the context of the various "isms" that are contributing to their problems. By identifying and focusing on the couple's strengths that have enabled them to successfully cope with situations that diminish their personal power, the therapist credits their struggle to survive. By conveying the message that the solutions they have sought to their problems indicate how determined they are to sustain their relationship in the context of their culture, the therapist affirms the couple's personal power (Pinderhughes, 1989).

Hardy and Laszloffy (1995) have written about the importance of cultural competency for family therapists. They maintain that knowledge of culture and ethnicity are crucial factors in working with clients. They advocate the use of a cultural genogram; the primary purpose of this tool is to promote cultural awareness and sensitivity by assisting therapists to understand their own cultural identities, and through this process develop a higher appreciation for the way culture influences the lives of clients in treatment.

COMMON ISSUES WHEN WORKING WITH PEOPLE OF AFRICAN DESCENT

Racism

While most of the racist laws that enforced segregation and discrimination throughout much of U.S. history have been repealed, the beliefs and attitudes that prompted and enforced those laws are still engrained in many members of the majority White society. Therefore, African Americans continue to face frequent, sometimes daily, encounters with prejudice and discrimination. The kind of racist violence that lead to the brutal murder of James Byrd Jr. in Texas in 1998 is viewed by most people in U.S. society as abominable and atrocious (White, 1999). Such crimes are noticeably less frequent than they used to be. Nonetheless, a crime like the Byrd murder has a profound impact on African American people. As Dr. Alvin Poussaint notes, "Blatant, life-threatening incidents of racism are less prevalent in this country, but the more subtle occurrences that happen every day are far more than mere minor annoyances. Racist incidents will always hurt because they remind us that we are still seen as second-class citizens by many people in this country" (cited in Jones, 1999, p. 59).

Everyday racist acts and comments are a form of aggression that reminds people of African descent to be ever vigilant against physical or verbal attack. It is not only the open insult that wounds, but also the subtle innuendoes and the assumptions that are expressed about an African American person's competence based solely on race. These experiences create a level of stress that is unknown in White society, and exacerbate most other problems that African Americans face. Exploring the impact of racism in the life of each member of a couple and in their relationship is an essential part of the therapy for African Americans.

"Perhaps Mother Wasn't So Extravagant"

Loraine and Edwin were in therapy to work on problems in their marriage. In one session Edwin decided to raise the issue of Loraine's spending habits. He complained that she had moved her car to a more expensive garage even though she now has to walk further to get to her job. He said, "You know, this is the same kind of extravagant behavior that my mother used to do that would piss off my dad." I asked Loraine if she could tell Edwin why she changed her parking place. She replied, "I just can't stand to walk by that construction site any longer. The sexist comments have become unbearable." She explained that when White women passed by the site, the workers made annoying and disrespectful comments. But when Black women walked by, the workers' comments became very explicit and included references to the women's "sexual appetites." Loraine told her husband, "All the African American women in my office have stopped walking by that site." Edwin then agreed that it was worth an extra $25 per month for parking to spare his wife the insults, but he also spoke about his pain and anger at not being able to shield his wife from such an experience. Then he added, "Maybe my mother wasn't so extravagant after all." Following this conversation, I encouraged Edwin to talk about how racism affects him in his work. At the end of this session, Loraine remarked,

"Even though we both know racism is with us daily, we seldom talk like this—some of our arguments make a different kind of sense now."

Skin Color

There is, of course, quite a wide range of skin tones within the African American community. Nonetheless, open discussion of skin color has been largely taboo until recently, despite strong feelings and attitudes regarding grades of color. African Americans will only discuss skin color with white people who demonstrate the appropriate understanding and sensitivity. It is important to understand some of the history that precedes this issue.

During the time of slavery light-skinned slaves were more "valued" than slaves of darker complexion by their white "owners," and the lighter slaves were given "preferential" treatment. Usually these lighter skinned individuals were the children of slaves who had been raped by their "masters" or the offspring of interracial relationships. Since the society at large considered European features to be the norm for beauty and an indication of intelligence, these people were considered "better Negroes." The dominant white society developed a complex rating system that graded the various skin tones and hair textures of the slaves.

The attitude that "whiter is better" has continued in U.S. society. To a degree, *some* African American families internalized this form of racism and gave preferential treatment to their children with lighter complexions (Watson, 1999). People of African descent who grew up in British colonies before they gained independence can still remember newspaper advertisements for jobs that stated required characteristics as, "good complexion and good hair," which was code for European features. The civil rights and the Black consciousness movements of the 1960s challenged these attitudes, but vestiges of this form of internalized racism still remain in many families.

"Ain't Nobody Gonna Diss Granny!"

Sometimes assumptions are made about people based on their skin tones. Let's look at the case of Allan and Dora. Allan is a dark-complexioned African American, and Dora is light complexioned. They fell in love while they were college students and planned to get married after they graduated. But they started having arguments because Dora refused to visit Allan's family. She complained that they treated her as if she was invisible and directed all comments to Allan. Furthermore, Dora said, Allan's father, Mr. Gordon, is always too busy to meet with her parents. Allan responded that she was overly sensitive and that his parents were just shy. Both young people denied having any idea what the cause of the problem might be.

When Allan's parents were invited to attend family therapy sessions with the couple they agreed to do so. In the first session, I asked Mr. Gordon how he felt about the relationship between his son and Dora. Mr. Gordon candidly replied, "I think Dora is a fine young lady." He paused, and then continued, "I can't pick my son's wife, I know that. But I've seen the picture of Dora's family and they are all kinda 'white looking.' I don't think they are gonna treat my son with respect."

After Mr. Gordon spoke, everyone became silent. I asked each person what their experiences had been with skin color distinctions. Allan replied that he had not given the issue much thought. Mr. Gordon just looked at the floor. Mrs. Gordon agreed that we should talk about this issue.

Then Dora took out a picture from her wallet and gave it to Mr. Gordon. "The picture you saw before was my Momma and Poppa," she said. "Now this is a picture of my Granny and she is just as dark complexioned as you. And ain't nobody gonna diss Granny."

Mr. Gordon quietly looked at the picture. He realized he had made a generalization that didn't apply to Dora and her family. With pain and hesitation, he began to talk about being a child with light skinned cousins who treated him as lower class and made disparaging remarks about his dark skin. "Now," he told Dora, "we all get along fine as adults, but I still remember the heartache of those days. So, you see, I was afraid your family would not respect my son." Both Allan and Dora assured him that her family had a high regard for his son. He then agreed to meet with Dora's parents.

It is important that we therapists address the issue of preferential treatment or prejudice based on complexion when we have reason to believe that issue may be contributing to the difficulties a couple is having in their relationship.

Conflicts over skin color are rarely discussed outside the African American community. Because this is such a sensitive issue for African Americans, White therapists need to approach this problem carefully, acknowledging that this issue might be difficult to talk about across racial lines. Useful questions include, "Do you think skin color differences contribute to your problems? If so, then I need you to help me understand this." Or, "Is the problem exacerbated by complexion dif-

ferences? If so, then we should talk about that." Or, "If skin color differences add a dimension to this problem, then I think we should be
discussing it." If the therapist shows respect and openness, the clients
will most likely respond in kind.

Importance of Spirituality

Two-thirds of the U.S. population acknowledge that religion is important to them (Bergin, 1991). Nearly three-fourths of African Americans
say religion is significant in their lives, and that they are affiliated with
an African American church (Billingsley, 1992). Most African Americans are Christians, even though they do not belong to a specific religious denomination (Moore Hines, 1998). Recently, increasing members of African Americans have embraced Islam.

Throughout their history in the Americas people of African descent have maintained their optimism by affirming their spiritual beliefs. Belief in a supreme power who expects a higher standard in
human relations is one of the foundations of African philosophy. Judaism, Christianity, and Islam were well established in Africa alongside
other indigenous religions. Timbuktu was an international center not
only for business, but for religious, philosophical, and cultural studies
from ancient times until the fall of the Songhay empire (Bennett,
1993). Christianity became the official religion of Ethiopia in the 5th
century (Bennett, 1993). The idea that the African continent was popu-
lated by godless heathens was concocted by Europeans to ease the con-
sciences of slavers and their investors. It was a way to portray Black
people as less human than Whites in order to justify slavery.

In the Americas these captives converted to Christianity and pre-
served their belief in God and faith in rewards in the afterlife. But their
spirituality also sustained their hope for a better life on earth. These
principles and beliefs are still meaningful to the African American community today. Their spiritual convictions are not just about going to a
better afterlife, but also about an enhanced way to live on earth. Spirituality promotes harmony in the community; regardless of specific religious affiliation, there is widespread support for what is "good and
true." It also promotes self-esteem and contradicts the negative stereotype promulgated by racists. The Black church was the first institution
that belonged exclusively to people of African descent, and it provided
them not only with a place of spiritual refuge and counseling, but also
with a location from which to organize their community (Boyd-Franklin, 1989).

It should also be noted that because of religious admonitions against homosexuality, the African American gay and lesbian population has not found the same level of support in some spiritual communities as heterosexuals have received. Studies of gay African Americans have demonstrated that "inner attributes, such as the partner's . . . spiritual energy, were significantly associated with satisfaction . . . and evaluating a partner higher on these personal qualities was linked to higher satisfaction" (Peplau, Cochran, & Mays, 1997, p. 33).

It is important to find those supportive religious/spiritual communities and direct clients to them because gay and lesbian African American people most often come from families and communities where spirituality and religion are crucial to well-being.

"Partake of What You Can"

Carlton and Joseph were two gay men who had been partners for more than 8 years. They lived in the Bronx. Carlton had AIDS, but Joseph was HIV-negative. I worked with them on issues of stress relating to AIDS, and cultural and family-of-origin differences. Joseph, a computer repairman, was from Jamaica; Carlton, a high school math teacher, was an African American from New York City.

During our work together spirituality became an issue for them. Joseph was a member of a church that was open to gay members and had an active ministry to people with AIDS. Carlton had not attended church for many years because he was an atheist. Joseph was upset because Carlton refused to go to church with him or to even attend nonreligious suppers at the church hall. Carlton argued that there is no such thing as a nonreligious function held on church premises.

We explored Joseph's reasons for attending church. He spoke about being raised Catholic in Jamaica and the feeling of security he enjoyed as a child knowing that all the saints were looking out for him. He also told us that the concept of God as the great loving father who takes care of all his children and forgives their sins was important to him. "You see," he said, "my sister and I never knew our Jamaican father. Our mother's father took care of us, provided for us, and played with us. You know, Grandpa and my mother's siblings raised us. So I grew up thinking of God as an old black gentleman looking out for all his children, and the saints are like my aunts and uncles." Joseph said that in New York he felt spiritually lost until he found this church where the minister did not stigmatize gay people and the congregation helped people with AIDS. He said, "I believe that it is the support of the church people that has given me the determination to protect my-self from HIV infection. So it is important to me to have Carlton meet these people."

Carlton allowed that maybe his reluctance to attend Joseph's church stemmed more from his own experiences with church and church people than from his atheism. He said his mother, Mrs. Ramsey, did not like Joseph because she thought that he had "turned" her son gay. Like some religious people, she believed that homosexual-ity is a sin and that AIDS was God's punishment for homosexuals' "sin-ful lifestyle and abominable sexual habits." While she believed that Jo-seph must be a "special kind of person" because he was not afraid to be in a relationship with her son, she would not permit him to enter her home.

Carlton said that when he became ill his mother asked the minister of her church to pray for him. The minister refused this request, and then proclaimed that the only way Carlton could return to the church was if he renounced his life of sin and ended his relationship with Jo-seph. Carlton's mother had attended this church most of her life and the minister had known Carlton since his birth. Carlton told us that he had stopped believing in God in his late teens, and now this minister's behavior turned him away from all religious people.

Joseph assured him that the minister and congregation at his church were different: they welcomed *all* people. I encouraged Carlton to attend a social evening at the church and to speak with the minister and some of the congregation so that he could learn more about these people who were so important to Joseph. He agreed to do that for Jo-seph.

The next time I saw the two men they reported that Carlton's mother, Mrs. Ramsey, had gone to the social with them. She asked the minister why his church was open to gay people. Carlton said, "The rev-erend told my mother that it was not his job to decide who is living in sin. His job is to work with all the children of God who come in peace and love. The mission of this church is to bring people to God, not to turn them away." Then Joseph added, "When the minister said those words, Mrs. Ramsey started to cry and I put my arm around her. She didn't push me away."

Carlton told me that they go to that church together now. Al-though he still does not believe in God, just seeing the happiness it brings to his mother and Joseph makes him happy too. He said he loved the music and the friendliness. He has started teaching an adult remedial math class for members of the congregation. "I like all the goodness. But, Mr. Black," he asked, "am I being a hypocrite, going to church when I do not believe in God?" I thought about this question, and then I asked him, "Suppose you invited me to dinner at your home and you provided soul food, Hispanic food, Chinese food, and seafood. What would you say to me if I looked at the buffet and said I could not eat at your table because I am allergic to seafood?" Carlton laughed and said, "I get the point. Partake of what you can and leave the rest for the other people."

Social Class Changes

African Americans have always known that education is their most powerful weapon in their struggle against racism and their strongest resource in their efforts to achieve success in this country. In the time of slavery, when education for slaves was forbidden, they secretly learned to read and write the language of this country.

As a result of the civil rights movement's success, the African American middle and professional classes have grown in numbers. With the removal of the segregation laws and the weakening of discriminatory practices in housing, economically successful African Americans have been moving out of the old inner-city neighborhoods and into the suburbs. Integration has had the effect of separating some of us from our cultural support systems. Indeed, our children sometimes have difficulty finding African American peers.

Coping with this form of isolation can also be a problem for an African American who is the only person of his or her race working in a firm, even if this person is in a position of some authority. It is important to maintain links to Black communities, institutions, and agencies where support, connections, and social interchange can be found.

The National Association for the Advancement of Colored People (NAACP) provides opportunities for African Americans to remain connected with each other and to link with other organizations such as the Coalition of 100 Black Men and the Coalition of 100 Black Women, where African American business and professional people can meet. Therapists should encourage African American clients to connect with these and other groups as a way of combating their isolation.

Historically, racism and discrimination blocked access to hard-earned and deserved positions and deprived African Americans of opportunities for advancement. In today's business world a more subtle system of prejudice often blocks the door to opportunity. Despite these obstacles, many African American have been successful (Gary & Leashore, 1982; Hacker, 1992). Their successes and achievements can be credited to individual and family resilience, the ability to rebound after setbacks and defeats, and the know-how to mobilize limited resources while "simultaneously protecting the ego against a constant array of social and economic assaults" (Daly, Jennings, Beckett, & Leashore, 1996, p. 191).

Networking with other Black professionals can help individuals devise strategies for dealing with the "tinted glass" ceiling and other racist practices that Black professionals experience. Jack and Jill and similar organizations allow African American children a venue in which to associate with each other and form peer groups and friendships.

Problems faced by young African American couples include the difficulties inherent in trying to straddle two worlds. The world of corporate America is as slow to change as the rest of the country. In many companies prejudice still bars some hard-working and talented African American men and women from deserved advancement. In this marketplace, the "world of the individual," personal competitiveness is often the *stated* ideal. African Americans have no problems being competitive and have proven this to be true by their accomplishments. But as minorities within some firms they might find themselves excluded from important lines of communication and overlooked for opportunities of advancement.

African Americans value feelings and emotions equally with logical and rational thinking. Friendship, compassion, sharing and cooperation, honesty, courage, and self-control are among the virtues held in high esteem by African American communities (Daly et al., 1996). For an African American to achieve and maintain a successful career requires a delicate balance while navigating between the two worlds. The difficulty in doing this sometimes cause problems in the lives of couples.

There are still too many occasions when African Americans experience frustration and anger generated by the realization that despite their abilities, education, and achievements, their race is still an obstacle to success. When working with these couples it is important for the therapist to help the couple understand the reverberating impact of the racist world on their relationship. The therapist needs to help such individuals to find ways that affirm their true worth, to connect with support systems, and when possible, to find some resolution to the injustice they face. Otherwise, the residue might create conflict in the couple's relationship.

"The Tinted Glass Ceiling"

Moses is a 30-year-old African American who came to see me because he was afraid that his drinking and his affairs with other women were ruining his marriage and might even destroy his career. His main concern, he said, was to preserve his marriage. His wife, Faith, declined couple therapy. Over the phone she told me, "Moses has to decide if he wants to be married to me before I will come to therapy with him. He needs to work out his issues—all of them."

I asked Moses to describe his marital problems. He said, "In the last 2 years I have had three affairs. I just seem to end one affair and move on to another." I asked what other issues were affecting his life and his marriage at this time. "I drink excessively and I smoke pot," he replied. He described "excessively" as "I drive home drunk from Westchester to Brooklyn at least three times per week and I smoke pot often with the people I hang out with." I asked him if he has ever had an accident or been stopped by the police. He said, "Never. I have either been very lucky or God is keeping an eye on me." I asked him if he really believed in God. He said, "I'm not sure, but I come from a religious family so I talk about God a lot."

I asked him to tell me about the family in which he grew up. He told me that his Uncle Joseph is an ordained minister and the family attends his church. His father, John, is a deacon in the church. Joseph and his wife have no children. Since Moses is his uncle's favorite nephew, the family hoped that he would take over his uncle's church. But when Moses went to college he majored in mathematics. He eventually earned a graduate degree in business administration, and now works in corporate sales. While the family and the congregation are proud of his achievements, they would rather see him follow the religious life. "But then," he added, "I was always the one to break the rules."

"What is the most important rule that you did *not* break?" I asked him. "Well, it is not exactly a rule, but when I married Faith I did what was expected of me. Her father is a deacon in the church, she is also a college graduate, a teacher, and she is a God-fearing woman. When we got married we made two families happy."

"But did the marriage make the two of you happy?" I asked him. Moses looked out the window and thought about his answer. "I'm not sure," he replied. "At first we were happy," he said after thinking about it, "but after our daughter, Andrea, was born things changed. Faith started spending a lot of time at my uncle's house, and she became much more active in the church. I started working longer hours because I wanted to be a vice president in the firm. I had a family to support and a career to build. Also, we planned to have more kids."

Moses told me that at age 27 he had been promised the next division manager's position that became available. However, a White man he had trained was given the promotion. Moses asked his boss why he had been passed over and was told that he needed to be more forceful with staff to make his unit more productive. They worked out some goals for him to achieve to gain the next promotion. The next year he received a substantial bonus because bonuses are based on profits earned, but again he was passed over for promotion. He realized then that he would only be making money for the company and that his bosses would never recognize his true value to the firm. This realization also caused him to question his own self-worth.

I asked him when the affairs started. He said that they began after he had been passed over for promotion the second time. He had gone to a party at the home of another department manager. He drank a lot, and he also started to smoke pot. He went home with a lady named Alice that night and they started an affair.

"So how did that affair end?" I asked. Moses looked a bit embarrassed. "That affair ended when Alice found out I was sleeping with Sofia, another woman from the office."

"How did Faith finally find out what was going on?" I wondered aloud. "Well, when Sofia found out I was sleeping with Susan, she called my wife and told her that I was sleeping with white women at the office." Only then did I discover that Alice and Susan were white. "Faith really lost it then. She waited up for me one night and told me she will discuss all this with the elders at church because I am behaving like an 'nigger.' We never use that word. I had never seen her like that before—she was raving."

"What did Faith mean when she said you were behaving like a 'nigger'?" I asked him. "Well, you know," Moses shrugged, "she means that I was behaving like the negative stereotype that white racists use to represent black people."

"Did she report you to the church elders?" I asked. "No. I agreed to come to therapy and she said she did not want to leave me because we have a child to think of."

I asked Moses what were his greatest fears for his future. He replied, "Substance abuse and office affairs will cost me my family and my job." At my suggestion, he agreed to attend Alcoholics Anonymous

(AA) meetings three times a week. The affairs, he said, had already ended.

When Moses achieved 6 weeks of sobriety and consistent attendance at AA meetings, Faith agreed to come to couple therapy. I asked her how she felt about her marriage. She immediately said, "I'm still very angry with him. This constant boozing and sleeping around with the white secretaries in the office is so juvenile." "I've stopped that," Moses replied.

"Yes, but I have not forgotten. It has only been a few weeks."

"Does it matter that the women were whites?" I asked her. "It's not that I have anything against white women as such," she replied, "but I know that he does not mean anything to them as a person—they are just sleeping with the boss hoping to get something out of it. And he is no better, because he doesn't care about them either—he's just using them."

"It's over," Moses said. "I'm sorry and I will never do that again." "Well, never is a long, long time. We will see if that is true," Faith replied.

"What can Moses do to show that he is serious about working to save this marriage?" I asked her. He quickly said, "Name it and I'll do it."

"You know what to do," she said. "Come to the church and take up your rightful position." Moses looked worried. "Faith, don't make me confess to the elders. And I don't want to be a minister."

"I didn't say confess," she told him, "I only said come to church. Moses, you are the only person who can decide what is your rightful position in the church, but you must be involved in some way. What you have been doing is keeping you from the support of the people who love and respect you. Your home is in the church."

Faith explained that she understands how unfulfilled and unappreciated Moses feels at work. But that does not excuse his promiscuous behavior. She understands that his career problems will not change until he is able to find a better company to work in or start his own business. She told him that the appreciation he does not receive at the office he will find in his church. "That has always been our way," she said, "our religious community sustains us."

"But I am not sure I believe there is a God. I feel like a hypocrite in church," Moses responded. "It's not just about believing in God. For people like us, it's about believing in our community. The community is where we find strength," Faith insisted. Moses agreed to attend church and join Faith in working two evenings per week with the youth program.

While the immediate crisis between Moses and Faith seemed solved with Moses's agreement to return to church, this was only the beginning of our work. A far larger issue to be addressed was Moses's position in his work context, and the impact of racism on his sense of himself as a man. Reconnecting with the African American fraternity he joined in college, and reaching out to other African American organizations and agencies, such as the Coalition of 100 Black Men, broadened his support base and increased his business contacts and opportunities for advancement. He continues to work on his substance abuse problems.

Definition of Family

African Americans and other people of African descent frequently maintain close connections with members of the extended family. This closeness provides support and resources. A person may be called "Uncle," "Aunt," "Mamma," or "Grandma," but the title denotes his or her functional position in the family, not necessarily an exact blood relationship to the family. A person called "Uncle" or "Aunt" may be the best friend of a deceased or otherwise absent parent. Such people maintain close contact and involvement with the family, and are important to the children and others in the household. Because of this particularly broad form of family construction, the standard genogram does not always accurately record the complexities of the Black family. Genograms should include other people that the family may name as being connected and supportive because they contribute to the strength and emotional life of the family (Watts-Jones, 1997).

When therapists work with families of African descent, they should keep in mind that the values of their culture and their struggles against oppression have made it necessary for them to draw wider and more encompassing family boundaries. A "family" is not always limited to blood relationships, and will often include other people who play an important supportive role within the family. A cousin or even the child of a family friend who is raised within the same household may be referred to as "my sister" or "my brother."

In Leonard and Shelly's case the definition of family needed to be explained and relationships clearly drawn. When one partner comes from a family with wide boundaries that include nonblood relatives and the other partner does not have these family traditions, problems and misunderstandings may arise.

"They Are All Our Children"

Leonard and Shelly came to see me because they were arguing continuously. Shelly said that Leonard was neglecting her and their children because of his obsession with finding Doug, the son of his former best friend, T. J., who was dead. "For the past 3 weeks," she said, "you have not helped our son with his history essay because you have been out every weekend trying to find Doug."

Leonard said that T. J. was more than a best friend, he was more like a brother because he had lived with Leonard's family since he was about 6 years old. Shelly asked, "Why did he live with your family when his father lived in the building next door?" Leonard explained that the two families were very close. T. J. moved back and forth between the two homes without restriction because of a strong friendship between the parents. When T. J.'s mother died, Leonard's mother became his second "mother," and thereafter he was like a big brother to Leonard and his siblings. T. J. was an only child and his father left him in the care of Leonard's parents while he was away at work. A trucker, he was often gone for many days at a time. So the boys grew up together as brothers. Shelly noted that these details had not been told to her before.

Leonard explained that while he was in college T. J. was hurt in a serious accident. He visited him regularly in the hospital. T. J. asked him to take care of his 2-year-old son, Doug, if he did not recover. Leonard promised to do this. T. J. did not survive, and thereafter Leonard became deeply involved in the lives of Doug and his mother, Lucy. He helped them financially and he was an "uncle" to Doug. But Lucy had a substance abuse problem and had to enter a treatment program. Doug came to live with Leonard and Shelly. He was 5 years old at the time, and he lived in their home with their two children for 5 years. During that time Lucy maintained contact with Doug. When she decided that her life was stable again and she was able to care for her son, Doug went back to live with her. Initially, Leonard kept in touch with them, and continued to help them financially. But the contacts became fewer as Leonard became busier with his own highly pressured life as a lawyer. Then Lucy moved to another borough and Leonard and Shelly lost contact with them. Shelly said she thought that Lucy and Doug were doing fine because if there had been problems Lucy would have contacted Leonard.

"So why are you out looking for Doug now?" I asked Leonard. He told us that 4 months earlier, while visiting his mother in the old neighborhood, he saw Doug. "He is a tall 15-year-old boy now, and he looks just like his father." Then, with tears welling in his eyes, Leonard said, "Doug didn't recognize me." He said that when he told the boy who he was, Doug said a cold hello and left after saying, "You stopped coming to see me."

At first Leonard felt hurt and angry, but when he thought things over he felt guilty and ashamed. "I broke my promise to T. J. and I abandoned my boy," he said. "But he is not your child," Shelly said, trying to comfort him. "They are all our children," Leonard replied, "that is why we give money to the high school at graduation time so that African American students in need can get assistance without sacrificing their dignity. But Doug is special. He *is* family." Shelly said that she had no idea he felt so strongly about this matter and that he should have told her. She did not come from a family with these kinds of connections.

I suggested that since he had seen Doug in the old neighborhood, his mother might have moved back and that reestablishing connections might be possible. Leonard said that was what he hoped for. Shelly told him that it is important that they talk about these issues together and he promised he would. I proposed that if they were able to reconnect, Lucy and Doug may agree to come to family therapy with them. They liked this idea and said they would find Doug and Lucy.

When the four adults and Doug met with me, the young man was able to express how he felt abandoned by his "uncle" Leonard. He described the anger he had carried for years. Leonard told him that he was sorry he allowed them to drift apart and he wanted to reconnect. I encouraged Doug and Leonard to talk about some of the good times they had together and what they missed. Doug said that he missed his cousins, Leonard and Shelly's children, because he felt like a big brother to them. Leonard told Doug that that was the role T. J. had played in his own life. Doug wanted to hear more about his father. They all planned to go out for dinner. Later, Leonard and Shelly told me that Doug was back in their life and they were happier.

CONCLUSION

As the problems faced by African American couples become more complex, the traditional sources of support such as the church or the elders of the family become overworked and sometimes inaccessible. Couples are turning to less traditional agents such as family therapists for the development of their problem-solving skills and assistance in working on relationship issues. To effectively work with people of African descent, the therapist needs to draw on a font of knowledge that includes an awareness of the strengths of the individuals and their community. Familiarity with the historical and cultural background that are the basis of these strengths will enable the therapist to be more effective in helping couples to achieve their desired goals.

REFERENCES

Bennett, L. Jr. (1993). *Before the "Mayflower": A history of black America*. New York: Penguin Books.

Bergin, A. (1991). Values and religious issues in psychotherapy and mental health, *American Psychologist, 46*(4), 394–403.

Billingsley, A. (1992). *Climbing Jacob's ladder*. New York: Simon & Schuster.

Boyd-Franklin, N. (1989). *Black families in therapy; A multisystems approach*. New York: Guilford Press.

Daly, A., Jennings, J., Beckett, J., & Leashore, B. R. (1996). Effective coping strategies of African Americans. In P. L. Ewalt, E. M. Freeman, et al. (Eds.,), *Multicultural issues in social work*. Washington, DC: NASW Press.

Gary, L. E., & Leashore, B. R. (1982). High risk status of black men. *Social Work, 27*(1), 54–58.

Hacker, A. (1992). *Two nations: Black and white, separate, hostile, unequal*. New York: Scribner.

Hardy, K. V., & Laszloffy, T. A. (1995). The cultural genogram: Key to training culturally competent family therapists. *Journal of Marital and Family Therapy, 21*(3), 227–237.

Jones, P. (1999, February). America in Black and White. *Woman's Day*, pp. 59–60.

Moore Hines, P. (1998). Climbing up the rough side of the mountain. In M. McGoldrick (Ed.), *Re-visioning family therapy*. New York: Guilford Press/

Peplau, L. A., Cochran, S., & Mays, V. (1997). A national survey of the intimate relationships of African American lesbian and gay men: A look at commitment, satisfaction, sexual behavior, and HIV disease. In B. Greene (Ed.), *Ethnic and cultural diversity among lesbian and gay men*. Thousand Oaks, CA: Sage.

Pinderhughes, E. (1989). *Understanding race, ethnicity, and power: The key to efficacy in clinical practice*. New York: Free Press.

Watson, M. F. (1999). Confronting the secret. *Family Therapy Networker*, September–October, 50–57.

Watts-Jones, D. (1997). Toward an African American genogram. *Family Process, 36*(4), 375–383.

White, J. E. (1999, March 8). Prejudice? Perish the thought. *Time*, p. 36.

CHAPTER 10

Men Together

Working with Gay Couples in Contemporary Times

Gary L. Sanders

Awareness, understanding, and acceptance in North America of issues of homosexuality have undergone a dramatic transformation in the last 100 years. Oscar Wilde, the great Irish writer, stood before a court in Dublin accused of sodomy after the discovery of his ongoing intimate relationship with Lord Alfred Douglas and declared:

> The love that dares not speak its name is such a great affection as there was between David and Jonathan, such as Plato made the very basis of his philosophy and such as you find in the sonnets of Michelangelo and Shakespeare. It is that deep spiritual affection that is as pure as it is perfect. It dictates and pervades great works of art. It is in this century so much misunderstood that it may be described as the love that dares not speak its name and on account of it, I am placed where I am now. It is beautiful, it is fine, it is the noble form of affection. There is nothing unnatural about it. That it is so the world does not understand. The world mocks it and sometimes puts one in the pillory for it.

Although Wilde's sentiments remain the same for men in relationship together today as they did then, the cultural understanding and acceptance of gayness has grown remarkably, particularly in the last 50 years. For instance, throughout Europe, being homosexual is now a protected human right. The Isle of Man, the birthplace of European elected democracy, was required to change its centuries' old antigay laws before it could officially become part of the European Union.

These changes are also occurring in North America. Sexual orientation is federally protected from discrimination in the Charter of Rights and Freedoms of Canada and now also in every province in the country. In a landmark case in 1998, the Supreme Court of Canada found against the Province of Alberta for not including "sexual orientation" in the provincial Human Rights Act and thereby failing to protect a gay man's job at a right-wing religious college where he was fired simply for being gay. In finding for the gay man and against the provincial government, the Supreme Court ruled that Alberta must include protection of sexual orientation in the Human Rights Act. Moreover, cultural acceptance of gayness is increasingly spreading throughout the United States—although there have been some recent setbacks in civil rights legislation in some parts of that country. Nevertheless, Savin-Williams (1989, 1996) points out that gay persons are coming to self-acceptance at ever younger ages, are being more open with those in their personal communities, and are becoming more visible in the community at large. The youthful proclamation of the 1980s, "We're queer, we're here, get used to it," is now giving way to gay and lesbian persons' inclusion in the larger North American society and a continual striving for access to the opportunities enjoyed by "every man and every woman."

It is the intent of this chapter to help readers certain relationship and sexual issues in their therapeutic work with gay male couples. The chapter is, of course, focused on gay male couples, but many of the issues, concerns, and solutions discussed here could also apply to lesbians in coupled relationships and even to heterosexuals in relationships. However, these other populations are more fully dealt with in other chapters in this volume.

In my view the most relevant determinant of outcome in working with gay or lesbian couples is the therapist's fundamentally held beliefs as to how he or she understands gayness itself. As a concept, gayness and lesbianism (or homosexuality as it has been clinically termed) can be metaphorically thought of as a "coat of many colors." The issue too often then becomes what "colors" are seen most predominately—either those that are favorites or those that are liked the least. The problem with either of these views is that the purpose of the coat (i.e., warmth in the cold) is lost. So it can be with homosexuality; the rhetoric of right or wrong, good or bad, moral or sinful can obscure the purpose of gay men's human efforts at generating and experiencing meaningful adult intimacy.

Many theories abound concerning why homosexuality exists, some of which offer a positive view of gayness and others of which offer a negative view. Negative views predominated in the recent past. By the early 1900s, some had begun to understand homosexuality as a normal biological variation, but this quickly gave way to notions of perversion, inversion, and "the third sex." It wasn't until the 1950s that a team of American sex researchers turned such negative notions on their head. The Kinsey Reports (Kinsey, Pomeroy, & Martin, 1948, 1953) not only revealed that homosexuality was for more common than had been previously imagined, they also showed that the divisions between homosexual and heterosexual *behavior* were not at all clear. For example, one of their major studies of American males revealed that 37% of adult men had had some homosexual experience to the point of orgasm since adolescence. But only 4% had been exclusively homosexual in behavior all their lives. So, sexual practices were not something fixed with such clear boundaries as once had been imagined.

Although the Kinsey Reports have been widely accepted and their findings have been often replicated, they have made only a limited impact on social attitudes toward homosexuality. In most parts of the world today women and men who live their lives as gay persons are still treated as freaks or outcasts, at worst subjected to murder,[1] at best pitied for their "abnormality." Why all this hatred?

The real issue appears to be that homosexuality seems to threaten traditional male domination (G. L. Sanders, 1988, 1993; M. Sanders, 1989; Sanders & Tomm, 1989). If men are to retain their so-called natural right to control women and the resources around them, the differences between men and women must be clearly defined and reinforced with heterosexualist practices. In Mozambique, for example, traditional initiation rights lay down the rules of how sex should be conducted: man on top, woman underneath. Men loving men and women loving women might throw this order into confusion.

Gay feelings, behavior, lifestyle, couplings, and culture are primarily a vehicle for human affiliation. When this understanding is held uppermost in mind, it comes as no surprise to discover that gay and lesbian persons individually and as couples have much more in common with their heterosexual brothers, sisters, and couples than many suppose. All clinicians would be wise to keep this in mind while looking at the unique differences that gay men struggle with in their efforts to find effective, meaningful, and fulfilling intimacy.

USEFUL DISTINCTIONS

I propose, like Oscar Wilde did so many years ago, that what we have come to call "homosexuality" has much less to do with sexuality than it does with the experience of human affiliation. Of course, by its very nature there can be a sexual component to that affiliation, in mind and/or in practice. However, it is my suggestion to view homosexuality through the lens of human affiliation. This affiliation is based on a preferential love relationship along with, perhaps, a hope for congruence of sexual activity. I suggest this view instead of that which sees homosexuality through the lens of genital activity alone. That is, rather than simply privilege behaviors and subsequently confuse those behaviors with a person's inner experience, I propose to view the inner experience as more fundamental and the behavior as either being congruent or incongruent with that experience. Further, it is my belief that the existence of a compelling invitation to keep one's love affiliation secret and the succumbing to that invitation is the "poison" that robs gay and lesbian persons of their joys in life and their hopes for the future.

If, however, the therapist subscribes to an understanding of homosexuality as primarily genitally based or simply as a "sexual identity" or "sexual orientation," she or he is apt to miss the mark in working with gay men. The couple's language of presentation may be around sexual concerns, or may be proffered in the traditional linguistic style of men, for example, with an emphasis on power and money. However, if the therapist is unable to see beyond these traditions of presentation and instead see that the client is actually in search of meaningful intimate human affiliation, then most therapists will have little positive effect or may even be inadvertently damaging in their clinical work with gay couples. For instance, this would certainly be the case in counseling persons to give up their primary and most effective affiliative orientation and try to "become" heterosexual.

The major impediments for gay men in developing, maintaining and promoting intimate relationships of value can be broken into what I have come to call the "triad of tyranny": patriarchy, heterosexism, and homophobia (G. L. Sanders, 1993).

In dealing with the issue of gay and lesbian love experiences, heterosexism is perhaps the greatest villain. *Heterosexism* is a culturally held belief, while *homophobia* is an individually internalized heterosexism expressed with negative intent (i.e., those negative feelings generated on becoming aware of gay or lesbian persons or experiences).

Heterosexism can be either conscious or non-conscious. For instance, a person may not feel that he or she is disturbed by awareness of gay or lesbian love, yet act in ways that minimize the opportunities to be aware of it. On the other hand, someone may in fact consciously believe that heterosexual love is more natural or "normal" without being obviously negative toward gay or lesbian persons.

The belief systems of heterosexism and homophobia operate at any of three levels. One level is that of a person's own inner experience. Most clinicians have seen someone who has experienced homophobia while reflecting on his or her own thoughts and feelings. These people, in fact, can include gay and lesbian persons who have come to believe the larger heterosexist discourse more than their own valued inner longings and experiences.

Another level of homophobic activity can take place in an immediate community such as a family of origin, among friends, or small social groupings such as church or place of work. Here, homophobia may be overt, such as gay and lesbian "jokes" that erase their subjects' humanity, disqualifications of valued relationships, or invitations to personal erasure for being different than the expected heterosexist stereotype. Or it can be covert, such as a refusal to acknowledge the importance of other persons of the same gender in a gay person's life, or a refusal to hear the beginning offerings of openness on the part of a lesbian or gay person, or the persistent invitation or expectation to the lesbian or gay person to follow a more heterosexual lifestyle.

Finally, homophobia can exist in social institutions where the conversations that have been generated through heterosexist values come to form rules, regulations, and expectations. Here, a parallel can be drawn with the experience of women in our patriarchal culture. Women have often been socialized into disbelieving their own experience, reflecting negatively on those experiences in which they do believe, seeing themselves as less than men, and accepting the status quo as somehow the norm to which they must submit, even though it is defined in deference to men. Similar experiences occur for lesbian and gay people except that for them the experiences often occur even more forcefully and less obviously.

Our culture has, over many centuries, come under the influence of an increasing "tyranny of sameness" (White, 1986). Certain fundamental cultural beliefs—for example, that we should be more similar than diverse, love through our genitals rather than through our souls, privilege property above experience, valorize rules rather than relationships, and so on—when inculcated by most individuals in our society are the true contagions supporting the problems clinicians see for gay couples and individuals.

Despite these problems, gay men have had some surprising opportunities for relational development. For instance, the 5,000-year history of patriarchal tradition for heterosexual union has been largely absent for male-to-male unions. Although Boswell (1980, 1994) has pointed out there were church-sponsored commitment unions for two men or two women for over 1,000 of the 2,000 years of Christian history, they have been lost to modern society for hundreds of years. The current dearth of available traditions allows a diversity of relational types for gay men including best friendship, lovership, mentorship, cohabiting, pluralships, and shifting allegiances. Second, the depth of affection and love felt by a gay man for another man can invite men to escape the yoke of patriarchal trivialization of affection. Some examples include the love of Alexander the Great and his general Haphestion (whom he publicly "married"), which is unmistakably recorded in history as rivaling that of Anthony and Cleopatra; or Michelangelo, who wrote all his sonnets to males; and even Oscar Wilde and his continuing relationship with an English aristocrat. Most importantly, however, these deeply felt affections can invite men into recognizing that individual experience is a more valid indicator of personal worth than is simple behavioral compliance or materialistic accumulation.

First, various intervention strategies will be offered, followed by a discussion of a number of common clinical concerns for gay couples.

INTERVENTION METHODS

Gay couples can, of course, suffer many of the same concerns as heterosexual couples, but they also struggle with the added burden of some problems associated with the fact of being gay. This section discusses intervention methods that I have found useful in my practice over the last 18 years.

Personal Reflective Skills

Effective Reflection

Fundamental in working with anyone of difference, particularly gay or lesbian couples, is an awareness of the unique cultural restraints that we all live with. By being self-aware of heterosexist assumptions, patriarchal beliefs, and even homophobic responses, and by making an effort to actively stand clear of them, we can develop what I consider to be the most important intervention of all: effective reflection. This allows a meaningful therapeutic alliance through respectful mutual acceptance. For instance, a therapist can ask, "How has society's antigay bias affected you as a couple and as individuals? How much have you been able to escape the effects of that bias to date? How much does the bias still trip you up?" Or, "How much do you worry that I, as your therapist, will fall victim to heterosexist assumptions as we work together? Is this something you as a couple have discussed? If you feel that I am acting in ways that colludes with an anti-gay bias, would you be comfortable in telling me?" "If not, can you help me understand how come not?"

By reflecting on and actually naming what is traditionally not commented on in therapy, the therapist offers gay couples the opportunity to see the therapist's openness to the issues of heterosexist bias. This practice invites greater trust and investment in the therapeutic process on the clients' parts.

Therapists can also help individuals reflect positively on their love experiences, for example, to see that these are based in human affiliation, and in the privileging of life over property, of togetherness over isolation, of connectedness over separateness. As therapists we must, through whatever skills and methods we use, invite our clients into siding with positive life-sustaining sentiments over beliefs that are unfriendly and self-erasing.

Therapists can help clients and their families make this distinction by asking questions such as: "Who do you believe recognizes most clearly that your relationship is based first and most significantly on your love for one another? You, your friends, your families, or someone else? If others who are important to you recognized and valued this love as the basis of your relationship, what difference do think this might make to your concerns? If society as a whole saw gay relationships as love-based rather than as genital-based, what difference do you think this would make for your future as a couple?"

Another way to help our clients—whether gay or straight—escape the trivializing effects of heterosexist assumptions of gay love is to see themselves as being victimized by inculcated ideas of heterosexism, homophobia, and patriarchy.

Externalization and Internalization

One way I do this is to invite the clients to externalize (White, 1986) these oppressive ideas. This involves "personifying" the tyrannizing belief, helping the clients to see how it has been "controlling" them, and, more importantly, how they have exercised occasions of being more "in control" of their lives than the ideas have been—that is, the idea of unique exceptions to the problem. By linguistically separating the problematic ideas from the person, I invite the client into experiencing greater choice over whether the idea participates in his or her life. This allows the person to have more conscious choice concerning what ideas and what values guide his or her life. When done in the context of positively affirming affiliation and negatively connoting erasing practices of one's self or others, therapists offer a more compelling invitation to escape the tyranny of heterosexist and homophobic beliefs.

Here is an example of externalizing in working with a gay couple.

Jason and Pierre, both 28, had been together for 3 years, and had lived together for 2 years. Although both sets of parents knew that their sons were gay, neither had invited them as a couple to family events such as Thanksgiving or Christmas. Both Jason and Pierre had kept up the tradition of attending their own family's events solo. They had come to therapy with each feeling the other was not taking their relationship seriously enough. After therapeutic engagement had occurred and their families of origin had been discussed, the therapist asked: "What ideas do each of you have as to how come the love that brought you together years ago remains unseen and unheard by your families?"

Pierre thought that his family just "couldn't handle it" and Jason believed that it was a needless provocation to "flaunt" their relationship at their parents. The therapist continued to ask a series of questions that invited the clients to see heterosexism as interfering in their lives like a meddling and unwelcome neighbor, to become aware of its influence over the people and practices in their lives, and to see the exceptions: "Who do you think has succumbed most fully to heterosexist [these beliefs were discussed so the term made sense to the couple] beliefs—one of you, your families, or others in your world? How fully has heterosexism silenced your love when you are with others? What exceptions can you tell me to Heterosexism's grip over your lives while with your families? If you were to stand together to counter heterosexism's grip on your future, would you have more or less success compared to trying it alone? If your successes started to grow, particularly with your parents, who would notice first? What effect would escaping heterosexism's erasing grip within your families have on each of your satisfactions in the relationship?"

Such questions help the couple to reflect on a future in which they, not heterosexism, control their lives.

Recognizing Differing Paces of Change

Additionally, in aiding our clients to escape the negative beliefs of the dominant culture and of the past, therapists need to be aware of the different paces that individuals use to escape the effects of tyrannizing convictions. Many gay persons are far ahead in their escape from these convictions when compared to their loved family members, since they have been on the journey of escape much longer than the family members have. This issue of timing is, in my opinion, highly important. What may appear to the therapist or to the client couple as an opportune time to confront erasing beliefs and actions may in fact not be the best time for the partner-in-life, the family of choice, or the family of origin. The experiences of these others and how their experiences may then affect the lives of the clients should also be considered, albeit not as the primary concern.

Linguistic Practices

Another important therapeutic resource is language use. By reflecting on and becoming increasingly aware of how language maintains the status quo, we as therapists can choose alternate language constructions that orient our clients to more respectful and accepting lives. For instance, by deliberately using the phrase "lesbian and gay persons" rather than the word "homosexual," one brings forth the experience of the persons being discussed (who see themselves as experiencing life through a primarily affiliative lens) rather than the experience of the persons traditionally doing the discussing (who historically see the relationship primarily through a sexual lens). Or, by using the word "invitation" to describe the social and interpersonal expectations of conformity with heterosexist values, the therapist can highlight the experience of choice that is implicit in such expectations. A therapist can help a client see such choices where that client may not yet have experience of them.

Being aware of linguistic assumptions and word usages can have a dramatic intervening effect. For instance, for gay men the word *lover* is taken to mean an affiliative investment, not the dominant heterosexist and patriarchal cultural view which commonly sees a lover as a sexual dilettante. The term *partner,* however, or *life-partner,* is acceptable and most often understood.

The simple use of *invitational language* rather than the traditionally used language of inculcation and objectification can offer significant therapeutic opportunities. For instance, on hearing of one partner in a couple saying he feels lonely, a common question is: "What makes you lonely?" The response could easily be something such as, "When my lover doesn't come home on time." A follow-up question may well be, "What could you do to reduce your loneliness?" The response could include "Convince him to come home earlier." In contrast to this implicit embedding of the "cause" of one's loneliness being the failure of the lover in coming home when wanted, another question could be, "What interpersonal situations invite loneliness into your experience?" Here the answer may be "When I am alone and missing meaningful company." In response to the question, "What could you do to reduce loneliness's grip on you?", he may answer, "Seek out company either on the phone or by visiting friends when my lover is away." In one scenario, it seems as if the lover is left responsible for easing the speaker's loneliness; in the other, the speaker can view himself as primarily responsible for the resolution of his own loneliness.

Celebration of Diversity

Simon, 41, had presented with his partner of 7 years, Paul, 29, complaining that Paul's interest in computers was damaging their relationship. They reported that they shared few interests in common outside of hiking in summer and going to the theater in winter. Otherwise, Paul spent a great deal of time on his computer and the Internet searching the web for things of interest. Simon, on the other hand, preferred to read novels and meet friends for coffee. Over the years, their lifestyles had become increasingly separate to the point that Simon suggested they attend therapy.

As therapist, I became very interested in their views of these differences: "I am curious, who believes more strongly that you have to be similar to have a better relationship?"

"We both do," they replied.

"How has the difference in your ages been an asset to your relationship rather than a deficit?"

"It has allowed me to help Paul with his job and family—things I had already dealt with" said Simon. "And it allows me to support Simon when he gets worried about the future being too short or about getting old as a gay man," replied Paul.

"What would happen if the two of you saw the differences in personal interests as a resource rather than a restriction? For instance, if Paul's computer interest and expertise was lauded and occasionally joined by Simon, and Simon's social activities could been seen as an opportunity for Paul to occasionally escape the house? If your resentment of differences was replaced with valuing differences, what would happen to your coupled experience?"

"Then there would be fewer upsets and less unhappiness." Paul stated. Simon agreed with him.

What Michael White (1986) has called the "tyranny of sameness" certainly is underscored in homophobic, heterosexist assumptions about homosexuality. However, it is not only a heterosexist view that sees difference as problematic. It can also be difficult for gay men themselves if differences between the two partners are seen as threatening rather than as celebratory. By openly inviting couples to reflect on the conceptualization of difference as enriching, as empowering, as an opportunity for celebration, one can help reduce the fear attendant to differences. This fear can include concerns such as outside friendships, different pursuits and interests, different religions, family-of-origin practices, cultures, ages, and so on. Too many couples see these as threatening the personally minted exclusivity of intimacy that the relationship offers them. Yet, by introducing the notion of celebration of difference, therapists offer their clients the opportunity to maximize coupled richness through sharing unique individual experiences.

Affective Primacy

It seems almost a truism these days to say that men in general (and, therefore, gay men in particular) enter into relationships with a habit of focusing on behavior and sexuality as methods of trying to unearth their intended emotional experiences of connection. Therapists can be of significant help to these men by helping orient them toward more congruent affective description, affective disclosure, and acceptance of affective communication.

Some men question the relevancy of these tender feelings, especially if they have been trained by patriarchal and/or homophobic conventions to believe that vulnerability is tantamount to a personal "death sentence." I often respond by inviting them to see feelings as an "emotional disposition toward action" which could have had evolutionary advantage for our species. Such a teleological rationalization appeals to many men. For instance, when one experiences fear, one can be seen as disposed to seek interpersonal safety; when one is experiencing sorrow, one is disposed to seek comfort; and when one is feeling loneliness, one is disposed to seek meaningful company.

Love, or happiness, interestingly, disposes one toward open sharing. The "Feeling Wheel" (see Figure 10.1) can be used to orient gay men toward the deeper meaning of their horniness, angers, or jealousies. For instance, when men tend to focus on anger, the wheel can be used to see what may be "under" the anger. Similarly, the central position of anger in the wheel can be exchanged for horniness, frustration, or any other emotion to see what vulnerable feeling is actually not being adequately addressed. Using this technique, therapists can go a long way toward inviting their clients into a deeper sharing and more intimate connection. Going even further by helping clients also develop effective language skills, active listening abilities, and nonblaming emotional disclosure can hasten relational improvement dramatically.

> Etienne, who was 38 when he and his partner of 2 years, Stephen, aged 37, came to see me, was originally from France. He had been living in North America for most of his adult life and worked in the airline industry. Stephen was from California and had met Etienne when he, too, worked in the airline industry. Now, however, he had his own computer consulting business. The concerns for the couple centered around increasing displays of anger by both. Etienne attributed this to the constant shift changes and potential layoffs in his work with the airline. Stephen thought his "temper" was more related to poor employee performance by the young people he hired at work and the subsequent difficulties he had fulfilling his contracts. Nevertheless, increasingly they were arguing between themselves and felt that they were "growing apart."

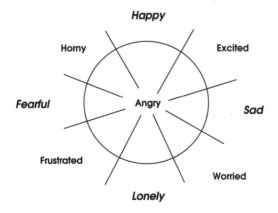

FIGURE 10.1. The "angry" feeling wheel.

I quickly chose to move the couple away from continued descriptions of anger and instead toward the more vulnerable underlying emotions for each.

"Etienne, what feeling do you think Stephen struggles with when he first becomes angry—do you think it is more related to hurt, fear, or loneliness? And Stephen, as Etienne thinks about this, what feeling do you think is underneath his displays of anger—more sorrow, fear, or loneliness?"

After thinking about it, both saw the other as struggling with fear.

"If each of you saw the other as trying to deal with fear rather than with anger, would you act differently at all? For instance, Etienne, what would happen if you looked under your feelings of anger at your more vulnerable feeling? Would you choose to privilege the anger with Stephen or the fear? If you were to "honor" the fear and then seek out interpersonal safety, would the fear grow or shrink? If it shrank, would you be more or less likely to continue to display anger?" And so on.

These types of questions can invite the clients' not only into recognizing their experiential choices, but more importantly, into seeing alternatives to their traditional nonhelpful habits.

Restorying Sexuality

Pedro, 25, and Rudy, 27, came to therapy to try and find a solution to their increasingly rare sexual activity and lack of fulfillment. In response to a few orienting questions about their love-making frequency (once every 3 weeks) and practices (mostly mutual masturbation and oral sexual contact), they indicated that they believed Rudy was less sexually desirous than Pedro. Both couldn't understand this change since 4 years earlier when they got together, Rudy had been the primary initiator of their sexual activity.

"Pedro, when you and Rudy are sexual, what percentage of the time do you believe he is being sexual out of real personal desire rather than because you want him to be sexual?"

Pedro guessed 70% of the time, but Rudy said his experience was more like 30%.

"What invites Rudy into trying to be sexual 70% of the time without actually having personal desire?"

Pedro was unable to guess, but Rudy suggested it was his love of Pedro and fear that if he wasn't sexual on a regular basis with him that Pedro would "dump" him and find another sexual partner, thereby inviting the relationship to falter.

"Rudy, which do you imagine it is that Pedro is primarily looking for, sexual release or heart-felt connection? In other words, is he looking for a 'penis-parkade' or a place to 'rest his heart' "?

Rudy replied that he thought Pedro was looking for heart connection but always expected to find it through sexual contact.

"Pedro, would you prefer Rudy to give of his body out of love for you when he is preferring not to be sexual or would you prefer he show his love in some way that he felt desire for, other than sexually?"

Pedro responded, like most partners would in such a situation, "I would want Rudy to follow his own heart—if he is not horny then he should not be sexual because otherwise he is actually misleading me. If he were to say, 'Here, use my body but don't mind that I am thinking of work, or the bills, or something,' I would turn him down. I am looking for love-making, not just a release."

How much difference would there be in your couple relationship if the two of you only had sexual contact when it was both mutual and freely chosen? Do you think sexual activity would grow in quality and quantity or not?"

Traditionally, sex is seen as something that is "done." This is the traditional understanding of gay men's sexual experiences. I have found it more useful, however, to reframe sex as something that is *felt*. I have called this way of viewing sexuality "The Five Sexy Words" (Sanders, 1991a). From listening more carefully to my patients (Sanders, 1991b), I distilled a series of five felt and shared experiences between two people that appeared minimally necessary before the activities the two engaged in could be considered by our culture as mutual sexuality. Although I have described these "Five Sexy Words" elsewhere (Sanders, 1991a), they are so fundamental that they bear repeating: volition, mutuality, arousal, vulnerability, trust.

By refocusing the gay couple's personal goals toward these shared sensual-erotic experiences rather than specific genital behaviors, therapists can help the men in a couple have a much more satisfying and rich relationship.

Thoughts Do Not Predict Actions

While working with gay couples, I have found that it is useful to help them to clearly understand the differences between thought and action. Although this sounds quite simple, when it comes to the area of sexuality, many of us, whether professionals or laypersons in the community, act as if the former is necessarily predictive of the latter. For instance, we often react with fear when one or both members of the couple express sexual fantasies and thoughts. We, as a community and as professionals, often become so alarmed at a person's fantasies out of fear that he will then act them out that we then act more like social control agents than as therapists. If each member of the couple can come to understand and accept his own and his partner's thoughts as simply "mindful events," rather than as "road maps" for action, the fears, jealousies, and acting out can be dramatically reduced.

> Stan and Randall had been living together for 3 years when they sought out therapy. Randall, a 29-year-old computer systems analyst, summarized the concerns the couple brought by describing Stan, 25, and a PhD student in biology, as overly possessive and jealous. A few questions by the therapist led to the disclosure that Stan would become inquisitional and blameful of Randall when he noticed Randall looking at an attractive man. Stan confessed that he feared Randall wanted to "step out" of their relationship. Events became even more problematic when, during a more open moment, Randall disclosed to Stan that he sometimes thought of these men when he was being sexual, either by himself or with Stan. Subsequent to this particular conversation, the jealousy and accusations increased. Randall felt increasingly guilty for his noticing of other men, and found that his sexual desire for Stan had begun to diminish.
>
> "Do either of you drive a car?," I asked.
>
> "Yes," each answered while looking as if I had lost my way therapeutically.
>
> "Do you drive faster or slower than the traffic around you?"
>
> Stan replied, "Faster."
>
> Randall added, "I go the speed limit, so I guess I am a bit slower."
>
> "Have either of you had the experience of becoming angry when trying to get somewhere quickly only to be blocked by a slow driver in front? If so, have you ever fantasized that you could somehow literally push his car onto the shoulder of the road, or make it vanish somehow? Or, maybe you have had the experience of upset and frustration when finding a driver behind you tailgating? Have you ever fantasized that you could actually stop your car quickly enough so that the tailgater smashes into your rear end, leaving his car disabled and yours, of course, magically untouched?"

Both men laughed and admitted they have had both experiences, although Stan said he was more likely to encounter the slow drivers and Randall said he was more likely to find the tailgaters.

"Stan," I asked, "how many of those slow drivers have you allowed yourself to actually push off the road?"

"None," he answered, "but I have certainly thought about it. My favorite fantasy at a time like that is that my car is equipped with one of those science-fiction 'phasars' and that I can simply push a button and the obstructing car and driver simply vanish in a cloud of molecules, letting me drive on through. But I have never crashed into anyone."

"And Randall, although many of us touch our brakes to alarm the tailgater behind, how many of these cars have you actually allowed to smash into your car?"

"None," Randall said, "but you're right that I do sometimes put on my brakes to tell the driver to back off."

"How are each of you able to do what you do? How is it that you don't just cave into your feelings?"

Stan replied that he finds that his anger dissipates more quickly when he plays the *Star Wars* fantasy. Randall said he found the same when he imagines the car behind being left disabled at the roadside as he merrily continues on.

"Do you find yourself more or less likely to drive in ways you would generally not value when you entertain these fantasies?"

Both answered that they felt they were able to drive more respectfully when they let the fantasies be than if they emptied their minds due to guilt for thinking in ways that they would never want to actually carry out.

I then told them a story of a couple much like themselves whom I had seen some years earlier. The man who seemed always on guard against his partner's "looking" habit had come to realize that his belief that what was thought would necessarily be acted on was more the problem than what was thought. He had had a sudden realization and said, "I think I understand this now. It doesn't really matter where you get your appetite, it only matters if you eat at home!"

Helping men to distinguish thought from action in such situations means that having thoughts about the attractiveness of those outside the relationship does not have to mean, in the mind of *either* of the partners, that those thoughts will eventually be acted on. It can, in fact, depathologize looking and fantasizing.

Family of Origin, Family of Choice

"No man is an island," wrote John Donne. Similarly, no gay couple can be an island either. Every gay couple belongs to a combination of families, friends, schools, churches, communities, societies, and each member of the couple is a citizen of a nation.

Families of origin are the family units most therapists first think about and therefore first focus on. Unfortunately, these families often lack pertinent and up-to-date information about gayness and their gay sons. They need to hear that there is no "blame" for their gay family member, particularly since blame was unfortunately too often a significant part of many therapies in the past. Once disclosure has occurred, therapists may need to encourage the family-of-origin members' relationship with his or her child through loving and accepting experiences. Promotion of acceptance of and comfort with the gay family member through information and reading is often of use for family-of-origin members.

The concept of *family of choice*, which was popularized by lesbian and gay people more than 30 years ago, is a very useful therapeutic distinction. Family of choice embodies the notion that the individual relationships in a person's life that are affirming and of value usually combine to make a better "family" than those traditional families that are sanctioned either through genetics (the biological family) or by law (such as a social services family). Although a biological family and/or a legislated family may have persons in it who become part of the gay couple's family of choice through experiences of value, the biological family may not simply by reason of its past history, be the most effective family.

> Marcos's family had emigrated from the Philippines when he was 6. He was now 35, and he had been to his native country only once some 15 years previously. It was, he said, in the Philippines that he actually came to truly know himself as being gay. Prior to that, he had feared he was gay but hoped he wasn't. However, while visiting extended family in Manila for a few weeks he had met a man with whom he had had a brief affair. This affair had confirmed his gayness in his own eyes. Over the years he had become increasingly self-accepting as a gay man, despite his Roman Catholic upbringing and his conservation cultural heritage. When he was 26, he met Peter, then 30. After a courtship of a few months, they had begun living together.
>
> Peter described how, at 19, his family had disowned him when

he disclosed that he was gay. They were members of a fundamentalist religious group who believed homosexuality was an unforgivable sin against God. They had chosen to cling to their religious beliefs and to reject their own son. Peter was terribly hurt by this rejection and described how, for some years, he had longed to repair things between himself and his family. He had even gone so far as to try to "renounce" his gayness. However, he had little success because his affiliative feelings for men were beyond his conscious control. If he succeeded in pushing his same-sex longings out of his experience, he found himself feeling empty inside, not filled with socially sanctioned heterosexual longings. Besides, he said, he had later fallen in love with another man and this had made a world of difference to him. Although that relationship did not last long, by the time he and Marcos had formed a relationship Peter was quite at peace with being gay but had minimal contact with his family of origin.

Marcos, on the other hand, had quite a different family story. After uncovering the undeniable experience of being gay in Manila, he had tried to hide the fact from his family for a few years. He had even persisted in the ruse of dating young women. However, he could no longer maintain his elusiveness when, at age 22, his mother confronted him about his marriage plans. Marcos chose to no longer lie to his mother and told her the truth. Apparently, she prayed for his being changed by God for the next few months, admonishing him not to tell his father or siblings. Yet, barely 2 months after he told his mother about of his gayness, she, herself, told her husband and Marcos's brothers and sisters. This created a crisis in the family. His mother and two of his sisters came to simply accept the fact that he loved men. Marcos told a story of how his mother made peace with him being gay by deciding it was God himself who had decided this for her son; Who was she to question God! However, his father and one of his brothers told him they could never accept him being "that way."

The couple had come to therapy due to increasing arguments about how to handle their families of origin. Peter, for instance, believed that Marcos should demand that his family accept him fully or do a "family-ectomy." Marcos, on the other hand, believed that Peter should try to make amends with his family, despite Peter's statements that he had no interest in resurrecting that area of his past.

"Who do you invite for Thanksgiving dinner?", I asked.

"We have some long-term couple friends with whom we almost always get together at Thanksgiving and Christmas. Also, every other year one of my sisters and one of my brothers and his wife come for Thanksgiving," replied Marcos.

"Sometimes we are invited to the home of one of these gay couples who we usually get together with," added Peter. "On occasion we have even gone to Marcos's sister's home. That is interesting because his whole family tends to be there then."

"Who do you invite to share other celebrations with, such a birthdays, anniversaries, and special events like promotions and graduations?"

"Again, it tends to be those same two couples, sometimes some of my family, and sometimes a single gay friend we have known for years," answered Marcos.

"What would it be like for the two of you if you decided to think of your 'family' as being those persons who have earned the right by being closest to you in heart rather than simply closest to you in blood? Do you think you would find greater peace and happiness or less?", I asked.

Both members of the couple reflected privately before answering.

Marcos asked, "Could that include some of my biological family?"

"It could, I suppose, include anyone in the world who had earned the right to be of your family by being closest to your heart," I said.

"I think I would feel less guilty when I don't automatically include all my biological family in special events," Marcos added.

"It is already like that, sort of," Peter went on. "I just haven't thought of it as a family since I have always thought of family as being who raised you. But if we thought of the people who love us as we are and who we love for who they are as family, I would be much happier."

By introducing this kind of language and the concept that persons choose family who are effective for them, rather than simply accept the family that was given to them by nature or law, a therapist helps open up opportunities for gay couples to immerse themselves in more supportive relationships. Even though a couple's extended family could, and most often does, include significant members of the family of origin, to openly speak of the possibility that the family of origin needs to "earn" the right to be part of a family of choice helps the individuals in a gay couple see opportunities for greater affirmation and resource in the future.

Stories of Others

Since gay couples are generally invisible to the community at large, gay men often lack gay role models and stories of the successful navigation of life's hurdles by other gay men. Public awareness of gay couples too often consists of the ubiquitous stereotypes of short-term, angst-ridden, and sexually promiscuous relationships. The stories of couples who have managed, despite extant social oppression, to forge successful relationships of meaning and mutual love are lost to most gay men through fear-induced invisibility.

Helping gay men hear others' stories so they can learn from them is both an elegant and an effective therapeutic intervention. Not only does it invite a sense of history and continuity that is simply "there" for straight couples, but it also can invite a sense of pride and hope since stories of success countermand the negative and disqualifying stereotypes that are prevalent in the community at large.

From time to time, I will tell a "clinical story" to couples who are struggling with current difficulties and appear to have problems anticipating the continuity of their relationship in the future. My intent in telling such stories is to bring a richer past into the present so that the couple can construct a more cooperative and wanted new future. The story is told as a method of informing rather than instructing, as in the following example.

> Larry and Ian have been together since 1961, when both were 25. They met while Ian was shopping for a car. Larry was his sales agent. Over the week or so that it took for Ian to purchase his new Chrysler, each recognized that he enjoyed the other's company. After some tentative and careful questions and answers intended to determine if each was gay, the two began an affair. Initially, it focused on the sexual domain. Neither had had a long-term relationship with a man before, although Larry had been dating a woman with whom he had broken up some months earlier. Each was acknowledging of self as gay but had not told their friends, family, or workmates. Both had only a few gay friends.
>
> Over the many years since their getting together, Larry and Ian had successfully negotiated significant upsets and enjoyed numerous special experiences. For instance, when the dealership when Larry worked went into receivership and he lost his job, Ian was there to help him by offering him a place to stay till he got on his feet again. Although Larry eventually found another job and got his own place, the two more or less had already begun living

together. The "pretext" of having a separate place would still last another year or two before they felt secure enough to live together in one place—although they kept up the appearance of separate bedrooms for a number of years more.

Ian, a veterinarian, made some lucrative investments. Together the two were able to purchase a failing auto dealership in the early 1980s. It was a wise investment because the auto maker took off in the late '80s, allowing the men to take early and comfortable retirement. Although other investments helped their financial independence, they routinely call the auto dealership "the money factory."

Time went on and the couple became more comfortable with being known as gay by family and friends. They faced the first major threat to the integrity of their relationship when Larry had a brief clandestine affair with a younger man at the dealership. This proved a crisis in their coupled experience, but they were able to negotiate it with the help of an acquaintance who happened to be a psychologist. Finding someone in the 1970s who could both work with gay men and who could work with couples was a stroke of good luck. By helping each member of the couple to be more open about his emotional needs and worries, and to work through the hurt and fear associated with the affair, the therapist enabled the couple's recovery. Indeed, they were even more committed to one another after the infidelity crisis.

Over time, Larry and Ian faced other crises. Larry required heart bypass surgery at age 43. Ian's parents died in an auto accident when the men were in their late 40s. Larry's father died from cancer, and so did one of Larry's sisters. Although the families had difficulty dealing with the fact that their sons were gay and living together in the beginning, by the time the men had been together for 5 years they were more accepting and inclusive. (It is often forgotten that this family scenario is much more likely than that of being rejected.)

Some years ago, the couple purchased a larger home and invited Larry's widowed mother to live in a suite in their home. They spoke of this being one of the more difficult decisions they had made because the new arrangement would be permanent and the other siblings resented her agreement to move in with "the boys." Nonetheless, the arrangement worked well enough that they were actually approached and questioned about their experience by other gay friends. Some of their friends also invited an aged parent into their homes, sometimes successfully and sometimes not.

I met the couple when the men are in their early 60s. They had requested couple counseling to deal with Larry's heart disease and the effect it was having on their intimate lives. Ian had pulled away and seemed forever immersed in their financial affairs. Larry had become increasingly depressed as he anticipated yet more heart surgery—perhaps even a heart transplant. However, in just a few sessions, the therapist was able to help the men address their fears of Larry's death and regain a joy in living whatever life was available to them.

Larry and Ian had now been together for over 35 years. They weathered life's adversities well, and can easily be a source of inspiration to younger gay couples. Yet, due to the invisibility of gay couples in community newspapers, television, movies, church bulletins, and other means of openness, few gay couples could know of Larry and Ian's rich life together. To provide gay men the opportunity to learn about successful gay relationships through real-life meetings with older gay men or by reading and storytelling can be immensely rewarding. The book *The Oldest Gay Couple in America* was a runaway best-seller in gay bookstores the continent over for just these reasons.

Ensuring Resources

The fact that this section is being written implies that therapeutic resources are available to gay couples. However true this may be in large urban centers where a concentration of gay and lesbian people has "brought forth" a cadre of professionals who are known to be available, it may not appear true in the vast majority of communities across North America. The cooptation of the term "family" by the heterosexist and homophobic right wing can suggest to gay men that they are not allowed or able to access resources that the dominant community has assumptive access to. For instance, I know in my own community that many gay and lesbian couples deselected our Family Therapy Program as a potential resource and instead called for help through our Human Sexuality Program. The latter was called, they say, because they assumed that the Family Therapy Program was only for heterosexual families.

As therapists, we can make a very important intervention on the larger systems level of community resources. That is, we can let the public in general and the gay subculture in specific know that couple and family therapeutic resources are open and accessible to gay men. Although we can do this via word of mouth, it would be much more effective to include the language of inclusion in the program and therapeutic descriptions that we offer to the general public. Also, we can list ourselves in gay and lesbian resource guides (most medium to large urban centers now have "Pink Pages" or "Unity Pages," a listing of gay-owned or gay-supportive businesses and establishments) as available to gay individuals, the couples they create, and the families they live in to increase the actual availability of therapeutic help for gay men.

CLINICAL CONCERNS

Gay men in couples, or as individuals, can present with any concern in the human realm of experience. Certain presentations, however, are more apt to be either seen in or brought up by gay men as a population than perhaps by other groupings of men. These can include loneliness, affiliative invisibility, unavailable couple role models, substance abuse, reliance on sex for intimate connection (genitalization of the heart), management of interpersonal boundaries, dealing with previous partners' sexual concerns, and availability of couple resources.

Loneliness

One of the more common presentations I see for men in gay couples is a sense of *anomie*. This is Durkheim's (1951) conceptualization of an existential loneliness and sense of isolation. Durkheim's concept refers to the demands of living failing to experientially reach the individual. One can certainly see how this problem could be applicable to gay men. Despite the recent civil changes and the emerging tradition of more respectful cultural understandings of homosexuality, particularly in the larger urban centers where a gay male presence in particular can be seen and felt, North American culture remains more pejorative and pathologizing of gayness than accepting and including.

As children who are in the process of uncovering the fact that their affiliative orientation is stronger toward members of the same gender enter into late childhood and the early teens, they become acutely aware of this pejorative view of gay and lesbian persons. In reflecting on their own affiliative leanings through such a disqualifying and pathologizing lens, these boys are apt to be less accepting of their own experience. Instead, as teens and men, they may then suffer from what I have come to call the "if you only knew" syndrome. Many gay clients have told me that they have felt unsupported and disconnected despite others' recognition of their personal, academic, familial and social accomplishments. It appears that these accolades are not sufficiently owned by the individual due to this "if you only knew" reflective stance taken by the gay person. Therefore, earned compliments seem simply not to "stick." They fail to touch or have meaning for the gay person due to his internal disqualification "if you only knew *(about my secret gayness)*, you wouldn't say such things."

Such practices, of course, lead to a sense of *anomie* and potential depressive experience that may easily be presented to a clinician either as couple dissatisfaction or as individual despair. Although many gay men will come to terms with this shame and begin to live a life that is more accepting and including of their homosexuality, the coping strategy of being "the best little boy in the world" can persist in other areas, particularly in coupling with a chosen and valued mate. Open conversation and disclosure of problematic experiences may be put aside in favor of pseudomutuality, leading, unfortunately, to a similar experience to that when the man was an early adolescent trying to "hide" his gayness. It is not at all uncommon, therefore, to hear one male speaking of feeling lonely in reference to his relationship with his partner.

Although most therapists have a plethora of interventions that can be used when dealing with this type of loneliness within the couple, I advise the use of interventions that I have discussed earlier in this chapter. Invite the men into more *effective reflection* and disclosure, to help them know what it is that they are actually feeling. By inviting the couple to reflect on their emotional reasons for being together (i.e., love, friendship, enjoyment, etc.), thereby creating a larger context for the concerns of loneliness or other problems, the therapist can help each of the partners to see the loneliness as having lesser substance. Therapists can orient the couple participants toward *affective primacy* in the relationship, that is, help each in the couple to disclose his vulnerable feeling of loneliness (and other vulnerable feelings) and to subsequently actively and affirmingly listen to his partner's disclosures. Using an intervention focused on *stories of others* can also be helpful here. It may allow the couple to see that the current state is not uncommon, and that others have recovered from such a state. Then the therapist can offer them some practical suggestions without being instructive.

Invisibility

It is now well known that the pejorative heterosexist stereotype of gay men as effeminate and weak, less "manly" than heterosexual males (i.e., gender atypical), is false. Gay men come in all shapes and sizes, ages, and ethnicities, with just as wide and diverse interests as men in the general population. There are no identifying gay stigmata. One of the most frequent complaints of men looking for relationships with other men concerns the actual difficulty of finding another (suitable) gay man to meet. When one adds together the facts that there are no visible signs to distinguish a gay man from a straight man, that the number of gay persons are approximately one-eighth to one-tenth the number of straight persons (Bagley, Bolitho, & Bertrand, in press; Bagley & Tremblay, 1997), and the still-extant pejorative view of gayness, it is no wonder that many gay men find it difficult to meet others who could become suitable mates.

"Ghettoization" in large urban centers is one attempted solution to this problem of invisibility. The Castro district of San Francisco, South Beach in Miami, Chelsea and the Village in New York City, Queenstown in Toronto, the West End in Vancouver, and West Hollywood in Los Angeles are well-known examples of dense, gay neighborhoods. Here there are opportunities for social interaction through work, community, church, and recreation that are more likely to include other gay men. But for the majority of North Americans, this is not the case. Although most medium to larger urban centers do have places where gay men can meet, they are intended primarily for drinking or sexual encounters. They are not set up to foster meetings that have the potential for openness or affiliative success.

Despite these impediments, the surprising fact is that a majority of gay men do find other men to have relationships with and do invest themselves in such relationships. Luckily, non-alcohol- and non-sex-based-opportunities for gay men to socialize and meet are emerging. For instance, many gay athletic associations, such as Front Runners, an international gay running group, or the Gay Games, are establishing chapters across North America. Additionally, efforts in some urban centers to provide social and recreational opportunities for gay and lesbian youth have resulted in the creation of youth groups for discussion and socialization as well as "juice bars," nightclub-like places that provide social opportunities without drugs or alcohol.

However, some gay couples begin their relationships in places or ways that are "unmentionable" in heterosexual contexts. I remember seeing one gay couple who had been together for over 30 years whose anniversary celebrations had never included members of their families of origin. This was due to their embarrassment at having met in a gay bathhouse, the only place for gay men to socialize in their small city many years ago.

It is not, of course, the work of therapists to introduce gay couples to others who can be affirming and supportive, but we can intervene in ways that help the men enlarge their worlds meaningfully. For instance, using the intervention of *stories of others* can be helpful. Not only can solutions such as community involvement, volunteerism, family involvement, and so on be imbedded in the stories, but other potential solutions can also be offered without being required. A therapist could also bring forth *family of choice versus family of origin*. The idea of family of choice may be much more appealing to the couple as a method to counter invisibility in terms of the family of origin. Therapists could use *externalization methods* as well. Invisibility itself could be externalized and shown to have influence over the couple's future. The couple can be invited into cooperatively countering Invisibility. Sessions can help search out examples of effective countering while inviting *reflection* on the connection between the escape from Invisibility and the well-being of the couple. Finally, *ensuring resources*, particularly awareness of resources of connection, can do much to counter invisibility. Most gay persons know of the available for-profit meeting places, such as bars and bathhouses. However, by orienting members of a couple to "experiment" with connecting through nonprofits, such as gay athletic groups, gay interest groups, volunteerism, and so on, invisibility can be escaped.

Role Models

Other than the "tyrannizing triad" of patriarchy, heterosexism, and homophobia, I would say that the most significant and ubiquitous problem for gay male couples is an absence of visible role modeling. Although the open presence of gay persons in popular culture has increased, it remains relatively rare to see depictions of gay couples in healthy and happy relationships, as is routine for heterosexuals. Additionally, although gay couples have existed since ancient times, openness about their lives and relationships within the community at large is still rare. Therefore the availability of role models to show typical developmental tasks, relational strategies, and problem solutions are seldom available. The recently popular gay book, *The Oldest Gay Couple in America* (Harwood, 1997), which chronicles the story of a couple who have been together for decades, is a testament to the need for such information. McWhirter and Mattison's (1984) seminal book *The Male Couple: How Relationships Develop* takes a detailed look at normative gay relationships in the 1980s in the United States. Other books, such as *The*

Male Couples Guide (Marcus, 1992), have updated this information. Nevertheless, the fact remains that this knowledge is not easily and readily available on a community-wide basis for the average gay man struggling to try to develop a meaningful relationship with his partner. Additionally, I know of very few family and marriage training courses where this information is routinely and effectively taught.

There are a number of interventions that a therapist can use in this area of concern. For instance, the therapist can introduce the notion of *celebration of diversity*, that is, that there are many ways to be a couple, not simply the heterosexual model. Again, *stories of others* can have a dramatic effect on couples struggling with absent or inadequate role models. *Ensuring resources*, particularly those that allow the meeting of other couples, can provide opportunities for role models that would otherwise be invisible.

Substance Abuse

As Don Clark (1987, 1992) pointed out in his classic book *Loving Someone Gay*, a further risk from the denial process that leads to anomie, loneliness, and even depression is substance abuse. It is common knowledge that males are demographically at greater risk for alcoholism and drug abuse than females. Therefore, it comes as no surprise that such abuse is even more problematic for gay males. Part of the tradition of alcohol use for coping with emotional discomfort derives from the urbanized gay male culture's heavy reliance on bars, discotheques, and nightclubs as places for socializing. Such commercial enterprises exist to make profits, and nowhere are there greater profits than in the sale of alcohol and drugs. Linea Due (1995), *Joining the Tribe: Growing Up Gay and Lesbian in the '90s*, shows that providing young gay and lesbian people with social opportunities that do not involve drugs or alcohol generates a significant difference in future coping habits. Also, many gay men do not fit the "youngman" stereotype of a hard defined body and handsome, well-dressed good looks (Flood, 1989). Yet, when gay men socialize in one of the few available places such as a bar or a dance palace, they frequently use alcohol or drugs in an effort to bolster self-confidence or to overcome natural shyness. This can lead to a potentially downward spiral of an increasing need to socialize yet also an increased reliance on chemical relief from anxiety and loneliness.

Additionally, the traditional patriarchal tradition of underverbalizing vulnerable feelings such as sadness, fear, and loneliness can leave men trying to "anesthetize" these very feelings via alcohol or drugs.

If these traditions are carried over into the men's intimate relationships, common experiential problems are then dealt with through the numbing effects of alcohol or drugs. Of course, then the dynamics of "enabler" or "codependent" often come into play. Luckily, these couples can be helped like any other couple struggling with substance abuse. The only major differences in working with gay males would be to acknowledge and work with the excessive "male" tradition of "bottling up" one's feelings and avoiding the possibility of open rejection. I find that inviting clients to see that they can be seen as "prisoners" of the dominant societal habit of silencing affective communication and then helping them learn an affective lexicon can make all the difference in the world.

Interventions in the area of substance abuse can include more *effective reflection*. The individuals involved can be invited into having greater awareness of what the "imprisoning" issues are. Heterosexism and homophobia often lead to internalized self-loathing. *Externalizing* homophobia, for example, can lend the individuals and the couple greater influence over the negative reflections and behavioral habits that support substance abuse. The therapeutic distinction that *thoughts do not predict actions* can help the individuals involved in the patterns of substance abuse to reflect on the difference between feeling an urge to drink, for example, and the underlying emotional invitation accompanying the urge.

Genitalization of the Heart

Patriarchal edicts have misled men for millennia in their search for affiliative fit. As a sex therapist, it often appears to me that many of my male clients, either gay or straight, appear to be "divining for their hearts with their genitals." This effort to "light up the heart by plugging in the penis" is omnipresent in our Western culture. One need only look at any downtown metropolitan center anywhere in North America or Western Europe and see the commercial establishments that exist to support this search method. Singles bars, "peeler" clubs, dance bars, "massage" parlors, not to mention "escort" agencies and personal classifieds, are ever present and readily available.

Unfortunately, this genitalization of the heart is often magnified for gay men's initial efforts at trying to find meaningful, human connection. Not only are gay men subjected to the prescripts of patriarchy (i.e., a man is always ready, willing, and wanting to have sex; Zilbergeld,

1993), but they are further culturally restrained from alternative methodologies such as dating, courtship, open introductions, and so on. Although some of these opportunities are increasingly occurring, especially in large urban "gay ghettos," the dominant discourse around homosexuality has traditionally been that "homosexuality" is carnal, impulsive, and trivial. These heterosexist assumptions are one of the greatest enemies to gay men's successful coupling and their development of personal esteem.

Although the AIDS epidemic of the 1980s and early 1990s temporarily interfered with the primacy of genital contact as a method of meeting for gay men, easy—and too often unsafe—sex now appears to be in resurgence for gay male youth in urban centers.

Sample interventions dealing with the habit of genitalization of the heart include helping each member of the couple to develop more effective *personal reflective skills* so that each man can see the emotional need he is actually trying to address. The therapist can invite the couple into using linguistic practices that are clear to each, descriptive of the emotional experience itself, inviting of the partner to join in with, and affirming of efforts made. It may seem obvious, but *affective primacy* is a major intervention for problems of genitalization. By aiding each man to see that what he is truly searching for is an "affiliative" experience rather than simply an orgasmic experience, therapists can invite their clients into truly being able to address and fulfill emotional needs. When a gay man, or, for that matter, any man, is able to address his emotional experience directly and effectively, a sense of liberated opportunity is brought forth. Through *restorying sexuality* and introducing the concept that *thoughts do not predict actions,* the men in the couple can be invited into literally "putting sex in its place." This means that sex is seen as part of the experiential celebration of unique intimacies that the couple can celebrate rather than as the "end all" or "be all" of the relationship. This latter view, of the indispensable nature of genital connection, rather than the experiential view of sex being for intimacy, is all too dominant for men and some women in our culture. Introducing *stories of others* who have been able to successfully escape the habit of genitalizing the heart can inspire not only hope, but also suggest without requiring methods that could be tried for the couple in treatment. Here, stories of how some men have found even better sexual connection by looking toward heartfelt experiences rather than simply genital activities can inspire. For instance, many gay men have had to confront simple behavioral efforts at sex by becoming conscious of the HIV epidemic. In rethinking their sexual practices and ensuring greater safety, some of these men have had an opportunity to actually discover that sex *is defined* less by the behavior and more by the mutual experience involved.

Boundaries

Much has been written about gay men's "permeability of boundaries." Johnson and Kieran's (1996) chapter, "Creating and Maintaining Boundaries in Male Couples," in the recent book *Lesbians and Gays in Couples and Families* edited by Laird and Green (1996) takes a detailed look at this issue. One of the most striking and potentially problematic boundaries is the sexual boundary. As Mattison and McWhirter (1995) point out, gay relationships can show a wide diversity of agreements in respect to sexual boundaries. Some relationships include explicit openness of sexual boundaries where either partner can have an outside sexual encounter as long as he does not "fall in love" with the third person. A variant on this agreement is practiced by those men who agree to have sex with an outsider only if that person is part of a "threesome" between the two committed men. However, others agree to implicit openness, where outside "dalliances" are accepted as a likelihood but never actually discussed; still others have clandestine openness, which is a contradiction of the either overt or covert expectation of monogamy; and yet others have agreed on and practice monogamy.

It appears in my practice that the sexually open type of relationship is more prevalent in younger gay couples than in older couples. It is my belief that this difference may be less a matter of one's generational cohort (e.g., middle-aged baby boomer vs. generation X'er), and more an issue of men growing emotionally and developing more effective intimacy skills over time. As one client in his 50s told me, "In my 20s I seemed to want to step out to taste the 'forbidden fruit,' now I have enough pleasure in looking at it and sharing the fantasy with my lover."

However, the discovery of an affair that had not been disclosed nor accepted can have the same damaging impact on gay couples that it has on any other couple in our community. Issues of betrayal, deceit, disrespect, sexually transmitted diseases, and self-esteem, as well as friendship circles and shame, can be consequences. However, it must be said that some men do develop loving and lasting intimate relationships that have permeable sexual boundaries. It depends, from my experience, on the "match" between the two individuals and their own value systems.

For these couples, the problem is often less with the couple than it is with the therapist. For instance, a heterosexual therapist raised in a "traditional" value system of dedicated heterosexual monogamy may erroneously believe that the issues the men are struggling with are primarily related to the permeable sexual boundaries rather than to whatever other concerns the couple may be dealing with. They may hold such erroneous belief despite the fact that up to 50% or men and women in such explicitly monogamous relationships sexually "step out" at some time or other.

Previous Relationships

Due to the comparatively fewer numbers of persons who are gay in relation to the community at large, and the concentration of gay culture in urban centers, gay communities can be relatively small. As such, a gay male couple may find themselves bumping into previous partners in the community in which they socialize, work, and live. This can also bring forth concerns of jealousy, abandonment, and personal inadequacy. Oddly, however, despite these potential concerns, it is not at all uncommon to find that previous relationship partners become part of the circle of friends of the current couple. This is not as frequently seen among gay couples as it is among lesbian couples, but it nevertheless seems to be more the case among gay men than it is among heterosexual couples.

However, in addition to these issues, the consequences of previous relationships such as children from heterosexual marriages, previous female partners from those marriages, biological family, extended family, and friendship circles further complicate the relational involvements of the current male partnership.

Many interventions are available to therapists dealing with the actual fact of multiple relationships. However, distinguishing *family of choice* from *family of origin* is perhaps the most valuable of them all.

Over the last 100 years, gay men and lesbians have pioneered the development of *"family of choice."* Centuries of hiding, pretending, and despair left gay people with little opportunity to be openly themselves with traditional family and friends. Luckily, this has changed for many in Europe and North America. Yet the emerging tradition of using positively experienced relationships as the definition of family rather than only the patriarchal biological line of inheritance allows many gay people to access greater value in their close relationships. These families of choice may include valued members from the biological family as well as other heterosexual people who are accepting and loving of the gay person. Additionally, however, they include other gay and lesbian people who have lent support and social help to the gay person and his partner. It is not unusual, therefore, to hear stories of Christmas, or Thanksgiving including some family-of-origin members but also gay friends and their partners and children. This mix of valued relationships is an incredible strength for gay couples—one that therapists too often forget when working therapeutically with gay persons. Intervening using *celebration of diversity* and *stories of others* will also invite the couple into recognizing their own resources and those that others have been able to use, despite the dominant discourses of trivialization of gay men's bonding.

Issues of Sexuality

In this section, I am describing not so much the issues of affairs or boundaries around the relationship, but sexuality in the relationship itself. This is an area that is often overlooked during therapy with heterosexual and homosexual couples alike. Nevertheless, it needs to be attended to as well—and not just from the usual disease-prevention perspective of safer sex. More importantly, this area needs to be addressed from the perspective of enabling affiliative celebration. Interestingly, as the writer Anne Rice (1999) stated:

> Gays are in the vanguard of that final divorce of sex from conventional notions of sin; the divorce of sin from mythology and religion. If we can carry this off—if we can take sex out of the realm of sin altogether and see it as something else to do with personal relationships and ethics, then we can finally get around to another phase of Christianity which is long overdue. That phase is the one which deals with the question of sin as violence; sin as cruelty; sin as murder, war and starvation.

Compared to other men, gay men are often able to have more diversity, self-expression, and personal enjoyment in their sexual contact. Nevertheless, they too can suffer problems such as desire discrepancy secondary to other life events, erectile dysfunctions, premature ejaculation, or other symptomatic concerns. These issues have been covered in other articles (Sanders & Tomm, 1989). The treatment strategies are very similar no matter the affiliative orientation and are based on promoting a "win/win" situation for both partners.

Couple Physical Resources

Without the usual strategies and role modeling, gay men have a variety of ways in which they can deal with individual physical resources being brought to an intimate relationship. Most usual is to maintain previously owned items separately and subsequently develop a "roommate style" with one another. However, over the years this often gives way to more joint endeavors, including joint ownerships of family homes, furnishings, and investments. As with heterosexual couples, inequalities in earning power, resource allocation, and family wealth can create significant problems of experience for gay men that the therapist will be asked to address.

Interventions here can include all those that the therapist has acquired in working with heterosexual couples. Additionally, emphasizing *affective primacy*, that is, inviting each member of the couple to, in essence, "see through" the money concerns to recognize the emotional issue that is underpinning the resource concern, can be very effective. Most often, the emotional issue is fear.

CONCLUSIONS

Gay men, like people the world over, strive to construct and maintain intimate coupled relationships. Rather than using outmoded and disrespectful understandings of gayness based primarily on sexual *behaviour*, this chapter invites the reader to use an experiential frame based on an understanding and acceptance of the notion of romantic affiliation. The disrespectful assumptions based on the "tyrannizing triad" of heterosexist, homophobic, and patriarchal concepts can be seen as impeding the development of secure and fulfilling couple relationships for gay men. However, it is not only the clients who suffer from this triad, since we, as therapists, need to escape our own subjugation by such unhelpful assumptions too.

The chapter detailed how a therapist can be of help to gay couples. The therapist can help clients develop personal reflective skills. These skills will help therapeutic participants to escape prejudice and therapeutic blindness, bringing forth a celebration of difference rather than relying on the "tyranny of sameness," aiding the couple in dealing openly and congruently with fundamental affective needs, restorying sexuality based on the experiential rather than on the behavioral, supporting gay couples' families of choice, and looking for and learning from successful stories of other gay couples.

Gay men can suffer any of the concerns that straight couples do, including issues related to money, power, job concerns, children, and so on. However, this chapter has looked at issues that tend to be more unique as concerns for gay couples: loneliness, invisibility, lack of role models, socialization through substance abuse, genitalizing vulnerable emotions, negotiating relational boundaries, dealing with previous partners, issues of sexuality and affection, and the management of gay couple resources.

Working with people who love one another can be one of the most rewarding professions in the world. Helping these persons open themselves to experiences of such loving is positive and affirming and is, to me, work well done.

NOTE

1. The October 1998 murder of 21-year-old Matthew Shepard in Wyoming dramatically demonstrated such risk. He was lured out of a bar by two men pretending to be gay, taken to an isolated country road, beaten unconscious, tied to a fence like a scarecrow, and left to die in freezing weather. He was found, still alive, 18 hours later by cyclists but died 2 days later never having regained consciousness.

REFERENCES

Bagley, C., Bolitho, F., & Bertrand, L. (in press). Mental health profiles: Suicidal behaviour and community sexual assault in 2112 Canadian adolescents. *Crisis: International Journal of Suicide Studies.*

Bagley, C., & Tremblay, P. (1997). Suicidality problems of gay and bisexual males: Evidence from a random community survey of 750 men aged 18 to 27. In C. Bagley & R. Ramsey (Eds.), *Suicidal behaviors in adolescents and adults: Taxonomy, understanding and prevention.* Brookfield, VT: Avebury.

Boswell, J. (1980). *Christianity, social tolerance, and homosexuality.* Chicago: University of Chicago Press.

Boswell, J. (1994). *Same sex unions in premodern Europe.* New York: Villard Books.

Clark, D. (1987). *Loving someone gay.* Berkeley, CA: Celestial Arts.

Clark, D. (1992). *The new loving someone gay.* Berkeley, CA: Celestial Arts.

Due, L. (1995). *Joining the tribe: Growing up gay and lesbian in the '90s.* Toronto: Doubleday.

Durkheim, E. (1951). *Suicide: A study in sociology.* Glencoe, IL: Free Press.

Flood, G. (1989). *I'm looking for Mr. Right.* Atlanta: Brob House.

Harwood, G. (1997). *The oldest gay couple in America: A 70-year journey through same sex America.* Secaucus, NJ: Birch Lane Press.

Johnson & Kieran. (1996). Creating and maintaining boundaries in male couples. In J. Laird & R. J. Green (Eds.), *Lesbians and gays in couples and families: A handbook for therapists.* San Francisco: Jossey-Bass.

Kinsey, A. C., Pomeroy, W. B., & Martin, C. E. (1948). *Sexual behavior in the human male.* Philadelphia: Saunders.

Kinsey, A. C., Pomeroy, W. B., & Martin, C. E. (1953). *Sexual behavior in the human female.* Philadelphia: Saunders.

Laird, J., & Green, R. J. (Eds.). (1996). *Lesbians and gays in couples and families: A handbook for therapists.* San Francisco: Jossey-Bass.

Marcuse, E. (1992). *The male couple's guide.* New York: HarperCollins.

Mattison, A. M., & McWhirter, D. P. (1995). Lesbians, gay men, and their families. *Psychiatric Clinics of North America, 18*(1), 123–137.

McWhirter, D. P., & Mattison, A. M. (1984). *The male couple: How relationships work.* Englewood Cliffs, NJ: Prentice Hall.

Persky, S. (1989). *Buddy's: Meditations on desire.* Vancouver: New Star Books.

Rice, A. (1999). You asked, Anne answered. www.annerice.com/ques-msc.htm.

Sanders, G. L. (1988). An invitation to escape sexual tyranny. *Journal of Strategic and Systemic Therapies, 7*(3), 23–35.

Sanders, G. L. (1991a). Sexplay—Five sexy words. *Calgary Participator, 1*(3).

Sanders, G. L. (1991b). Personal reflections of a man who practices sexual therapy. *Dulwich Centre Review.*

Sanders, G. L. (1993). The love that dares to speak its name: From secrecy to openness, gay and lesbian affiliations. In E. Imber-Black (Ed.), *Secrets in families and family therapy* (pp. 215–242). New York: Norton.

Sanders, G. L., & Tomm, K. T. (1989). A cybernetic–systems approach to problems in sexual functioning. In D. Kantor & B. Okun (Eds.), *Intimate environments.* New York: Guilford Press.

Sanders, M. (1989). Homosexual acts—Are they natural, moral, or either? Philosophy 224.3 (01), University of Saskatchewan, Calgary.

Savin-Williams, R. C. (1989). Coming out to parents and self-esteem among gay and lesbian youths. *Journal of Homosexuality, 18*(1–2).

Savin-Williams, R. C. (1996). Self-labelling and disclosure among gay, lesbian, and bisexual youth. In J. Laird & R. J. Green (Eds.), *Lesbian and gays and couples and families: A handbook for therapists* (pp. 153–182). San Francisco: Jossey-Bass.

White, M. (1986). Negative explanation, restraint, and double description: A template for family therapy. *Family Process, 25*(2), 169–184.

Zilbergeld, B. (1993). *The new male sexuality: A guide to sexual fulfillment.* New York: Little, Brown.

CHAPTER 11

Lesbian Couples Entering the 21st Century

Caroline Marvin
Dusty Miller

$\mathbf{A}$t the millennium, the form of intimate life represented by the lesbian couple is becoming more and more evident. Although there have always been women partners, these couples did not enjoy the visibility they do today. As the lesbian couple becomes a more stable cultural form, and therefore more likely to enter therapy, traditionally trained therapists accustomed to seeing two-gendered couples will surely find that their familiar maps and rules no longer apply.

What has changed in the psychotherapy of lesbian couples in recent years? Perhaps the most dramatic change is that lesbian couples appear for treatment at all. In times past, lesbian couples were more closeted and more likely to assume that a psychotherapist, trained to think of homosexuality as a pathology, could not offer them any support or understanding. More recently, politically oriented lesbians feared that the male dominance embedded at the heart of psychotherapy theories would cause them to be actively harmed by any treatment process. Today, however, when Ellen De Generes's coming out can be featured on national television and a lesbian couple can appear on the cover of *Newsweek*, many lesbians are no longer leading hidden, ashamed, or secretive lives. As they accept themselves fully, they can imagine receiving support from psychotherapists, some of whom are gay and lesbian themselves. Furthermore, feminism has influenced theory profoundly, such that psychological theory is truly less hostile toward lesbian clients.

A second profound change in the reality of lesbian couples today involves the continuing development of reproductive technologies and the increased availability of adoption. Whereas in the past never-married lesbians were probably childless, today every permutation of parenting dilemma can affect the lesbian couples we treat.

COMPARING LESBIAN AND HETEROSEXUAL COUPLES

Lesbian couples are *unique* when viewed through the lens of gender or the lens of female/lesbian oppression. But lesbian couples should be seen as *similar* to two-gendered couples when viewed in terms of commonalities such as life stage, class, ethnicity, or race. In the chapter that follows, we will consider this continuum of similarity and difference and make suggestions to therapists who are treating lesbian couples at the millennium.

The one overarching message we would like to send to therapists who have seen many straight couples but who are just beginning to work with lesbian couples is: *Avoid generalizing similarities or emphasizing differences, but be sensitive to both.* Perhaps the most reliable way to understand any lesbian couple is to ask them to share their own ideas about lesbian couples and to describe how they see themselves in relation to other couples (lesbian, gay, and heterosexual) they know. Therapeutic questions about similarities and differences can be enormously helpful in developing the complex portrait necessary to accurately represent the rapidly evolving experience of any lesbian couple in today's culture. From our own perspective, an attitude of *celebrating* the differences, the freedom, and the lack of cultural constraint lesbian couples may experience is often the most helpful way to approach problems and enjoy gifts.

Lesbian Couples as Unique

Green, Bettinger, and Zacks (1996) report that same-sex couples as a group are "cohesive, highly flexible, and receive meaningful support from friends" (p. 222). In addition they report that *lesbian* couples are "*functioning exceptionally well*" (p. 222; italics in original). These investigators discuss the misconception "based on family systems literature's depictions of lesbian couples as fused and gay male couples as disengaged" (p. 198) that same-sex couples are struggling and unhappy. They comment: "If you only have dark lenses, you will have a dim view!" (p. 223). To counter this dim view, they report that the lesbian couples in their studies report "*significantly more satisfaction*" (p. 198; italics in original) in their relationships than heterosexual married couples do.

Psychotherapists treating lesbian couples today should also be informed about the work of theorists from the feminist psychoanalytic and the relational schools. We especially recommend the collection of writings edited by Glassgold and Iasenza, *Lesbians and Psychoanalysis* (1995), and the work of Julie Mencher and others at the Stone Center at Wellesley College. Mencher (1997), like Green et al., reexamines the notion of fusion in lesbian relationships, focusing on the positive and constructive qualities these "fused" relationship patterns bring to bear. Unlike traditional theorists who describe relational maturity as the distinctiveness or differentiation of the two selves, Stone Center theorists are more interested in the *quality of the processes* between the two individuals. These writers and researchers focus on relational authenticity, and on mutual empathy, engagement, and empowerment as the criteria of health and maturity.

When seen from the Stone Center perspective, some characteristics of lesbian relationships that have been described pejoratively as "fusion," are viewed simply as the natural and healthy outcome of the meeting of the relational styles of two women. Lesbian relationships have been described in terms of their intense intimacy, high degree of sensitivity to the emotional world of the other, and the embeddedness of the two identities within the relationship. Perhaps lesbian couples simply show us what the intimacy patterns of women are like when unfettered by male relational styles and patriarchal assumptions about women. As Mencher (1997) puts it, "In a relationship in which both partners, as women, are consistently directed toward connection, there can exist a full range of possibility for mutuality, empathy and authenticity" (p. 324)—the fundamental processes of a healthy relationship.

Lesbian Couples as Similar to Other Couples

If we want to consider how lesbian couples are much the same as the other couples we treat, we might look at developmental stage as a unifying frame. For example, in the courtship stage we would expect to look at sexual and romantic issues, regardless of gender. In her invaluable book *The Lesbian Family Life Cycle* (1995) Suzanne Slater provides a frame to consider lesbian couples as a group needing special consideration, and simultaneously as a group with the same ordinary and normal developmental needs as the two-gendered couples we treat.

> Because our culture still withholds the profound, if simple, message that lesbian family life is normal, our families don't have markers to normalize our passages through a normal lesbian life cycle. . . . We must provide lesbians not with some unique support, but with the same support automatically issued to heterosexual families. (Slater, 1997, p. 6)

Slater (1995) suggests that we normalize and contextualize lesbian relationships by looking at the tasks and accomplishments of five life-cycle stages: couple formation, ongoing couplehood, the middle years, generativity, and couples over 65. In our view, this alternative life cycle might be an improvement for heterosexual couples as well, evolving beyond the traditional family life-cycle paradigm of weddings, births, divorce, and midlife angst.

Slater's developmental frame will be useful in organizing the observations that follow concerning contemporary lesbian couples, in therapy, and approaching the millennium.

COUPLE FORMATION

Lesbian couples in the first stage of the couple's life cycle are not always chronologically young. The several couples we will discuss in regard to their "formation" have members who ages differ as much as 40 years. Like other couples, lesbian couples may form at almost any life stage. Caren and Ellen's story illustrates dilemmas common to lesbians across the life span, but particularly acute in the couple-formation stage.

Love, Marriage, and Homophobia: Caren and Ellen

Caren's family of origin's refusal to accept her relationship with Ellen came as no surprise to her. Her affluent family had been unable to accept Caren's sexual orientation since she first came out to them 10 years earlier. Now, at age 28, Caren had been deeply hurt by the family's resistance to her attempts to bring her two worlds together. About midway through the course of couple therapy, Caren and Ellen had an elegant wedding, complete with a sunset ceremony on a beautiful beach. Although Ellen's Irish Catholic family were shaken by her decision to marry a woman, they did attend the wedding. The painful contrast of Caren's absent family has been an ongoing issue for this young couple.

Like many other young couples at the stage of couple formation, Caren and Ellen are also working out how to make a life together that allows for the differences they bring to the relationship. Class differences are significant; political differences are sometimes explosive. Each woman is learning the intricacies of joining with the other's friends and work colleagues. Negotiating time—time alone, time as a couple, time for work—is an arena of struggle and compromise for many new couples. But the complete refusal by Caren's family to accept their marriage makes Ellen and Caren's couple-formation challenges sharply different from those of most heterosexual couples.

Unfortunately, except in major cities and a few "gay ghettos" like Provincetown and Northampton, Massachusetts, coming out is still an enormous concern for lesbians. In a recent study of lesbian life conducted by the National Lesbian Health Care Survey (NLHCS), only 27% of lesbians reported being "out" to all family members (Alexander, 1996). Furthermore, the absence of legally sanctioned marriage for gays and lesbians continues to cast a troubling cloak of invisibility over the marriage and commitment rituals many lesbian couples do celebrate. Because Caren and Ellen are not legally married, it is much easier for Caren's family to continue to deny or dismiss the couple's existence.

Interestingly, and contrary to many therapists' common assumptions, Green et al. (1996) did not find a significant link between lesbian partners' outness to family-of-origin members and the couples' own relationship quality. In their words, "Satisfaction of lesbian couples in our study is entirely unrelated to whether partners are out to their mothers, fathers, siblings or a combination of the three" (p. 200). This finding should comfort therapists who have wondered if it is necessary to urge coming out upon clients who are reluctant to do so.

The therapist who worked with Caren and Ellen focused on the challenges they faced from cultural homophobia as they worked to solidify their relationship. The therapist's own acceptance and appreciation of this couple helped to balance the rejection experienced from Caren's biological parents. The therapist also focused on the political disagreements these two women had, helping them to understand that these stemmed from the family-of-origin values each brought to the relationship (like any new couple). In therapy these women came to see that the differences between them had seemed more threatening because of the cultural oppression they shared.

At one point in the therapy the therapist suggested that the couple search for salt and pepper shakers for their home, a task that might teach them how they are alike and different at the same time. This search became a great adventure for them and they found several . . . the beginning of a collection that continues to this day.

Because this couple's commitment ceremony took place during the course of therapy, preparation for the ritual became a vehicle the therapist could use to help them think deeply about their relationship and their commitment to one another. The women wrote vows that came directly from the meanings they had developed together in therapy. Privately, each woman wrote the vows that she considered most essential for her own commitment to her partner. They then presented them to each other in the session. Both women and the therapist were surprised and ultimately delighted when the final version of the vows was different and unique for each woman. Caren and Ellen also used the therapy to prepare letters for each family of origin, explaining what they were doing and why. Because they had come to see the relationship as a "container" for their own personal growth and development, their therapist suggested that they find or purchase a container within which to place the vows they had written. Together they selected a beautiful Shaker wood box to serve that function.

Heterosexism and Invisibility: Judith and Ann

Judith and Ann were a relatively "new" couple although their relationship began when both women were in midlife. Judith had no children and was delighted at the ease with which she and Ann's daughter, Jodi, connected. This was no surprise to Ann, since Jodi had been raised in a lesbian household. But when Jodi married her male partner, the couple *was* surprised to discover how stressful Jodi's wedding was for their relationship.

While none of the wedding participants displayed obvious homophobia or disqualification, both women felt the power of heterosexism. Despite Judith's involvement in planning for and financing the wedding, she felt throughout the wedding festivities that her role was unacknowledged. This became particularly painful during the taking of the wedding pictures when she was not invited to be in them. Thus her role as Ann's partner was rendered invisible.

At Judith's insistence, the couple entered therapy. Both women commented about how validating it felt to be recognized at that time as a legitimate couple by their therapist, especially given the invalidation they had experienced at Jodi's wedding. It is important for both lesbian and straight therapists to recognize how deeply meaningful their own attitude of appreciation and validation can be for a couple who are so profoundly invalidated by the culture at large. By the same token, both lesbian and straight therapists must also realize how devastating their unexamined homophobia, unconsciously expressed, can be.

Shortly thereafter Judith and Ann had an important conversation with their heterosexual friends Bonnie and Jack, who told them about Jack's daughter's wedding. Bonnie was Jack's second wife. Although she had been involved for years with Jack's children, at the wedding she too felt invisible because her role as stepmother was not recognized in the various wedding rituals.

Therapeutically, what seemed most important was for the therapist to be sensitive to Judith and Ann's perceived differences from straight couples in how they experienced this heterosexual ritual. Judith's pain and disappointment were validated both by the therapist and by her partner. But it was also comforting to her to know of Bonnie's heterosexual experience of marginalization because she was a *stepmother*, a role that both Judith and Bonnie shared. Judith revealed in therapy that knowing about Bonnie's comparable experience helped to restore her faith in Ann. She admitted that she had felt betrayed by Ann, doubting her lover's capacity to resist the disturbing power of heterosexism. Now she could reframe the event, to some extent normalizing it as "just the nutty stuff that happens around weddings."

Judith and Ann's therapist used this opportunity to help the couple explore the way their *own* "internalized oppression" had led *them* to lose a little faith in their own strong relationship, given the actual or perceived slights from Ann's extended family. Both women felt that the wedding experience ultimately strengthened their coupling by unearthing some of their own doubts and insecurities about the relationship, which they were projecting onto others.

The issue of "internalized oppression" or "internalized homophobia" is an important one for the lesbian couple therapist to understand. Whether gay or straight, it would be very difficult to grow up in our culture without absorbing the culture's attitude, prejudice, or even disgust at homosexual life. If a woman absorbs that attitude and is homosexual herself, then self-disgust or self-loathing could result. Gair (1995) defines internalized homophobia as unexplored and unresolved feelings of shame in relation to one's sexuality that interfere with the recognition, verbalization, and exploration of intimacy. In her words, "Internalized homophobia takes something life-affirming, sexuality, and makes it bad" (p. 111).

The couple therapist can help by encouraging the couple to explore their feelings about sexuality, to appreciate the joy they feel, and to normalize any shame they feel as something any oppressed group experiences because of the way the culture is represented "inside them." Simply becoming conscious of these negative feelings can do much to alleviate their destructiveness. Furthermore, the therapists' own positive attitude toward the couple has a strong mitigating influence. Thus, many lesbian couples prefer to work with a lesbian couple therapist. However, others may choose a straight therapist in order to find a supporter within the heterosexual world.

Sharon Klineberg and Patrica Zorn (1995) recommend couples group treatment as a preferred form of therapy for lesbian couples, particularly because of issues of internalized homophobia. A group can provide the intense holding, safety, and validation necessary to discover and begin to dissolve inner constrictions. Furthermore, witnessing the ways that homophobia is expressed in other couples can help each couple to discern it in themselves.

Ex-Partners as Friends: Charlotte and Margaret

Another factor that distinguishes lesbian couples from two-gendered couples is how frequently ex-partners are incorporated in the new lesbian couple's life. In many lesbian communities, ex-partners remain members of the same social network. Perhaps because of the need to seek support from other lesbians in a hostile world and/or because les-

bians often experience very close friendships in their couple relationships, lesbian ex-partners may have an unusually strong need to stay
close.

For Charlotte and Margaret this issue became a source of pain. Although each woman had former lovers in her social network, Charlotte
and her most recent "ex" had had difficulty dissolving their sexual relationship. This cast a shadow at the beginning of Charlotte's courtship
with Margaret. Margaret was understandably reluctant to accept the
"ex" as simply another of Charlotte's friends. But Charlotte had energetically embraced ongoing friendships with her ex-partners in the past
and found Margaret's resistance to the recent ex-lover difficult to accept.

Charlotte and Margaret first discussed the dilemma with their
therapist, then they discussed it with lesbian friends. For more isolated
couples the support to talk this out might not be available within the
community at all and a therapist might be the only one available to
help them. If the therapist understands that there is a pattern in which
many lesbians remain friends with ex-partners, she could help the couple normalize this experience. Charlotte and Margaret's therapist was
able to help them decide that, in this particular case, the presence of
Charlotte's most recent lover was simply too painful for Margaret. In
the end, Margaret did not have to accept Charlotte's desire to include
this particular "ex" among her friends, but the therapist was able to
help the couple a great deal by contextualizing their situation and exploring the general pattern in the subculture.

As can be seen from Margaret and Charlotte's story, an issue lesbian couples frequently bring to therapy is the predictable jealousy that
arises when ex-partners remain involved or outside friendships seem
"too intense." Although jealousies are faced by heterosexual couples
when an "ex" remains involved or an opposite-sex friendship becomes
important, the intense closeness experienced by many lesbian couples
may make such jealousy feel considerably more intense. Although the
therapist of heterosexual couples may help them to exclude the problematic third person, the therapist of lesbian couples needs to understand both the intense jealousy and the norm to stay engaged with previous partners. Frequently, the therapist can be of assistance simply by
helping the couple create clearer boundaries around when and how an
ex-lover or close friend is to be involved. What are the boundaries that
each woman in the couple can accept? It is also important for the therapist to help the couple normalize the insecurity and jealousy they may
feel. The therapist can help both women understand that in a society

where the lesbian couple has no legal rights and no socially sanctioned marriage rituals, it is understandable that the relationship may feel more fragile and more susceptible to intrusions and violations. In this case, the therapist helped Charlotte and Margaret to think of their relationship as a vessel that held them both safely and allowed each of them to be challenged and to grow. They could both see that the vessel of their relationship should not be too porous; it did require some boundaries in order to sustain them well.

Coming Out of Heterosexual Marriage: Andy and Emily

As lesbian couples become more visible and more accepted in our culture today, some women who married in response to social pressure or the desire for children at a time when marriage seemed the only route to childbearing are coming out at midlife.

Andy and Emily were each with other partners when they met and fell in love. It is, of course, difficult for any couple, gay or straight, to form a new relationship when a prior relationship is ending simultaneously.

Emily's former partner was female. Although Emily and her former partner had never lived together and had remained closeted in a very conservative community, they had jointly raised the several children of two previous marriages during their 10 years together. Emily and her former partner had had an intense but stormy relationship. The effects of living in a closeted way wore on them, and their children lived with the secret of their relationship. For many years they had seen a couple therapist but had been unable either to settle the many disagreements between them or to separate from each other.

Andy, who came from a fundamentalist Christian family, had been married for nearly 20 years and was the mother of a son. Although she had always secretly yearned for a lesbian relationship, her realistic fear of being shunned by her family kept her firmly identified with heterosexuality.

Both women experienced great relief and delight when they met and fell in love. However, neither woman left her prior relationship easily. Making the transition for each of them was very difficult. Both women struggled to balance the joy and excitement they felt about what was beginning with the grief and guilt they felt about what was coming to an end.

Stepfamily issues were a challenge for Andy and Emily. Each of the three adolescent children involved had his or her own grief and anger about the losses and changes they were experiencing. One turning point occurred when Andy's son came back from a college campus visit proudly bearing a lollipop he'd been given at a campus festival. It bore the tag: "There's a lesbian in your life; lick homophobia!"

A complicating factor for Andy was the enormity of the change in her sense of identity. Although she held an intense desire to share her life with a woman, she grieved the loss of "herself" in the life that had become so familiar to her. She was astonished at how much of her life had been organized around her heterosexual identity and her heterosexual privilege. As she had feared, her conservative and religious family of origin refused to validate her decision or even to meet Emily. When Andy and Emily moved in together, Andy's parents refused to telephone her or even to correspond with her at their new home. Since Emily's family was supportive of the new couple, Emily felt understandably hurt and confused to be so explicitly rejected, and feared that Andy would ultimately choose her family over the new coupling.

Although Andy's women friends were immediately supportive of the couple, each old friendship changed in some significant way and eventually became more distant. It seemed that Andy's needs for feminine support had been great when she had been married to her husband, but now her needs had changed. A few friends felt abandoned and jealous, "sidelined" by Emily's presence. One straight friend even confided that she too had felt sexual and romantic pulls toward Andy and that those feelings had formed part of the unspoken foundation of their friendship. For many straight women, the erotic tensions in their friendships with other women are unnamed and unspoken. As the therapist remarked, "It can be threatening to watch an old friend come out."

Andy and Emily did not enter therapy immediately. It would have been too difficult to admit that their new relationship had problems, given how emotionally costly the decision to come together had been. Later, after therapy had been helpful, they were able to describe how they had feared (or projected) that a therapist might be judgmental, advising them to separate or chastising them for abandoning their former partners. As it happened, the therapist was able to help them appreciate the strengths of the new coupling and to find language to articulate the ways in which the old partnerships had in fact become untenable. At the same time, the therapist could agree with the women themselves, who felt that much about how they had left their former partners had been sudden and wounding to others and had not happened "in the best way." With the therapist's support and Andy's as well, Emily eventually wrote a letter of apology and accountability to her former partner. This act helped her to experience some emotional relief simply because of her own honesty. Andy made various attempts to communicate with her parents and for a time imagined that they would eventually soften. Finally her mother wrote, "I will *not* give up what I have always believed about 'God's plan for families.' " The therapist gently supported the two women in relinquishing their hopes for connection in that family. Andy was eventually able to move beyond her own anger, disappointment, and grief and simply respect herself for her courage to come out at all, given the religiously bound, homophobic climate of her family.

Many lesbian couples lack simple social support for their relationships. The context of therapy can be invaluable as a "safe harbor," where the relationship and its struggles can be appreciated and validated by another, in ways that the culture offers so automatically to a new heterosexual courtship and marriage as it forms and develops.

ONGOING COUPLEHOOD

At this stage, the couple is beginning to negotiate a more committed relationship. A multitude of issues may arise, from living arrangements and financial sharing, to learning how to sustain closeness, make room for friends and family, and compromise around leisure activities. Some of these issues may pose special challenges for the lesbian couple.

According to the NLHCS (Alexander, 1996), the most common concern for lesbian women under age 55 was money. This finding should not surprise us when we recall that women are still paid considerably less than men for their work. Women also comprise a disproportionate number of those Americans living below the poverty level. It follows, then, that a couple comprised of two women might struggle with money. Furthermore, heterosexual couples can more easily fall back upon cultural norms about how money will be managed or shared, while in lesbian couples precedents are less available, and issues such as dealing with highly discrepant incomes between two women can be troubling and difficult to negotiate.

Sharing Income: Alison and Lea

Alison and Lea came to therapy complaining that they had drifted apart. Alison was angry at Lea for what she saw as her overinvolvement with work. Lea, who had endured many losses in her own life, worked as chief social worker on the children's ward of a cancer treatment center. She loved her patients and her social work staff, but was frustrated with the hospital setting in which she worked. She had many serious political disagreements with hospital management. Some of her late-night and weekend work related to dying children, and some of it stemmed from administrative and policy impasses within the hospital that she felt compelled to address. She made a good income, but had no savings or investments.

Alison was a highly paid manager in a corporate setting. She earned an excellent income and also benefited from a small trust fund. Alison loved her work but she could easily leave it behind her at night. She had weekends and vacations free to travel. She wanted more companionship from her partner and yearned for a more playful and spontaneous relationship. Both women were gifted with intelligence and a witty sense of humor. Their therapist could see that the energy between them was potentially very vibrant.

Lea admitted that she wanted the same changes in the relationship that her partner did, but she also noted that she could not begin to imagine limiting the time she worked because of the number of people who depended upon her and because of the life-and-death nature of the work itself. She confessed that she was exhausted and beginning to become somewhat depressed.

In the first session, the couple easily agreed to a simple goal of committing to a certain evening in the week to devote to the relationship, which would involve cooking and eating a meal together, then simply talking, making love, or reading side by side. They planned to spend some weekend time together as well, attending a film festival they were both enthusiastic about. Since they wanted the same thing, it seemed that they had simply needed the support of a therapist to talk it over and make a plan.

But 2 weeks later they arrived for their second session angry and frustrated. None of the scheduled activities had taken place: Lea had been busy with a crisis at work, had worked most of the weekend, and seemed to be coming down with a cold as well. Alison blamed Lea for not carrying through with the plan. Lea blamed Alison for not being more understanding, particularly given the unexpected death of an apparently recovering child on her unit over the weekend.

The session ultimately became a moving one in which Lea explored her difficulty separating from job demands and both women began to see how unresolved losses in Lea's life led her to lose her boundaries in the work setting. She cried as she told again stories of her brother's lingering and painful death a few years earlier and the loss of both parents in her young adulthood. The couple left the session with the original problem as yet unsolved, but feeling closer. Alison seemed relieved simply to feel more deeply connected to Lea again.

In the third session, Alison spoke first, directing her remarks to her partner: "I want to know if you would consider resigning from your job and letting me support you while you think through what you want to do next. I think you need time off for a rest. I think the political problems at your work are chronic and unsolvable, and I think the work is too emotionally draining. If, after some time off, you find you want to go back to school to study something new, I will help you pay for it. Are you willing?" Lea was stunned. She could not comprehend her partner's generosity. She wasn't sure she believed it! The two women had always kept their money entirely separate. They had two separate checking accounts and split every bill exactly in half. It had been a sort of political decision, aimed at ensuring equality within the relationship.

For the next several sessions the therapist helped the women talk through the implications of this radical proposal. How would it change the relationship? Would it somehow give Alison more power to determine the couple's direction? Would Lea feel like the "wife," the "kept woman"? Would Alison grow to feel resentful of Lea's financial dependence? Would Alison be judgmental of Lea's wish to spend money, for example, on gifts for her family? The women and their therapist wondered aloud how this dilemma might feel different if the couple were a man and a woman. Would a man support a woman more easily, and would she accept such support as a matter of course? Would they worry about the power implications of the arrangement? Or if the woman was offering to support the man, would the relationship be more threatened?

In the seventh session the couple ended therapy. Lea had decided to take at least the summer off and had submitted her resignation at work. They agreed to return to therapy if problems arose from the new plan. A follow-up call 2 years later revealed that Lea had taken almost a year off. Subsequently, she graduated from a yoga teacher training program that Alison paid for and began to teach yoga in their home. Alison was still providing most of the couples' financial support and they both reported that they were doing well and feeling comfortable with their financial arrangement.

Sex: Good News/Bad News

Lesbian sexuality has been viewed across extremes of sexual caricature: from the male fantasy world of lesbian erotica where lesbians are nymphomaniacal sex bunnies, to the endless dirge of "lesbian bed death" in the lesbian literature.

The myth of lesbian bed death is one commonly held by therapists who treat lesbian couples, as well as by many lesbian couples themselves. According to this belief, sexual activity diminishes greatly or disappears altogether after the early years of a lesbian relationship. Seeming to confirm this idea was a study by Blumstein and Schwartz (1983) who found that lesbian couples report having "less sex" than heterosexual or gay male couples and that "frequency" declines as relationship length increases. But as Suzanne Iasenza (1995) notes, "Perhaps the most problematic element in sex research discourse is the definition of sex as a measurable unit of some sort of genital contact usually including orgasm of at least one of the partners, a definition that is much more user-friendly for males" (p. 357). In other words, in measuring frequency of sexual contact between lesbians, what exactly does the researcher count? Marilyn Frye (1991) comments, "Do lesbian couples 'have sex' less frequently than heterosexual couples? I'd say that lesbian couples 'have sex' a great deal less frequently than heterosexual couples; by the criteria . . . most heterosexual people use to count 'times,' lesbians don't have sex at all. No male orgasms, no 'times' " (pp. 2–3). Frye goes on to recommend that we develop new nonheterosexist language to describe sexual activity between women.

We do need to create a vocabulary for lesbian sexual expression that captures its frequently sensuous, flowing, rather continuous nature, in contrast to the episodic, more orgasmically punctuated lovemaking of heterosexual couples. The concept of lesbian bed death may have arisen in part from the imposition of heterosexual definitions of "sex" upon the experiences of women couples. Unfortunately, the concept itself may have led to resignation on the part of temporarily sexually inactive couples.

In contrast to the negative findings of Blumstein and Schwartz, other studies are more optimistic. Coleman, Hoon, and Hoon (1983) reported that lesbians experience a *higher* frequency of sex and are more sexually arousable than heterosexual women. Iasenza (1995) found lesbians to be more sexually arousable as well as more sexually assertive. Bressler and Lavender (1986) found that lesbian women and heterosexual women experience equal frequency of orgasm.

Iasenza (1999) has argued that the concept of lesbian bed death should be abandoned entirely. Certainly, the promulgation of this idea creates a kind of self-fulfilling negative prophecy, harmful and discouraging to any couple who might be suffering a temporary diminishment of desire.

Nonetheless, as the couple enters the "ongoing couplehood" stage, the task of developing a sustained sexual commitment may challenge the sexual understandings of each woman. Now that they have passed the falling-in-love stage, what kind of sexual closeness will be maintained? How does real life alter the delicious love and romance of the courtship period? Which member of the couple is the first to say she's too tired after a long day of work to make love?

Our advice to therapists working with lesbian couples who have become celibate is to gently suggest that the couple resume their love making, planning a day and time to do so, and using the safety of therapy to explore any specific emotional content that emerges from the process. In our clinical experience, an intervention as simple as suggesting that the couple resume their love making and then return to therapy to talk about it has cured the difficulty for many couples. In these cases the pleasure itself seems to be a significant enough reinforcer to keep the couple sexually engaged. In more complicated situations, it is still important that the therapist avoid reinforcing the myth that celibacy is inevitable and instead communicate the idea that the couple is entitled to as full and rich a sexual experience as they desire. The book *Lesbian Sex* by JoAnn Loulan (1984) has long been a standard guide for assisting couples in resuming sexual activity and includes homework exercises that many couples have found helpful.

Bisexuality: Leslie and Sara

Leslie and Sara told their therapist that while they were still very committed to each other, they were in crisis. Leslie was experiencing a strong sexual attraction to a man she worked with and was feeling very tempted to act on these feelings. Sara was angry, hurt, and afraid that their relationship was ending. "But it's not about you," Leslie reassured Sara repeatedly in their therapy sessions. But both the therapist and Sara felt that it was, to some extent, "about" Sara—or at least about their relationship.

"Is it because we don't make love as often as we used to?" Sara asked. "The sexual part of our relationship hasn't been the center of things like it used to be," Leslie replied, "but I love you more than ever. My feelings for Roger are just about me, my bisexuality. At least I'm not attracted to other women. Can't you just accept that I have these sexual feelings for men and that I even might have to act on them once in awhile. It's not about us."

The range of sexual feelings and preferences that women experience are not dichotomously "lesbian" or "heterosexual," but rather form a continuum from exclusively lesbian to exclusively heterosexual. The work the therapist did with this couple was to help them become more mindful about their sexual identities, desires, ethics, and practices. They had come to a stage of relationship in which some decisions had to be made. What kind of commitment were they each ready to make to each other? What kind of sexual life were they going to shape together? Would they agree to be monogamous? Would they compromise on the frequency and range of sexual activities? And what did it mean to them as a couple that Leslie was so clear in identifying her bisexual desires?

There is an intense debate in the gay–lesbian political community as to whether gays and lesbians really have a choice about their sexual orientation. Some research indicates that gay men, and possibly lesbians too, have clear biological differences from heterosexuals that may determine their sexual orientation from birth. Many lesbians, however, believe that for them the choice is more determined by nurture than by nature. The issues are complex, but what seems relevant now is how contemporary lesbians couples are affected by the bisexual option. For the therapist, it may be very important to determine whether each woman has the same political views about bisexuality. Unlike a heterosexual couple, where men tend to be either titillated or at least not deeply threatened by the woman's bisexual potential, for many lesbians the bisexual option is threatening and shameful. The shame may be connected to internalized homophobia: "She'd rather be with a man—I'm not as good as a man, I'm not a legitimate partner. . . . "

For Leslie and Sara, the central question in this stage of the couple's life cycle is whether or not Leslie's bisexual desires will be enacted and whether or not her attraction to a man is related to what is happening in the couple's sexual life. Sara needed to explore what Leslie's sexuality meant for her. Did this diminish her desirability? Did she need to be more "butch" in their sexual activities? Was it really true—for her—that Leslie's feelings about the man at work had nothing to do with the couple's degree of love and commitment?

Sex and Childhood Trauma

As their conversations deepened, it seemed that Sara brought challenging issues of her own into the couple's sexual life. Sara was a survivor of childhood sexual abuse. At the beginning of their courtship, she had felt more sexually open with Leslie than with any previous partner (Sara was exclusively lesbian in her previous intimate relationships). But as the couple moved into this stage of ongoing couplehood, more of her sexual inhibitions returned. She felt less like making love and became more restrictive in the types of sexual activities she was able to enjoy.

As in many lesbian couples, Leslie and Sara's female socialization to be other-oriented caused a powerful mutual sensitivity to the sexual wishes of each other. Leslie did not want to push Sara sexually and so she silently acquiesced to what she perceived to be Sara's sexual schedule and behavioral restrictions. This, of course, left more room for her sexual desires to grow in another direction. Because she knew about Sara's history of sexual abuse, she felt that it would be wrong to talk to her about either their own diminishing sexual activity or to confide in her about her own heterosexual fantasies.

Another difference between heterosexual and lesbian couples is the impact of sexual trauma upon intimacy. Since young girls are more frequently violated than young boys, and since a lesbian couple is comprised of two women, the statistical probability that one or both members of a lesbian couple may be survivors of sexual abuse (Kerewsky & Miller, 1996) is high. In the NLHCS mentioned above, 37% of the lesbians surveyed reported having been harshly beaten or physically abused in childhood at least once and 19% reported a history of incest (Alexander, 1996). This prevalence matches the average rates of abuse and incest among all women (Kerewsky & Miller, 1996). Thus, an individual lesbian is no more likely to have been abused as a child than an individual heterosexual woman, but the relationship of two women is more likely to bear trauma than the relationship of a man and a woman.

The picture is even more complex then the above figures suggest. Being more likely to bear the scars of abuse upon intimacy, lesbian couples may suffer. However, in heterosexual couples the woman replicates sexual intimacy with a male, a person likely to be of the same gender as her abuser. Thus, the lesbian couple with trauma may have the liberating advantage in sex and intimacy.

Fortunately, their therapist was able to help Leslie and Sara talk about all of these issues. For at least the period of time it would take to work out their future commitment, they agreed that Leslie would not act on her heterosexual desires and that they would remain sexually monogamous. They also made a commitment to work on talking more openly about their sexual relationship and trying to understand more together about how Sara's abuse history influenced their sexual life.

Cultural Prohibitions, Isolation, and the Closet: Gloria and Maria

It is much harder to stay in the closet when you are with a lover, and now partners have to negotiate how and whether they will be out to family, friends, colleagues, etc.

—SLATER (1997, p. 21)

Gloria and Maria, a Latina couple, don't live together because they are forced to be very closeted. Maria's family could not accept her orientation because of their devout religious convictions. And Gloria is equally fearful of being outed because she is a teacher in a predominantly Hispanic school.

Being forced to remain in the closet at this stage of their ongoing relationship creates many hardships for these two women. Maria has to take care of an aging parent by herself because the couple believes that they can't risk the visibility of living together. Living by herself is also very hard for Gloria because she would like to be an equal partner in sharing Maria's sizable burden.

At this stage of ongoing couplehood, a closeted couple may become so isolated that they develop an insular "you and me against the world" life that doesn't allow them to draw on the support of a community. The tasks of working out intimacy issues, living arrangements, the integration of each other's families and friends, and the like are complicated by the degree of isolation the couple faces. Gloria and Maria are not completely at peace with their sexual orientation. A lifetime of cultural prohibitions continue to take their toll. Any couple, but especially closeted couples, may be struggling with internalized homophobia.

Therapists need to help clients sort out what may be a distinctly gay–lesbian couple issue, that is, being visible in a same-sex couple, versus the issues that could affect any couple where one person (or both) fears a deeper commitment.

THE MIDDLE YEARS

For many lesbian couples in the third stage of the couple life cycle, the primary issues may be very similar to those faced by heterosexual and/or gay couples. Many are buying houses, planning vacations, working out financial arrangements, deepening friendships with other couples, and settling into life as a couple. Many lesbian couples are concerned with issues of childbearing or childrearing.

At this stage of life it is important for lesbian couples to consider legal planning to ensure that their rights as a couple are fully protected. Will one woman take out a life insurance policy and name her partner as the beneficiary? If one woman dies prematurely, will she leave her estate or some part of it to her partner? Who owns the home? Is the surviving partner entitled to live there? In the case of accident or terminal illness, who makes decisions about life-support measures? Is a woman even permitted to visit an ill or dying partner if the family of origin or offpring disagrees? These and many other questions can trouble the lives of same-sex couples with no legal standing as life partners. In the case of breakup, how will assets be divided with no formal divorce process to structure the decisions? Therapists would be wise to encourage lesbian couples to take legal measures to ensure that their rights are fully protected. Legal agreements are critical to the lesbian couple, for nothing will be automatically assumed by society about the women's entitlements. Lesbian couples should have wills, health-care proxies, and all the rest.

Choosing Children

Becoming Pregnant: Gina and Fran

Many lesbian couples are choosing to have children. Certainly, the basic fact that the lesbian parental team is comprised of two women makes this enterprise significantly different from the parenting of heterosexual couples. One might assume that it must be much easier for two women to coparent—after all, women have been coparenting with their sisters, aunts, and mothers throughout history. Indeed, this is another significant strength of the lesbian coparenting couple, that two adults both socialized to caretake children can often do this very well.

Another strength of the lesbian couple with children can be that they are making a conscious choice to adopt or become pregnant, and often making this choice at a later age than the average heterosexual couple. And there is also the possibility that both parents can become pregnant, eliminating some of the issues associated with the potentially disengaged father.

Gina and Fran, a couple in their mid-30s, chose alternative insemination as the method of creating their family. The fact that Gina is the biological mother has been a difficult issue. Fran fully expected to be as completely involved in parenting as her partner. But after their daughter, Beatrice, was born, Fran began to feel excluded from the mother-child dyad despite what Gina did to try to prevent this. Fran told friends that she felt an alienation or envy similar to any male parent; in fact, she thought she felt a little worse because she didn't even have the role or status as "father." What would Bea call her? As time passed, issues arose about how Fran was viewed by teachers, pediatricians, and other parents in relation to the child. According to the law, Fran did not even have the right to pick up their daughter at school. (In most states only one woman in the couple can legally adopt a nonbirth child; when there is a father in the picture, the lesbian partner may not be able to adopt the birth child of her partner).

Just before Bea entered first grade, Fran and Gina consulted a lesbian family therapist about their complicated issues around parenting. With the therapist's help they made some simple decisions about how they would deal with the public schools. They decided to meet with Bea's teachers before the beginning of each school year, specifically to introduce their family and make suggestions to the teacher about how their family form could be acknowledged positively in the classroom. They committed to follow up informally with the teacher throughout the year. It seemed to the therapist that Gina and Fran's decision to deal with the schools in such a proactive way helped to unify the couple and soften some of the more subtle feelings between them about how to feel equally involved with Bea as two moms.

Adopting: Pam and Sue

When Pam and Sue adopted two little girls, aged 5 and 6, there were many issues to consider. There was much careful planning and preparation to help the children negotiate the heterosexual world, as well as to adjust to their new home, new community, and belonging to a family. It wasn't until the girls were a few years older that the fact of their living in a lesbian family actually became of interest to them. Both seemed to easily accept the knowledge that the majority of children in school with them had heterosexual parents while they had lesbian parents. The younger child went through a phase of proudly announcing to complete strangers at every opportunity that she had two mothers. What has become painful for the girls and their mothers are those occasions when other children tease them about having lesbian parents.

This version of societal homophobia creates stresses for the couple. In their efforts to protect the children, they work harder than most parents to make sure that their children are well adjusted, well socialized, and well behaved. Parenting older children who came into the family with serious attachment issues becomes even more complicated when enactments of homophobia are added to the picture. Many lesbian parents are raising the most challenging children (older children, addicted babies, children from other cultures) because healthy American infants are adopted by heterosexual couples, whom most agencies continue to prefer.

Pam and Sue are strong parents to their two daughters, but they desperately needed consistent support from their families and their friends. Many lesbian couples raising children are less fortunate because they lack the support of family because of family rejection. Lesbian parents raising children in isolation face double the challenges of most heterosexual couples. Yet they can also be viewed through the gender lens as having (potentially) double the resources: because both partner parents are adults who have been socialized to raise and nurture children. As more and more lesbian couples openly raise children together, researchers will be able to give us more answers about how these couples and their children fare.

GENERATIVITY

The lesbian couple at the stage of generativity is generally less focused on dynamics within the couple and more concerned with dealing with external events. For example, career changes may introduce geographical or financial challenges. And if the couple enters the generativity stage during the midlife years, they may also be facing biological changes, such as menopause, the aging process in general, or the impact of serious illness. If they have raised children, the couple may be concerned with the wellbeing of their young adult children. All of these issues would seem to be the same for heterosexual or even gay couples at this life stage as well. Even the fears of aging and mortality that lead to affairs at this stage may be common to all three types of couples. Only by applying the gender lens do the differences become more visible.

Affairs: Alice and Mary

Alice and Mary were always the most glamorous couple at lesbian gatherings in their community. Alice, the slender boyish blond, and Mary, the dark voluptuous femme, consciously accentuated their stylistic differences. They were "the beautiful people," always up on the latest hairstyles, clothes, music, and dances. They were entertaining. They were charming in their visible devotion to each other. Their condominium was large, beautifully decorated, and in the most up-and-coming, gentrifying neighborhood. Each woman was well established in her career. Over the years they had been politically active, supporting the local women's health center, serving on boards and committees of various gay and lesbian causes. They had long-standing friendships in the community. It would seem that this was the proverbial couple who "had it all."

The community was shocked when Mary suddenly began a very public affair. After a flurry of confusion about who was to blame, the community sided with Alice. The affair became everyone's business. "How could she have done this?" was the indignant question circling at lesbian dinner parties.

Why did this affair become everyone's business? Why did a normally open-minded community take one woman's side against the other? Why, indeed, did Mary have an affair when she and Alice appeared to have come so far in establishing a successful couple relationship?

When a lesbian couple reaches the stage of generativity and then splits apart, it can be threatening to other lesbians. This may be due to the female ideal of remaining mutually attuned to the needs of the other. An affair threatens the belief that women will always protect each other within the relationship. There is also a yearning among many lesbians to believe that our relationships are as strong, healthy, and long lasting as those of the dominant heterosexual culture. Without the sanction of marriage and the presence of children, the lesbian couple has to work harder to legitimate its union. There are not the same external supports to keep the couple protected as a unit. Thus, when a couple splits up after all that has seemed to establish its permanency, it is shocking and threatening to other lesbians. The role models have fallen from grace.

Perhaps this "classic" midlife crisis was not so different for this lesbian couple than it would have been if Mary had been partnered with a man. Mary may have felt that an affair would make her feel younger, less aware of her mortality. But what makes this scenario *different* for the lesbian couple? There is the likelihood that both women are feeling the impact of menopause. This hormonal storm can certainly create stress that threatens a couple's serenity. Another more positive difference is that there may be less possibility that one woman will leave the other financially devastated, since the earning power of two women is often roughly equivalent. The woman who has the affair is also less likely to leave her partner for a much younger woman, unlike the classic midlife heterosexual couple where the wife is supplanted by a young "trophy" bride.

At the urging of their friends, Mary and Alice agreed to consult a therapist. The therapy was brief, and helped the women to clarify with each other that the relationship was indeed ending. In the first session, Mary took the lead. She used the safety of the therapist's office to tell Alice more about the details of her infidelity. She spoke with sadness and regret but with firmness about her own conviction that the relationship with Alice needed to end. Alice, who had expected the session to initiate a new beginning for the couple, was devastated. She seemed shocked and stunned. At first it seemed that she would flee the session, but with the therapist's help she was able to remain. She gradually began to express the anger that was now consuming her. The therapist struggled to contain the growing intensity of the session. With 20 minutes remaining, she directed the women to plan a temporary separation. Alice elected to move to the home of a mutual friend until some plans could be worked out about living arrangements, and Mary agreed not to use the home she and Alice had shared for any contact with her new lover. A second session was scheduled in 3 days' time.

In the second, third, and fourth sessions, the therapist helped the couple settle more of the details of their separation. In addition, she gradually helped them to tell the story of how they had grown apart emotionally. As with any divorcing couple, they could recall turning points, fights that had been allowed to go underground. In addition, it seemed that alcohol had been a factor in weakening the connection between them during the early years. Although both women were now nondrinkers, they could see that the early foundation building of their relationship had been compromised. The work was sad and painful but also somehow oddly relieving. As the couple came to terms with the necessary ending, their community seemed to begin to accept the breakup as well, with less "splitting" or taking sides.

In the fifth session, the couples work ended. It seemed that for each woman, the personal emphasis needed to be on her own next steps and personal understanding of what she had learned about herself from the relationship. The therapist offered to see each woman once individually to work on integrating what the couple therapy had taught her, and did so. Alice had already begun a new individual therapy relationship, and the couple therapist provided a referral for Mary so that she could do the same.

Couples over 65

While many of the issues affecting older lesbian couples are the same as those affecting older heterosexual or gay couples, there are likely to be a few significant differences. As noted earlier, because of the legal and cultural non-recognition of the relationship, there are often disastrous consequences in regard to property, hospital visitation privileges, and a variety of "next-of-kin" decisions related to medical procedures, life supports, and funeral arrangements.

Celebrating a Life Together

Phyllis Lyon and Del Martin are a well-known lesbian couple, now living in San Francisco, who are enjoying a full and wonderful life together. Both are in their 70s, and continue to work together as writers and political activists just as they have done for decades. As young women in the 1950s they founded the first national lesbian organization in the United States (and perhaps the world), the Daughters of Bilitis. They published an early, important nonfiction book about lesbians, *Lesbian/Woman* (Martin & Lyon, 1972/1983), and changed the image of lesbians from that of sad lonely sisters of the "love that dare not speak its name" variety to positive, healthy women who enjoyed their lives.

Their social activism has not been only on behalf of lesbians. Del Martin (1976) also wrote the first book about battered women, a book that brought the battered woman out of her closet of shame and fear. Currently Phyllis and Del are very busily engaged in social justice activities concerning ageism, focusing especially on the oppression of older lesbians and gay men. They work at both the local and the national level, writing, speaking, and helping to develop social structures that support the needs of these elders.

When Paki Wieland and Dusty Miller interviewed them for a planned book on resilient elders and social activism, they were touched and inspired by their profound connection. The interdependence of their lives is as visibly sturdy as the roots of trees that have grown together. When we asked them questions, their sentences flowed together with the grace of a seasoned dance team. We videotaped our second meeting with them, and noticed how much they also move together in nonverbal synchrony. When we asked Phyllis and Del what kept them so energetically involved in all their work projects, they both said, "Because it's fun!"

And this may be the secret of joy for many lesbian couples who make it through to this life stage together: two women can, with luck, grow into old age together and remain physically, sexually, mentally, and emotionally vibrant. Because of the difference in how men and women tend to age, the lesbian couple may live on longer and be less likely to face a long period of bereavement. And because of women's capacity for vitality in old age, they may experience the retirement years together as a long wonderful adventure.

CELEBRATING DIFFERENCE

For those of us who are in lesbian couples and/or who provide help to them, it is important to be sensitive to and informed about the continuum of similarity and difference between this group and the two-gendered couples many of us see more frequently. As the "rules break" and we discard our maps "out of date by years," we must be attuned to the new patterns and forms as they emerge, while remembering that much about intimate life will be the same, regardless of gender. For example, we must be able to discern those couples for whom race or developmental stage or class is more salient than sexual orientation or gender. We must appreciate the powerful impact of homophobia and heterosexism.

In closing, we offer again the observation that an attitude of *celebrating* the differences, the freedom, the empowerment, the lack of cultural constraint lesbian couples may experience is often the most helpful way to proceed.

REFERENCES

Alexander, C. (1996). The state of lesbian mental health. *In the Family, 1*(3), 6–26.

Blumstein, P., & Schwartz, P. (1983). *American couples: Money, work, and sex.* New York: Morrow.

Bressler, L. C., & Lavender, A. D. (1986). Sexual fulfillment of heterosexual and homosexual women. In M. Kehoe (Ed.), *Historical, literary, and erotic aspects of lesbianism* (pp. 109–122). New York: Haworth Press.

Coleman, E. M., Hoon, P. W., & Hoon, E. F. (1983). Arousability and sexual satisfaction in lesbian and heterosexual women. *Journal of Sex Research, 19*(1), 58–73.

Frye, M. (1991). Lesbian "sex." In J. Barrington (Ed.), *An intimate wildness: Lesbian writers on sexuality.* Portland: Eighth Mountain Press.

Gair, S. R. (1995). The false self, shame, and the challenge of self-cohesion. In J. M. Glassgold & S. Iasenza (Eds.), *Lesbians and psychoanalysis* (pp. 107–123). New York: Free Press.

Glassgold, J. M., & Iasenza, S. (1995). *Lesbians and psychoanalysis.* New York: Free Press.

Green, R., Bettinger, M., & Zachs, E. (1996). Are lesbian couples fused and gay male couples disengaged?: Questioning gender straightjackets. In J. Laird & R. J. Green (Eds.), *Lesbians and gays in couples and families* (pp. 185–230). San Francisco: Jossey-Bass.

Iasenza, S. (1995). Platonic pleasures and dangerous desires: Psychoanalytic theory, sex research, and lesbian sexuality. In J. M. Glassgold & S. Iasenza (Eds.), *Lesbians and psychoanalysis* (pp. 345–373). New York: Free Press.

Iasenza, S. (1999). Myth of lesbian bed death. *In the family.*

Kerewsky, S., & Miller, D. (1996). Lesbian couples and childhood trauma: Guidelines for therapists. In J. Laird & R. J. Green (Eds.), *Lesbians and gays in couples and families* (pp. 298–315). San Francisco: Jossey-Bass.

Klineberg, S., & Zorn, P. (1995). "Rekindling the flame." In J. M. Glassgold & S. Iasenza (Eds.), *Lesbians and psychoanalysis* (pp. 125–143). New York: Free Press.

Loulan, J. (1984). *Lesbian sex.* Minneapolis: Spinster's Ink.

Martin, D. (1976). *Battered wives.* San Francisco: Glide.

Martin, D., & Lyon, P. (1983). *Lesbian/woman.* New York: Bantam. (Original work published 1972)

Mencher, J. (1997). Intimacy in lesbian relationships: A critical reexamination of fusion. In J. V. Jordan (Ed.), *Women's growth in diversity: More writings from the Stone Center* (pp. 311–330). New York: Guilford Press.

Rich, A. (1978). *The dream of a common language.* New York: Norton.

Slater, S. (1995). *The lesbian family life cycle.* New York: Free Press.

Slater, S. (1997). Normalizing lesbian relationships. *In the family.* October issue.

CHAPTER 12

Remarriage

Redesigning Couplehood

Anne C. Bernstein

More than 200 years ago, Samuel Johnson summed up the traditional view of remarriage, an attitude that prevails into our own times: On the one hand, the widower who takes a second wife "pays the highest compliment to the first, by shewing that she made him so happy as a married man, that he wishes to be so a second time" (1769). On the other hand, Johnson opined, the remarriage of "a gentleman who had been very unhappy in marriage" (in our own day presumably one whose first marriage ended in a divorce) demonstrates "the triumph of hope over experience" (1770). Whether for good or ill, whether wise or foolish, both such views—besides ignoring the experience of the wives in question—frame marriage as a fixed, unitary phenomenon, with clear and specific roles, rules, and normative expectations, which one successively attempts to reproduce irrespective of the personhood of one's partner.

But remarriage, even more than first marriage, involves a deconstruction of the institution of marriage itself. First marriages that do not endure teach their participants that cultural ideas about the ideal marriage that ignore context, time, and place—a one size fits all off-the-rack style of being married—may not fit the changed conditions of contemporary life. Instead contemporary remarriage is and can be a more improvisational endeavor, with successive marriages differing from one another as developmental, sociocultural, and economic forces alter the contexts in which they occur.

In *Brave New Families*, Judith Stacey (1990) describes the decline of the modern family as a response to postindustrial economic conditions, including the shift away from productive employment and the failure of most jobs to pay a "family wage." Without this economic base, the gendered roles that are the linchpins of the modern family cannot be sustained, making the "modern" family "old-fashioned." Stacey describes the "postmodern" family as "a normless gender order . . . in which parenting arrangements, sexuality, and the distribution of work, responsibility, and resources are all negotiable and constantly renegotiable" (p. 258). The postmodern perspective embraces uncertainty and doubt; old patterns or ideas are implicitly discarded or radically transformed, while the shape and significance of what is to follow remains unfathomable. In employing this concept to characterize changing family and gender arrangements, Stacey's ethnography illustrates that "no longer is there a single culturally dominant family pattern to which the majority of Americans conform and most of the rest aspire" (p. 17).

Think back to the days of our grandparents and great-grandparents, nearly midway between Samuel Johnson's times and our own: Grandpa wanted a wife, and everyone knew what wives did. Grandma wanted a husband, and everyone knew what husbands could be expected to do. For most couples, those who had to work for a living, wives and husbands were busy all the waking day earning their bread, keeping the house, raising children, and tending to aged and ill family members. Friendships were often centered within kinship groups and were confined to same-sex cohorts. Marriage was the only socially acceptable context in which to relate sexually, at least for women. Happiness and personal fulfillment, while always appreciated, were considered an added blessing, not a bottom-line requirement.

Fast forward to the dawn of the 21st century: wives and husbands are each juggling multiple roles in two-paycheck households in which housekeeping and child care, while still falling disproportionally on women's shoulders, are frequently subject to negotiation, and assumptions about who is expected to do what are increasingly challenged. Residential patterns include frequent relocations, with 16–21% of Americans changing domiciles each year for the past 50 years (U.S. Bureau of the Census, 1997). Friendships that develop in the workplace cross sex lines, and socializing with kin, while valued, consumes less leisure time. Sexual relationships outside of marriage are talked about openly and without shame, both in ordinary daily life and in the media. The ideology of marriage has shifted from a spiritually sanctioned utilitarian contract to a means of personal fulfillment. Marriage is for "love" and when one is no longer "in love," neither economic necessity nor social sanction has the tensile strength to bind together couples whose members may yearn to try again to realize their romantic ideal.

Therapy with remarried couples is not so much a question of technique as a way of engaging with the discourse about family life that "disrupts or relaxes ... the complex network of presuppositions" (James & McIntyre, 1989) that create distress and foreclose possibilities. This chapter examines the social changes that contextualize remarriage (shorthand for recoupling, with or without legal sanction), examining how demographic changes alter the cultural meaning of recoupling, how mate selection differs when prior unions have ended in separation and divorce, and how changing gender roles get revised in the remarriage roulette. Family therapists need to take into consideration how remarriages differ based on whether it is the second or subsequent partnership for one party or both, and whether one or both bring children—minor or grown—to form a stepfamily. The "new extended family" created by serial marriage, and continuing relationships among the formerly coupled and their kin, create still additional therapeutic challenges, inviting clinicians to question traditional beliefs about what constitutes a family and how to be a couple whose kin networks radiate in multiple concentric circles.

THE SOCIAL CHANGES

Change: Remarriage as Normative

The last U.S. Census results indicate that 56–60% of all first marriages end in divorce, and an additional 5% end in separation (Bumpass, Martin & Sweet, 1991; Norton & Miller, 1992). About 72–75% of divorced individuals go on to remarry, most within 2 to 3 years, with the result that 40% of all marriages in the United States are a remarriage for one or both adults (Bumpass, Sweet, & Martin, 1990). Of these, 60% will go on to redivorce within 5 years (Norton & Miller, 1992). On average, these remarriages that end in divorce are of shorter duration than dissolved first marriages (7.25 years vs. 11 years; National Center for Health Statistics, 1995). When we count the number of couples who live together without marrying, either because marriage is unavailable for same-sex couples or because heterosexuals elect not to marry again or ever, we are looking at more than half of the committed couples sharing a household in a second or later such arrangement.

Thus, it has become "normal" to remarry. Statistically speaking, the "norm" is the mean, the average in a numerical distribution; in sociological language, "norms" refer to expectations about behavior. With the demographic increase in remarriage, serial monogamy has become normal in other senses: "usual, routine, ordinary, typical, standard, customary, prevalent." Can the remaining meanings, "sane" and "healthy," be far behind? A *New Yorker* cartoon depicts this destigmatization of remarriage in popular culture: a woman talking with a man at a cocktail party tells him, "Oh, I've had a few failures, followed by a string of successful marriages."

This is not to say that the experience of couple dissolution is not profoundly painful for most and that many do not see the end of a committed relationship as a failure—whether one's own, one's partner's, or a mutual defeat. Be that as it may, the power of numbers, specifically the knowledge that legions of others have made similar steps and missteps, exponentially reduces the social stigma of divorce. Increasingly, despite widespread cultural ambivalence about this being the case, couples even in first marriages may repeat their wedding vows with an unspoken coda: "If it doesn't work out, we can always try again."

Couples and their therapists confront a diverse universe of competing values about divorce and remarriage in disentangling how these themes are constructed in both personal and shared narratives. In the life story of the remarried individual, how does the cultural context, the weltanshauung of oneself and one's demographic cohort, commingle with beliefs about personality and individual accountability to make sense of these biographical events? With changing expectations of marriage as an institution and the increased plasticity of gender expectations about how "husband" and "wife" are framed as marital roles, the permutations abound.

Change: Optional Marriage, for Companionship, Not Survival

With increased social acceptance of divorce, the question of whether to stay together when distressed and conflicted about the relationship presents couples and therapists with increasingly ambiguous choices. When persevering in marriage is experienced as discretionary, how does one sort out whether to stay or to go, to work through issues in couple therapy or to try to meet one's relational needs elsewhere? When divorce no longer connotes moral failure or irresponsibility, how then to understand its meaning for a couple and the individuals who are its members?

Just as divorce and remarriage have become normative, marriage is increasingly seen as optional, a "lifestyle" choice rather than the only viable way to be an adult in society. As noted earlier, there has been a shift away from instrumental and role-governed definitions of marriage to models that center on companionship, relatedness, and emotional connection. These changes in how marriage is conceptualized, both culturally and by its participants, raise questions of purpose, meaning, and functioning for which there are no easy answers: Why get married? What is marriage for? How does it work, and for whom? And, central to the focus of this chapter, How is marriage different when there is a change in partner? While the extent to which these questions are part of interior monologues or couple dialogue may vary from community to community, across cultural groups, and among social classes, the need to define the new collectivity and to negotiate among systems of social and personal meaning is part of the remarital contract.

Therapeutic Task: Creating Another, Different Marriage

Most of the remarriage literature focuses on those couples with children from prior relationships for whom remarriage creates a stepfamily. But even without children, remarriage differs from a first marriage. It is difficult, however, to differentiate among maturity, having a different partner, and having been married before as factors in creating that difference. Being older, and often wiser, having worked through personal issues identified in the past as problematic, can contribute to one's preparedness for a more reciprocal partnership. Being partnered with a different spouse may elicit different aspects of self, evoking alternate relational capacities that bypass past pitfalls. And having been socialized as a spouse can help to make accommodations that were abrasive the first time around more easily negotiated—as one wife said of her former husband, "I trained my first husband to be a decent second husband."

First, and most universally, there is the loss of the belief in marriage as "happily ever after." While an enduring marriage remains a goal, forever-ness is no longer seen as inevitable. For the widowed, the fragility of life itself underlines the finiteness of any human relationship. For the divorced, losing a marriage emphatically illustrates that affective bonds can be mercurial; those feeling betrayed by a former partner may face great difficulty in trusting another, while searching for assurance that it can be different this time.

The altered state of consciousness known as "being in love" may itself be suspect, viewed now as a transitory state rather than as an enduring basis on which to build a life together. Determined to learn from experience, the formerly married sometimes deliberately set about to take a radically different course than their previous one. Those who married for love that later soured may choose a new partner according to more pragmatic and reasoned criteria, whereas those whose practical or expedient matches left them feeling empty may look to romance and passion in their selection of a partner. John, for example, described having a great deal of ambivalence about entering into his first marriage at 28: when his then-girlfriend had insisted they break up or marry, he had decided to go ahead because they got along, had similar backgrounds, and "it felt like time to marry." Twenty years later, he contrasts his former marriage to the relationship he has with his fiancée, a passionate connection that has taught him, he says, "what the relationship between a man and a woman is all about." Conversely, "Married Prince Charming," as one woman signed herself in writing to "Dear Abby" (Van Buren, 1998), tried to console a fellow reader who had complained of a marriage to a decent man who was not and never had been her "soul mate" by reporting that her own "soul mate," married decades earlier as "the greatest love in the history of the world," was now someone she neither loved nor liked.

Perhaps most pivotal in terms of making a remarriage more satisfying than its predecessor, the formerly married know some things about living with a partner: what it is like to share space and to confront differences in needs, wants, and preferences about how to live. They may be more able to distinguish how they themselves contribute to marital dynamics, having learned something about self-in-relationship: after all, when a change of partner does not bring with it a change of fortune, it is more difficult to consistently blame one's partner for life's disappointments. And they may be more ready to dispense with the romantic ideal that one person can fulfill every interpersonal need and complement every facet of oneself; instead they may be more ready to prioritize among their needs in selecting a new mate.

In revisioning love stories to create more fulfilling marriages, the formerly married invariably contrast their former partners with their present ones. Comparisons, while odious, are also inevitable, a means of discriminating among options and protecting against further loss. If anything, perception heightens contrasts, as differences are exaggerated by the determination to have them so. If a former spouse was seen as too clingy and dependent, a new partner who seems strikingly independent may be chosen by a suitor who selectively ignores any evidence to the contrary.

What Therapists Need to Know

1. Revisionist histories of former marriages are inevitable and universal, not "true" or "false." Narratives about relationships that have ended are stories told in the present about the past. As such, they entail what Michael Bernstein (1989) has called "backshadowing," a retrospective account of the past "in which the shared knowledge of the outcome of a series of events by narrator and listener is used to judge the participants in those events *as though they too should have known what was to come*" (p. 16; emphasis in original). In narratives of terminated marriages, the narrator was one of those participants, and the sequence of events is selected to confirm the inevitability of dissolution. With the outcome a foregone conclusion, antecedents are searched for, and located, that confirm a story that begins "I always knew . . . " or "I should have known. . . . " Called "self-narratives" by Gergen (1994), these accounts of the "relationship among self-relevant events across time . . . do not reflect so much as they create the sense of 'what is true' " (pp. 187–189).

2. The telling of the story of the former marriage reveals the extent to which ex-spouses are emotionally, as well as legally, divorced (McGoldrick & Carter, 1999). Narratives replete with simmering anger, resentment, envy, jealousy, or guilt mean that attachment, although negative, is still strong. Ahrons (1994), summarizing how to integrate a divorce "in a healthy way," emphasizes the need to remember the good as well as the bad parts of the relationship, accept the inevitable ambiguities in how it unfolded, face loss without becoming immersed in pain, let go of anger, and forgive both one's ex-partner and oneself. Therapeutic work with remarrying or remarried individuals who have not yet worked their way through these challenges requires moving beyond "splitting." This object relations term refers to the inability to locate both "good" and "bad" in a single attachment figure. It results in caricatured versions of the former partner that interfere with disengaging from the old relationship. It is impossible to rehabilitate one's sense of oneself as a good enough person without finding some re-

deeming personal value in the partner with whom one had chosen to share one's life. Accepting ambiguity in the marital history, and one's own ambivalence about who each member of the couple is and what both have done, helps each become available to connect with a new partner.

3. Working with both past and present marital narratives involves a shift in focus from the partner's character to the self as partner, from placing blame to understanding the relational dynamic. Each person has a wider repertoire of thoughts, feelings, and behaviors than are demonstrated in any single relationship. One marriage may differ from the next not only in having a different partner, but also in being different *as a partner*, whether because one has learned from experience and developed maturity, or because the relational dance that elicits varying aspects of self is played out with different instruments and in different keys with a new partner. A pursuer in her first marriage, for example, who had complained about her husband's psychological unavailability, criticizing him as afraid of intimacy and barraging him with unwelcome plans for joint activities, may discover her own needs for solitude and "space" in remarriage to a husband whose need for togetherness exceeds her own. Each partner's psychological makeup—the confluence of temperament, personality, character, and history—exercises a tidal pull on the other, inviting participation in old scripts by inducing assigned roles through behavior and communication patterns that tend to elicit certain responses. Family systems theory describes this process as "complementarity," and object relations explains it as "projective identification."

Clinical Examples

When dealing with conflicts or relational impasses in remarriage, it is helpful to revisit how comparable issues were addressed in prior pairings. This allows therapists to assist couples in creating a more workable relationship. Changing partners may not be the hoped-for balm to relational distress, and even when a more felicitous pairing has been made, patterns learned in the old partnership may inadvertently be carried over to the new. As Mark Twain (1897) tells us, a cat who sits on a hot stove will never do so again—but she won't sit on a cold stove either.

Steve, an African American professional in his late 30s, expressed a great deal of resentment toward his second wife, Ellen. Though her complaints that he was not available for the intimacy she desired caused him discomfort, he prided himself on his independence and knew that he was not especially trusting. At one point in the therapy, his anger that he produced 80% of their income came to the forefront. In exploring his relationship with his first wife, whose disabling history of substance abuse had left her unable to parent their son, he spoke of his bitterness about her irresponsibility: how she had "messed up" her own life, hurt him and their child, and taken advantage of him financially in a divorce settlement that had brought her little benefit and him much pain. Anticipating seeing his first wife the following month, he was concerned that his anger would be overwhelming, but as he began to acknowledge how angry he still was at his former wife, his resentment toward Ellen—a respected professional, whose earning capacity could not match his—began to dissipate. He could identify that feeling taken advantage of did not originate with or belong to their relationship, and he found that he could talk with Ellen about finances without any of the emotional charge that used to accompany such discussions, reinforcing the therapeutic hypothesis that his resentment had been transferred from his prior marriage.

Recognizing that one responds to a different spouse in much the same way one has before can help put the brakes on the urge to flee. Sally, an Anglo American woman of 42 and Tony, an Italian-born 45-year-old, were both remarried; it was her second marriage and his third. Referred by his individual therapist for couple therapy, they initially presented with stepfamily issues: his angry criticism of her parenting and the children's behavior and her defensive protection of the children and simmering resentment toward his negativity and efforts at control. It soon became apparent, however, that triangular stepfamily tensions ebbed and flowed with how close the couple were to one another. When Tony experienced Sally as avoidant and unapproachable, he felt terribly lonely. Rather than address his desire for closeness directly, however, he found fault with the children, trying to make contact through angry criticism, which, of course, only increased her withdrawal. When the therapist worked directly on their differing needs and sensitivities with respect to closeness, Sally expressed her profound discomfort with getting close. A woman whose own childhood had persuaded her she could depend on no one but herself, she disclosed that she had never felt close to her previous husband, who was an alcoholic. Tony's own history as an abandoned child for most of his youth complemented Sally's history so as to form a pattern of interlocking sensitivities about being close and interdependent that became the heart of the clinical work.

Identifying the similarities in the trajectories of past and present relationships can underline the need to work through repetitive issues. It is not unusual for people to discover that they run into problems at the same point in the development of successive relationships. Carol, a mid-30s social worker in couple therapy with her lesbian partner of nearly 3 years, knows that the 3-year mark is a pivotal one for her: each of her previous two relationships broke up at 3 years, when she begins asking herself "Is this what a relationship should and can be? Are the ways in which I'm dissatisfied particular to this partnership or are they more individual issues that need to be addressed?" Similarly, Alice, a 44-year-old attorney, recognized a similar pattern with a different interval: she had been married for 7 years during her 20s, then had a 7-year-relationship with her daughter's father, and now was at the 7-year mark in the relationship that had brought her and her partner to couple therapy. For each of these women, as for many other people of both sexes, particular issues emerge at different stages in the development of their couplehood. Recognizing the pattern allows them to make choices about how to address the distress or dissatisfaction: knowing that changing partners will only postpone the problem encourages them to seek therapeutic solutions.

Change: Reinventing Gender Roles

Changes in gender roles figure prominently in "rewriting love stories" that have ended and in distinguishing past from present marriages. Recapitulating roles from past marriages that were ended by choice, whether individual or mutual, is often seen as a less-than-attractive option, because such roles are associated with dissolution: "wife" and "husband" roles become identified with the prior occupants of those roles, providing a disincentive to their wholesale reproduction in remarriages.

With the second wave of American feminism in the late 1960s and 1970s, the negotiation of gender roles in marriage became increasingly subject to marital bargaining. When a marriage ends because one spouse demands changes that the other either refuses to make or submits to begrudgingly, remarriage often entails a reactive attempt at reparation. In discussing how he and his second wife planned to divide child care responsibility for their mutual child, one man was emphatic that "it was not going to be 50/50. I was not interested in 50/50 anymore. I'd seen that movie." If the prior definition of marital roles has been traditional, adhering to stereotypical notions of masculinity and femininity, refugees from such role-based unions tend to be more improvisatory in remarriage, tailoring the division of labor and expectations about how partners interact to who they are and who they want to be to one another. There are, however, many lessons that can be drawn from aversive experiences: partners who identify previously unworkable gender arrangements as a source of marital dissolution may seek to take the opposite course—either more traditional or more innovative patterns—in remarriage.

While it is always important for couples to question their assumptions about how gender organizes expectations of one another, making explicit their assumptions about how to be a couple and negotiating arrangements that honor the values of the couple and the talents of both individuals, for remarried couples it is also important to recognize that the needs of children be respected in creating the spousal division of labor, for both logistical and emotional tasks. This topic will be explored more fully in the section on stepfamilies.

Change: Development Is Not Just for Children

The late 20th century saw the emergence of a new area of psychological study. The idea that people continue to develop beyond adolescence, facing a series of adaptive challenges, with transitional periods that disrupt the status quo ante and require significant personal change, has given rise to the field of psychological studies in adult development.

When it comes to remarriage, there are a number of developmental considerations that therapists should bear in mind when assessing and intervening clinically with couples. First, marriages that are remarriages for both members of the couple are qualitatively different than marriages in which one party is marrying for the first time. For the divorced or widowed spouse, the changes in consciousness discussed above qualitatively alter the experience of marriage. Whether happy or unhappy, a prior union remains a salient part of his or her experience, a hook that snags associations, inviting comparisons for good or ill.

While the losses for the widowed and divorced—loss of a spouse or a family unit—are apparent and acknowledged, the losses for the first-time marrier may be invisible and unspoken. These include the loss of a sense of mutuality in embarking together on a new endeavor as a shared adventure and the loss of the opportunity to create a life together without the "ghosts" of former partners, unbidden images of one's predecessor at each step of the way, and without the necessity to balance obligations to children and negotiate with ex-partners.

This asymmetry may be compounded when partners have a sizable age difference, which is more characteristic of second or later marriages than those in first matches (Dean & Gurak, 1978). Where each partner is in her or his own developmental lifeline may be less congruent than in first marriages. Experience in having been married before may not be the only source of décalage: there may be large gaps in what each has accomplished in work roles and community involvement, and differences in their obligations to provide care for aging relatives. Although age is not the only basis for these differences, partners may be at very different phases of family formation. One may be a long-time parent while the other aspires to parenthood. One may have preschool children and the other grown children and even grandchildren. Synchronizing life plans between partners who are at strikingly different points in their lifelines can be a challenging task, in life and in couple therapy, one made more complex by accelerating possibilities in assisted reproductive technologies. As collaborative reproductive possibilities proliferate—the use of donor ova or sperm or gestational surrogates to create offspring—family formation options previously foreclosed by age, previous sterilization, or infertility confront remarrying couples whose reproductive histories diverge with decisions that require further negotiation.[1]

Developmental issues in adulthood intersect with changes in gender roles to make finances another challenging issue for remarried partners. The "one-pot" model typical of young couples starting out with few assets and obligations may not be the best fit for couples coming together when one or both has considerable property and/or financial obligations to children and former partners. Therapists can assist couples in working out whether "two-pot" (each managing his/her own income and expenses) or "three-pot" (your, my, and our bank accounts) models for managing family finances are the best fit for the emotional needs of the partners.

Change: Stepparents as Helpmates, Not Replacement Parents

For many, remarriage means becoming a stepparent to one's partner's children as well as a spouse to a new partner. It is projected that soon, 30–40% of children in this country will have lived in a stepfamily by age 18, and that currently at least 14% are living in stepfamily households

(Hetherington & Jodl, 1993). One out of every three Americans is now a stepparent, a stepchild, a stepsibling, or some other member of a stepfamily, and more than half of Americans today have been, are now, or will eventually be in one or more "step" situations during their lives (Larson, 1992). Taking as our definition those families in which one of the adult partners enters the relationship already a parent—including first marriages of single parents and long-term cohabitation with heterosexual or lesbian and gay partners—we are talking about stepfamilies as the single most prevalent family form for the 21st century.

Despite their increased prevalence, "stepparent" continues to connote a stigmatized identity. The legacy of the Brothers Grimm, the tales of Cinderella, Sleeping Beauty, and Hansel and Gretel, provide strong cultural programming associating "stepmother" with "wicked," "stepfather" with "abusive," and "stepchild" with "mistreated," "unhappy" or "not-as-good-as." These stepfamily stories—those we are told and those we tell ourselves—shape our experience and our relationships. The dominant discourse on families continues to frame stepfamilies as deviant and, by implication, deficient, emblematic even of "not good enough parenting" and deprived or abused childhood (Whitehead, 1997; Poponoe, 1993; McLanahan & Sandefur, 1994).

For the recently remarried, becoming a stepparent presents the challenge of reinventing the role to fit the times and the needs of children, and adults, in their new families. While pre–World War II stepfamilies more frequently resulted from marriages cut short by the death of a spouse, the rise in the divorce rate since 1970 means that most contemporary stepfamilies supplement rather than replace the parental figures in a child's life. Families that have produced children do not end when parents divorce. Instead, they inaugurate a reorganization of the procreative family. Ahrons (1987) calls postdivorce families "binuclear": when children divide their time between parental households, there are two centers of the family, not a single nucleus. Proposing African American family structure as a model for European American postdivorce families, Crosbie-Burnett and Lewis (1993) label this structure "pedi-focal," including everyone involved in the nurturance and support of a given child, regardless of household membership.

Although national studies show that divorced fathers tend to have limited contact with children that decreases over time (Stephens, 1996), and that 90% of children reside with their mothers (Furstenberg & Cherlin, 1991), there is a countermovement toward continuing coparenting following parental divorce. In California, referred to as "the vanguard of the family law revolution," there has been a significant shift to joint custody, both legal and physical. A northern California study reported that, in the mid-1980s, 80% of the families studied had joint legal custody, presumed to encourage shared decision making between parents and "frequent and continuing contact" between nonresidential parents and their children; 20% shared both physical and legal custody (Maccoby & Mnookin, 1992; p. 113). While less widespread in other areas of the country, changes in divorce and custody laws and guidelines that start in California tend to radiate across the country, providing a model for later changes elsewhere.

What Therapists Need to Know

1. *Feeling like family takes time.* Patricia Papernow (1993) has described the stages by which a group formed by remarriage begins to feel like family, establishing its own culture, different enough from what went before that the stepparent feels at home, but not so different that each biological unit feels cut off from its own history. Papernow estimates that it takes 5 to 7 years—and courage, understanding, and lots of support—for stepfamilies to reach the stage of family development when intimacy and authenticity in stepfamily relationships have been achieved, so that stepparent and stepchild both can feel like family insiders, and the solidity of the couple bond provides a strong center to the stepfamily.

2. *Family membership is not a zero-sum game.* Parents are forever. Children's loyalty to their parents leads them to protect fiercely an absent parent's place in their hearts. While parents tend to think that the impact of divorce and remarriage is minimized once children are grown and have left home, adult—even middle-aged—children have intense reactions to parental repartnering. Only stepparents who are marrying a widowed parent with *very* young children can be said to replace those children's parent. Becoming a stepmother to children who already have a mother, a stepfather to children who continue to see their father, involves creating a different kind of relationship, rather than attempting to replicate the deeply internalized cultural ideals of what it means to be a parent. The first, most important, consideration in figuring out how to stepparent is for all family members to be absolutely clear that the stepparent is not a replacement for the parent of the same sex: all must acknowledge parents are irreplaceable, and that the stepparent cannot and does not wish to compete for primacy in the children's affection.

This means creating a place in the family for the stepparent that is not occupied by anyone else. While stepparent roles are necessarily ambiguous and very dependent on the age of the children, some roles seem to work better than others. James Bray (1992) and others have found that parental monitoring, being aware of where and what the children are doing and upholding the rules set by the parent, much like any childcare provider, yields better results than other stepparent styles (e.g., another coequal parent), especially in the first few years and especially with older children. This requires that each parent take primary responsibility for decision making and limit setting for his or her own children, who must also receive a clear parental message about what is expected and that the stepparent is deputized to see to it that expectations are met in the parent's absence.

It is important here that stepparents be imbued with a sense of what they can do effectively, rather than have it impressed upon them what they should not do. The goal here is a parental system in which the partners may have differing responsibilities, but neither is powerless over the conditions of their own lives. The challenge here, to paraphrase Jamie Keshet (1989), is to work out a role division that respects *and* challenges both the biological ties of the parent and children and the gender roles for which men and women have been socialized. Expecting stepfathers to discipline because they are men and stepmothers to nurture because they are women sets up both to be miserable and to be experienced as "wicked" by the children.

Clients are invited to question what they expect of themselves, what family members expect of them, and what cultural expectations they have absorbed. Are they facing demands and asking of themselves feelings and behaviors that are more appropriate to first families? How do these expectations fit current opportunities and inclinations? Which beliefs are remnants from ill-fitting hand-me-down fashions and what might they design to fit their lives as they are living them? (Bernstein, 1999).

3. *Take a "both/and," not an "either/or," approach to cultivating stepfamily relationships.* A great deal of the pioneering work on stepfamily therapy emphasized developing a solid couple bond (Visher & Visher, 1989, 1979). By definition, stepfamilies are those in which the couple relationship is more recent and less developed than the parent–child relationships, making strengthening couple intimacy more difficult (McGoldrick & Carter, 1999). Remarried couples get to know one another while parenting, missing out on the one-to-one courtship and honeymoon periods during which first-marrieds solidify their commit-

ment and work out their differences to create a shared way of being and doing together. The myriad challenges of early remarriage, such as running a household and helping children adjust to stepfamily life, make it difficult for adults to take the time and energy to nourish their own relationship as a couple.

Strengthening the couple bond is an essential focus for therapy with remarried couples. A stepfamily will not endure if the adults whose marriage brings it into being do not build a cohesive, resilient relationship. Indeed, research on stepfamily therapy identified improving the couple bond as the single most effective intervention to ensure family stability (Pasley, Rhoden, Visher, & Visher, 1996). While essential, therapeutic messages to build a strong couple relationship in order to ensure the stability of the family, model effective adult intimacy, and create a lasting marriage have, however, sometimes been distorted into prioritizing the couple relationship over other deserving and valuable bonds.

Privileging one relationship over another can set up the (erroneous) impression that there is not enough love to go around. Grace and Eric, both parents of adult children, invited friends and family to an engagement ceremony in which they made vows to one another, among them one that stated "Eric will work on holding the boundaries with his children." His son seemed to take this in stride, but his daughter, 24-year-old Jeannette, expressed her distress during a family outing the following day, recounting how hurt she had been in what the couple described as an "outburst" that had precipitated the crisis that delayed the wedding and brought them to therapy. Acknowledging that the public declaration of limiting his accessibility to his adult children may have been a "red flag," Eric was nonetheless relieved that the resulting crisis allowed them to put the issues—how to be a couple whose relationships with their adult children was not a subject of marital contention—on the table.

To explore this issue clinically, a therapist would first explore with the couple what they had intended to convey and whether it matched what his daughter understood as the message to her and her brother. Did "boundary making" mean the same thing to all? Or was Grace wanting to assure herself that she would come first in her new husband's life, while Jeannette envisioned the boundary as a moat around a castle, with her stepmother-to-be in charge of the drawbridge? Each member of the marrying couple comes to the altar with extensive histories and long-standing relationships with significant others. The focus of the clinical work is on how each thinks and feels about how to be a couple in midlife, how to protect the intimacy of their special bond without hurting beloved children, and whether and how their individual needs can be reconciled. What might Eric say or do, for example, to assure Grace of her importance to him? What might she need to feel secure that his continued closeness to his children is not competitive with his love for her?

Every stepfamily dyad is reciprocally influenced by every other. Indeed, the survival of the marriage itself is contingent on cultivating workable steprelationships. Researchers and clinicians have repeatedly confirmed that the quality of the stepparent–stepchild relationship is a better predictor of overall family happiness than the spousal relationship (Crosbie-Burnett, 1984; White & Booth, 1985; Visher & Visher, 1988; Fine & Kurdek, 1995). And while there are no significant differences in marital satisfaction among those in first marriages, single remarriages, or double remarriages (whether one or both partners is remarrying), those remarried couples with stepchildren in the home report more negative marital quality than those without (White & Booth, 1985). Couples are especially well served in therapy by helping them to achieve consensus about child rearing and the role of the stepparent, preventing child-related issues from destabilizing the remarriage or detracting from marital quality (Kurdek & Fine, 1991; Bray, Berger, & Boethel, 1994).

Parent–child relationships must also be nurtured. Children must be reassured that their place in their parent's affection is secure, even as their parent's intensity of involvement, time available, and singularity of focus are often diluted. In striking contrast to first-marriage families, in which child adjustment correlates with marital adjustment, research into the relationship between marital quality in remarriage and the psychological adjustment of the stepchildren shows a curious twist. Hetherington (1987) found that in stepfamilies a close marital relationship was associated with high levels of conflict for the children, especially stepdaughters with their mothers and stepfathers. Brand and Clingempeel (1987) come to a somewhat different conclusion, finding this negative association between marital quality and child outcome only for stepmother families with stepdaughters.

Daughters typically experience more of a sense of loss than sons when a parent remarries. They have more often been close confidantes of their single mothers. The greater the intimacy in the mother's new partnership, the less access the daughter feels to her mother, and the more she misses the exclusivity she had earlier enjoyed. Talking with Debbie, the teenage daughter in a lesbian stepfamily, conveys this sense of loss: "You really feel like your mother's gone, that the person takes your mother. She spends more time with my mother; my mother sleeps with her. We used to spend time watching TV together, and now she spends time with Susan, alone in the room, and she goes out more."

Newly partnered parents who see the establishment or return to a two-parent household as a normalizing improvement in the child's life may need a gentle therapeutic reminder that change, however beneficial, always requires a period of adjustment: children are more likely to feel abandoned than grateful if the intimacy of the parent–child relationship, usually more intense in single–parent households, is preempted by "family time" that always includes a quasi-stranger. In a session with mother and daughter, Debbie could tell her mother that she felt abandoned; her mother could assure her that while she now had to share more of her time, she had not lost any of her love; both could then address how to preserve the closeness with each other that both valued.

When it is a father who remarries, a stepdaughter's loss may be still more bitter. Not only are single fathers more indulgent and more permissive with their daughters than with their sons, but daughters of single fathers are more apt than their brothers to cast themselves in a partnership role in their father's households, making the entry of a stepmother more of a usurpation (Santrock & Sitterle, 1987).

All this underscores the importance of taking a "both/and," rather than an "either/or," approach to cultivating stepfamily relationships rather than hierarchically privileging one dyad over another. A child who feels abandoned by her parent will not be accepting toward the stepparent she sees as her rival for her parent's love. The parent who feels he is not free to adequately care for his child will resent his partner for making him feel torn asunder in a lose–lose loyalty struggle and will be angry at his child as an obstacle to marital happiness. And feeling unpartnered in a remarriage that lacks intimacy will deplete the emotional resources, strain the resilience, and disincline a stepparent to extend himself or herself to a partner's children.

All stepfamily relationships need attention, especially intimate couple time and protected parent–child time. Although it lacks the emotional urgency that makes these the relationships that people struggle hardest to protect, the stepparent–stepchild relationship also needs the one-to-one time without which relationships that are truly personal do not develop. When stepparent and child are not competing for the attention of the child's parent, their relationship, which is both the most fragile of family bonds and the linchpin to remarital happiness, can deepen into a connection that is valued for itself as well as for the benefit of their shared loved one.

4. *Detriangulate detoured conflicts.* Another important component

of the therapeutic work with stepfamilies, both within and between households, is sorting out and working through conflicts by proxy, whereby family members take on others' emotional work, with women typically more expressive of men's unvoiced issues, and children carrying their parents' pain, resentment, and guilt. When presented with any stepfamily dyad experiencing conflict, it is vital to look at whether another twosome is avoiding conflict. The stepparent can be a "free-fire zone" in families, diverting children's anger from their parent, like the young adult stepdaughter who saw her stepmother's hand in everything, picturing her father as a pushover to a manipulative and demanding woman and underestimating his ability to make his own choices, or the 13-year-old boy who openly enjoyed getting his stepmother worked up as a safer alternative to provoking his stricter and more beloved father. For their part, stepparents may act out their anger toward their stepchildren, avoiding conflict with their partners.

Detoured conflicts between remarried couples often present as stepparent–stepchild issues, as with Sally and Tony, described above, whose difficulties in feeling intimate were obscured by myriad complaints about steprelationships ("Your children walk all over you," "My children are afraid of you—whenever they ask for anything they expect that you'll interrupt and say 'no' ") and resentments toward ex-spouses. Similarly, 14-year-old Julie was initially referred because of stepfamily tensions in her remarried father's household. In working with the family, all the adults—mother, father, and stepmother—seemed to identify the primary problem as marital. Although Julie had made the initial decision not to return to her father's house until things changed between her and her stepmother, all but her stepmother seemed now to think that the decision was the stepmother's to make. Although he continued to see her frequently away from home, her father was loath to press the issue. For the stepmother, the central problem was that her husband seemed uninterested in discussing anything *other* than his daughter; he seemed to try not to talk about Julie and then did so only when he was too upset to contain his distress.

The initial therapeutic work consisted of detriangulating the mother from Julie's relationship with her father and stepmother by working with the parents to change communication patterns between households, interrupting a confusing and distressing game of "telephone." For example, Julie would hear from Mom, who had heard it from Dad, that Stepmom could not cope with her. Or Stepmom would tell Dad, who would tell Mom, who would then tell Julie, that Stepmom was planning an outing with Julie; then, when the invitation did not arrive, Julie felt let down. Julie complained about Stepmom to Mom, who complained to Dad. And when Stepmom wrote a letter to Julie, explaining her position and why she felt the way she did, Julie gave her response to Mom to send and then never received a response.

In therapy, Mom was encouraged to support Julie in working out her relationships with her father and stepmother, rather than trying to intervene directly (to no avail and much tumult), and to refrain from passing on hearsay about the other household. Julie was encouraged to speak with each adult directly about what she wanted and needed from each. Dad was supported in dealing directly with both his daughter and his wife. Indeed, as Stepmom had stated in her letter to Julie, conflict was being detoured away from the remarriage and displaced as step-mother–stepdaughter issues. Marital therapy for Dad and Stepmom was a prerequisite to significantly altering Julie's integration into Dad's remarried life. "Therapy with my wife is the priority now," Dad concluded, "and I'm ready to insist on it."

Change: Growing Acceptance of Quasi-Kin Relationships with Ex-Spouses and Their Families

No longer are ex-spouses seen as inevitably antagonistic, never amicable, unable to sit down at the same table to celebrate a family rite of passage. With the spread of no-fault divorce, there is increasing variety in the range of ex-spousal relationships. In her groundbreaking research into postdivorce relationships, Ahrons (1994) found that only half of the families studied fit the prevailing stereotypes of the divorced as archenemies. Those that do divide almost equally into "Angry Associates," whose anger, bitterness, and resentment continued to fester, infecting their coparenting and involving their children, and "Fiery Foes," whose rage is the stuff of which headlines, B-movies, and lawsuits are made.

The other half of the families studied remained amicable and cooperative following divorce. Of these, the majority were described as "Cooperative Colleagues." Constituting about one-third of the total group, these couples were able to separate their parental responsibilities from their marital discontents, coping well with their anger so that their children did not get caught up in their conflicts. A "small but significant minority" of couples, labeled by Ahrons "Perfect Pals," remained best friends who continue to enjoy an intimate, nonsexual, caring relationship.

In her ethnography of working-class families in Silicon Valley, Stacey (1990) observes "people turning divorce into a kinship resource rather than a rupture, creating complex, divorce-extended families" that she labels "recombinant" (p. 16). Family arrangements are diverse and fluid; the "new extended family" can include ex-spouses, their new partners, and one's children's grandparents, erstwhile in-laws—all of whom may be participants in a network of exchange of services that add to the quality of life for each. While it may still be experienced as "a little bit unusual" for a former husband to serve as the wedding photographer for his ex-wife's second marriage, for example, "the increasingly warm relationships that had been developing between . . . divorce-related couples and their respective kin," who frequently celebrated birthdays, anniversaries, and "an ecumenical array of Christian, Jewish, and secular holidays," was a source of both pleasure and social support for its participants (p. 77). A gift beyond measure to the children of such families, cultivating relations with "optional relatives . . . those with whom one never had blood ties and no longer has marriage ties," can be beneficial to all, reducing stress about inclusion/exclusion at family rituals and providing for an exchange of services. Ms. Manners (Martin, 1989), reviving a little-understood kinship term, offers them the opportunity to refer to themselves as relatives "once removed" (p. 176).

What Therapists Need to Know

1. In working with remarried couples, clinicians who can extend the strategy of inclusivity to relations between households help create the basis for a parental coalition among all the adults that reduces conflict and improves child outcome (Visher & Visher, 1989). Uncooperative parental households, on the other hand, exacerbate loyalty conflicts for children, preclude effective parenting, leave adults feeling out of control of daily life, and lead to frequent uproar.

Benign relationships between ex-spouses also promote remarital happiness. Subsequent marriages work better when former partners are neither idealized, as when a beloved, deceased spouse becomes an unrealizable standard for comparison, or demonized, as when conflict between former partners long outlasts the marriage itself.

The most unstable and difficult ex-spousal relationship occurs when the man has remarried and the woman remains unpartnered, statistically a more frequent constellation (Ahrons & Rodgers, 1987). One difficulty in reassuring mothers that stepmothers are not out to replace them is fathers' dramatic devaluation of their former wives (Schuldberg & Guisinger, 1991), so that mother often correctly perceives that father fantasizes that his remarriage can re-create a family in which mother plays no part. He complains to his new wife, who gets angry both at his ex-wife on his behalf and at him for the passive resignation that frequently accompanies his extreme negativity. By focusing on the "outrageousness" of an ex-wife, stepmothers misdirect their energy and attention from the unresolved issues within the new marriage. Similarly, mothers who target their ex-husband's new wives as responsible for his uncooperativeness or for their disappointment in how their children are cared for in his home are diverting accountability from where it belongs: with the children's father. Frequently, both women find it less dangerous to scapegoat each other than to risk an open confrontation with the man who occasions their participation in each other's lives.

Building empathy between a mother and a stepmother can be a challenge, but the payoff more than rewards the cost. The higher the regard in which stepmothers and their husbands hold his ex-wife, the happier both are with the current marriage (Guisinger, Cowan, & Schuldberg, 1989). And the more respect a mother has for her children's stepmother, the easier it is for the stepmother to be open-hearted and openhanded to her stepchildren.

The same principle holds for fathers and their children's stepfathers. Although less frequently a source of marital tension, perhaps because fathers are more likely to reduce their own role in their children's lives when their ex-wives remarry, ongoing tension with an ex-spouse, male or female, compounds the tensions, both marital and parental, for any remarried couple.

The goal, to the extent that it can be a reasonable construction of the data, is for both partners in a remarriage to see ex-spouses as benign noncompetitors. Most often, jealousy or possessiveness over a new partner's relationship with a prior mate reflects insecurity in the new marriage. Tony, for example, took issue with Sally's friendliness with her ex-husband, whom she would talk with about how his life was going. Frequently, her response was to get angry at how her ex was managing his personal life, repeating patterns that had led to the dissolution of his prior marriage, to her. She would then come home and vent her anger to Tony, who became resentful about the amount of time and "space" that her ex was taking in their life together. She, in turn, complained that he blamed her for her former husband's nonpayment of child support, although she saw herself as doing everything possible, including taking legal action. When, however, Tony felt that Sally was attentive and accessible to intimacy with him, his resentment about her prior partner waned from a cause célèbre to a minor irritation.

2. Good fences *and* good bridges make for workable "new extended families" created by remarriage chains. By addressing issues of power and control, therapy can help in working out permeable yet protective boundaries between households, allowing for communication and cooperation while safeguarding against intrusiveness.

There are probably nearly as many "solutions" to the problem of creating flexible but protective boundaries as there are remarried families. For some, it is a stretch to have an ex-spouse come to the front door and wait on the stoop while picking up a child. For others, it is "no big deal" for a remarried couple to come home to find a child entertaining her other parent. Each couple must negotiate how to respect the needs of all family members for both privacy and connection, untangling the threads of attributed meanings in emotionally "knotty" situations, like who is welcome in whose home and when. Is the living room OK, but the bedroom area off-limits? Do the same rules apply to ex-spouses as other guests of one's children, or does special clearance have to be obtained first?

His stepchildren's relatives visiting them in their home was a thorny issue for Tony, who felt invaded when he came home to find his stepdaughter visiting with her paternal aunts. For Sally, having her former sisters-in-law in the house was a nonevent; familiar and well liked, they were always welcome. For it to be otherwise felt like telling her daughter that the family home was not her home, too, and she could not bear to bar the door to them, however much she worried about Tony's angry tirades should he learn of their presence. But what most galled Tony was not the aunts being there, but his being surprised to find them there. After talking through what each needed in order to feel at home, he was able to come to terms with entertaining his predecessor's kin as long as he was "in the loop." Like Tony, most remarried people have an easier time accepting that boundaries must be permeable when they feel participant in their creation and feel confident that the boundaries will be protective.

While overrigid boundaries may invite stretching, underprotective boundaries may require bolstering. It is never worth it to punish a child, for example, by attempting to restrict their time with the other parent. Each household may invite the cooperation of the other parent in developing consequences for problem behaviors, but inflicting punishments that impact the other household without consent invites strife and benefits no one. Similarly, remarried couples must feel that they have some say over the structure of their own lives.

Alice's husband, Raoul, also an attorney and a few years her senior, was intensely resentful about what he perceived as the subordination of their needs as a couple to making arrangements for his 10-year-old step-daughter to spend time with her father, Marc. In the years before remar-rying, Alice had easily accommodated to Marc's comings and goings: he lived thousands of miles away, and whenever he came to see their daugh-ter was fine with Alice. More flexible than many new spouses, Raoul ac-cepted Marc's staying in their house when he was in town, or even spend-ing *some* vacation time traveling together with Marc. But he resented that Marc would walk into their bedroom to talk with either him or Alice and feel at home, and he protested always putting their own plans on hold, waiting to hear what Marc wanted to do and then accommodating him. While Alice knew that Marc never presumed he was welcome, always in-quiring whether Raoul was agreeable with whatever plan he proposed, that part of the transaction never made it back to Raoul.

For Alice, announcing the plans as a fait accompli was a necessary prioritizing of her daughter's needs, and, in an illustration of how each stepfamily dyad influences the process of each of the others, an indi-rect criticism of Raoul as a stepfather. Seeing Raoul act with her daugh-ter in ways that seemed unloving to her, she felt the need to compen-sate by doing everything possible to maximize Marc's involvement as the more nurturing father. Therapy focused on working out more pro-tective boundaries between the remarried household and Marc, and in detriangulating Marc from Raoul's relationship with his stepdaughter, so that their relationship could develop without constant comparisons with Marc, by either Alice or her daughter. While it was hard for Alice to explain to Marc why making arrangements had to be more formal now, requiring her and Raoul to tell Marc both what they would like and what they were open to, it was also enormously helpful for her and Raoul as a couple. And as Raoul was liberated from the no-win position of never measuring up to Marc as a father, he was able to get Alice's recognition that he was an essentially benign and beneficial part of the girl's life, and his relationship with his stepdaughter improved as well.

CONCLUSION

Thinking about how to engage therapeutically with clients who seek the assistance of family therapists in recoupling to better effect is more a question of ideology—how we are thinking about what it means to be a couple and what makes second, third, or later attempts at couplehood different from the first time around—than of methodology. Even more than in first marriages, remarriage involves deconstructing what it means to be a couple and recontextualizing relational possibilities: the therapist invites the couple to personalize their marital contract, to create inclusive and democratic solutions to family membership, and to redistribute the emotional and logistical division of labor, both within a stepfamily household and between households linked in the remarriage chain. Rather than rebuilding from old architectural plans, constructing a more rewarding relationship demands going back to the drafting board to redesign couplehood in ways that enable clients to discover ways of thinking, feeling, and behaving that are both more personally satisfying and more congruent with the changed context of family life.

ACKNOWLEDGMENT

I would like to thank Ruth Rosen for sharing her thinking about remarriages when neither partner is a parent, and Peggy Papp, Constance Ahrons, and Conn Hallinan for their generous editorial assistance and excellent suggestions for revising earlier drafts of this chapter.

NOTE

1. An in-depth examination of what clinicians need to know about these issues is beyond the scope of this chapter. For further discussion of decision making about having children in remarriage, see Bernstein (1990). An exploration of late-life pregnancies and assisted reproductive technologies can be found in Chapter 5 (Scharf & Weinshel) of this volume and in Bernstein (1994).

REFERENCES

Ahrons, C. R. (1994). *The good divorce: Keeping your family together when your marriage is coming apart.* New York: HarperCollins.

Ahrons, C. R., & Rodgers, R. H. (1987). *Divorced families: A multidisciplinary developmental view.* New York: Norton.

Bernstein, A. C. (1990). *Yours, mine, and ours: How families change when remarried parents have a child together.* New York: Norton.

Bernstein, A. C. (1994). Women in stepfamilies: The Fairy Godmother, the

Wicked Witch, and Cinderella reconstructed. In M. P. Mirkin (Ed.), *Women in context: Toward a feminist reconstruction of psychotherapy* (pp. 188–213). New York: Guilford Press.

Bernstein, A. C. (1999). Reconstructing the Brothers Grimm: New tales for stepfamily life. *Family Process, 38*(4), 415–429.

Bernstein, M. A. (1989). *Foregone conclusions: Against apocalyptic history*. Berkeley and Los Angeles: University of California Press.

Brand, E., & Clingempeel, W. G. (1987). Interdependencies of marital and step-child relationships and children's psychological adjustment. *Family Relations, 36*, 140–145.

Bray, J. H. (1992). Family relationships and children's adjustment in clinical and nonclinical stepfather families. *Journal of Family Psychology, 6*, 60–68.

Bray, J. H., Berger, S. H., & Boethel, C. L. (1994). Role integration and marital adjustment in stepfamilies. In K. Pasley & M. Ihinger-Tallman (Eds.), *Stepparenting: Issues in theory, research, and practice* (pp. 69–86). Westport, CT: Greenwood Press.

Bumpass, L., Martin, T. C., & Sweet, J.A. (1991). The impact of family background and early marital factors on marital disruption. *Journal of Family Issues, 12*, 22–42.

Bumpass, L., Sweet, J. A., & Martin, T. C. (1990). Changing patterns of remarriage. *Journal of Marriage and the Family, 52*, 747–756.

Carter, B. (1988). Remarried families: Creating a new paradigm. In M. Walters, B. Carter, P. Papp, & O. Silverstein (Eds.), *The invisible web: Gender patterns in family relationships* (pp. 333–367). New York: Guilford Press.

Crosbie-Burnett, M. (1984). The centrality of the step-relationship: Challenge to family theory and practice. *Family Relations, 33*, 459–464.

Crosbie-Burnett, M., & Lewis, E. A. (1993). Use of African-American family structures and functioning to address the challenges of European-American postdivorce families. *Family Relations, 42*, 243–248.

Dean, G., & Gurak, D. T. (1978). Marital homogamy the second time around. *Journal of Marriage and the Family, 40*, 559–570.

Fine, M. A., & Kurdek, L. A. (1995). Relation between marital quality and (step) parent–child relationship quality for parents and stepparents in stepfamilies. *Journal of Family Psychology, 9*, 216–223.

Furstenberg, F. F., & Cherlin, A. J. (1991). *Divided families: What happens to children when parents part*. Cambridge, MA: Harvard University Press.

Gergen, K. J. (1985). The social constructionist movement in psychology. *American Psychologist, 40*, 266–275.

Gergen, K. J. (1994). *Realities and relationships: Soundings in social construction*. Cambridge, MA: Harvard University Press.

Guisinger, S., Cowan, P. A., & Schuldberg, D. (1989). Changing parent and spouse relations in the first years of remarriage of divorced fathers. *Journal of Marriage and the Family, 51*(2), 445–456.

Hetherington, E. M. (1987). Family relations six years after divorce. In K. Pasley & M. Ihinger-Tallman (Eds.), *Remarriage and stepparenting: Current research and theory* (pp. 185–205). New York: Guilford Press.

Hetherington, E. M., & Jodl, K.M. (1993). *Stepfamilies as settings for child develop-ment*. Paper presented at the National Symposium on Stepfamilies, Pennsyl-vania State University, University Park, October 14–15.

James, K., & McIntyre, D. (1989). A momentary gleam of enlightenment: To-wards a model of feminist family therapy. *Journal of Feminist Family Therapy, 1*(3), 3–24.

Keshet, J. K. (1989). Gender and biological models of role division in stepmother families. *Journal of Feminist Family Therapy, 1*(4), 29–50.

Kurdek, L. A., & Fine, M. A. (1991). Cognitive correlates of adjustment for moth-ers and fathers in stepfather families. *Journal of Marriage and the Family, 53*, 565–572.

Laird, J. (1989). Women and stories: Restorying women's self-constructions. In M. McGoldrick, C. Anderson, & F. Walsh (Eds.), *Women in families* (pp. 427–450). New York: Norton.

Larson, J. (1992, January). Understanding stepfamilies. *American Demographics*, pp. 36–40.

Maccoby, E. E., & Mnookin, R. H. (1992). *Dividing the child: Social and legal dilem-mas of custody*. Cambridge, MA: Harvard University Press.

Martin, J. (1989). *Ms. Manners guide for the millennium*. New York: Simon & Shuster.

McGoldrick, M., & Carter, B. (1999). Remarried families. In B. Carter & M. McGoldrick (Eds.), *The expanded family life cycle: Individual, family, and social perspectives* (3rd ed., pp. 417–435). Boston: Allyn & Bacon.

McLanahan, S., & Sandefur, G. (1994). *Growing up with a single parent: What hurts, what helps*. Cambridge, MA: Harvard University Press.

National Center for Health Statistics. (1995, April 18). Advance report of final di-vorce statistics, 1989 and 1990. *Monthly Vital Statistics Report, 43*(9, Suppl.).

Norton, A. J., & Miller, L. F. (1992). Marriage, divorce, and remarriage in the 1990s. *Current Population Reports* (Series P-23, No. 180). Washington, DC: U.S. Government Printing Office.

Papernow, P. L. (1993). *Becoming a stepfamily: Patterns of development in remarried families*. San Francisco: Jossey-Bass.

Pasley, K., Rhoden, L., Visher, E. B., & Visher, J. S. (1996). Successful stepfamily therapy: Clients' perspectives. *Journal of Marital and Family Therapy, 22*, 343–357.

Poponoe, D. (1993, October 14–15). *The evolution of marriage and the problem of stepfamilies: A biosocial perspective*. Paper presented at the National Sympo-sium on Stepfamilies, Pennsylvania State University, University Park.

Santrock, J. W., & Sitterle, K. A. (1987). Parent–child relationships in stepmother families. In K. Pasley & M. Ihinger-Tallman (Eds.), *Remarriage and step-parenting: Current research and theory* (pp. 273–299). New York: Guilford Press.

Schuldberg, D. & Guisinger, S. (1991). Divorced fathers describe their former wives: Devaluation and contrast. *Journal of Divorce and Remarriage, 14*(3–4), 61–87.

Stacey, J. (1990). *Brave new families: Stories of domestic upheaval in late-twentieth-century America.* New York: Basic Books.

Stephens, L. S. (1996). Will Johnny see daddy this week? An empirical test of three theoretical perspectives of postdivorce contact. *Journal of Family Issues, 17,* 466–494.

Twain, Mark. (1897). Puddinhead Wilson's new calendar. Chapter 11 in *Following the Equator.* Hertford, CT: American Publishing Co.

U.S. Bureau of the Census. (1997, March). Annual geographical mobility rates, by type of movement, 1947–1997. Website at http://www.census.gov/population/socdemo/migration/tab-a-1.txt

Van Buren, A. (1998, April 9). "Dear Abby." *San Francisco Chronicle,*

Visher, E. B., & Visher, J. S. (1979). *Stepfamilies: A guide to working with stepparents and stepchildren.* New York: Brunner/Mazel.

Visher, E. B., & Visher, J. S. (1988). *Old loyalties, new ties: Therapeutic strategies with stepfamilies.* New York: Brunner/Mazel.

Visher, E. B., & Visher, J. S. (1989). Parenting coalitions after remarriage: Dynamics and therapeutic guidelines. *Family Relations, 38*(1), 65–70.

White, L. K., & Booth, A. (1985). The quality and stability of remarriages: The role of stepchildren. *American Sociological Review, 50,* 689–698.

White, M., & Epston, D. (1990). *Narrative means to therapeutic ends.* New York: Norton.

Whitehead, B. D. (1997). *The divorce culture.* New York: Knopf.

CHAPTER 13

Reflections on Golden Pond

Ruth Mohr

The mental health field has gradually come to recognize the emergence of a unique stage in the developmental life cycle, a stage relatively unknown to previous generations, a stage beyond the commonly held profile of later life. Because of increased longevity, a favorable economy, and a supportive social attitude toward living, older people have been offered a new life experience for which there is no precedent.

In spite of the plethora of medical, technological, and economic advances intended to make life easier and longer, getting old is getting more complex. There was a time in the not-too-distant past when couples raised their children, launched them as young adults into either marriage or career, and did their bit as grandparents; simultaneously, they worked until they died. These transitions were accepted as normal and inevitable.

Marriages today are lasting longer than in the past because of our increased life spans. In addition, remarriage is occurring more often and later in life, blended families include as many as five generations of related and unrelated members, and unmarried coupling is increasing. Partners are going through developmental stages for which there are no scripts either for the people living this phenomena of healthy longevity, where options and stresses unknown to earlier generations abound and confuse, nor for therapists trying to treat these couples.

A key concept for working with this population is that older couples, unlike their younger cohorts, need less a future they can aspire to, and more a reasonable narrative they can believe in—a different story they can comfortably invest in. No one knows this better than those couples who find themselves without a script useful to and congruent with their time of life. Reacting and interacting around this bleak reality may effect their relationships in unique and sometimes troublesome ways. It is the task of the couple therapist to unearth the biological, sociological, historical, and spiritual context in which each couple operates since these factors form an experiential collage determining the quality of life and death being shared during the last stage of their experience together.

RENEGOTIATING THE MARITAL
CONTRACT AROUND RETIREMENT

The marital contract is the cornerstone of the coupling unit and the subsequent family structure. The ability to accommodate to the transitions indigenous to life partnering requires many renegotiations of the marital contract. Indeed, most couples perform the task many times during the life of their marriage. But as the couple age, different kinds of negotiations around different issues are required. Statistics show that divorce is an option few older couples choose as a solution to their problems, regardless of how painful or how dull their marriage has become.

One of the most difficult life crisis to negotiate is retirement. Many of the problems facing older couples have their roots in unresolved issues concerning retirement, whether retirement be from a career, from a role, or from a commitment. This effects every member of the family but particularly the spouse.

Many couples on retirement enter what is known as "the honeymoon period," that first phase on the continuum of retirement. They often enter this transitional period by traveling for adventure or to research areas for possible relocation; by taking up sports, hobbies, and academic pursuits; and by entertaining ideas they had not previously time for. True to its name, the honeymoon stage is a period for dreaming about possibilities. This stage may, however, be followed by disappointment, disillusionment, and even depression for the couple, or it may be followed by a period of settling down, accepting the limitations of aging, a mellowing out, and a letting go.

While some women look forward to retirement as an opportunity to spend time with husbands formerly engrossed in outside work-related pursuits, others are unwilling or unable to reorganize their lives to accommodate the reentry of the retired male. The "I married him for better or worse, but not for lunch" syndrome is particularly acute when the retiree retreats to the home, impinging on what previously had been the woman's domain. Many women suffer with and for their spouses as retirement changes the quality of their marriages and lives in ways they neither want nor anticipate. Other women find themselves freer to pursue new individual interests at this time, when responsibilities for home and dependent family members have lessened. Still others are beginning to peak in their social or career lives and may experience their husband's retirement as a burden or an interruption, or at least as a shift in roles.

Such shifts are not necessarily incongruent with the emotional and biological makeup of the different genders. There is a tendency toward a natural androgyny in later life, with men becoming more reflective, inner-oriented, and home-based. Women may become more aggressive with age and orient themselves to matters outside the couple venue, or choose to take a one-down position, hoping to force their husbands' return to their original construct of male dominance.

These postures come out of caring positions; fearing change and the vulnerability that attends change, they seek to restore a prior contract in which the relationship involved predictable roles, boundaries, and behaviors. The process of letting go of a life's occupation that organized and stimulated one's day-to-day experience while staying connected to and retaining the vitality of involvement in a meaningful existence is a universal and sometimes overwhelming task for those entering the later life cycle.

Letting Go and Staying Connected

One of the major dilemmas for the aging couple is how to let go *and* stay connected. This runs counter to the normative developmental process of investing in life through the building of attachments and the accumulation of objects and relationships. With aging, the process of divesting begins. Estates are downsized, networks get smaller, everything from status to stature shrinks. Emotional changes begin, too, with consequent changes in behavioral patterns as the cycle of investing and accumulating reverses, and control over personal and financial issues is increasingly delegated to others. Interest in a future-oriented society wanes.

Letting go is a slow and natural progression toward death, one that is sometimes easy, sometimes not, but easier when the pace of the couple is congruent.

The need to let go and the need to stay connected is the hallmark of the later life cycle stage. If the couple processes this dilemma congruently, resolution will be easier. Retirement is a phase where often the couple is not on the same wavelength and needs to renegotiate their individual positions. It is a period during which letting go and staying connected is particularly stressful since it invades all areas of the couple's life: work, family, community, and their collective and individual identities. With this shift in identity comes a shift in the way the couple relates to each other, requiring an evaluation and renegotiation of their contract with each other.

In the case of Sam and Miriam, the process of letting go and staying connected consisted of several stages. Their retirement was not the result of a carefully mapped-out plan for entering the last stage of the later life cycle. The crisis that brought them into therapy was the result of an impetuous, unilateral act by Sam. "Unilateral decision making" were words not to be found in their particular marital agreement. Theirs had been a traditional marriage. Each had their role and had performed it well.

As a young man, Sam started the business that would make him his fortune and provide him with status in the community. Miriam had been the woman on his arm, yet capable of running interference and fixing situations when necessary. Together, they discussed issues, made their plans, put them into action, and dealt with the consequences. Miriam was proud of their partnership and of her contribution to Sam's success. She'd felt important.

Sam had retired 15 years earlier at age 65, with Miriam's blessing. After selling his business, he started a second career almost immediately as a philanthropist, becoming the president of a large and prestigious charitable organization. Miriam supported this move, and became heavily involved in the organization. As wife of the president, she enjoyed the esteem and privileges of that position, around which all their social and intellectual lives revolved.

Now, at age 80, wanting to make room at the top for younger men whom he feared might begin to think of him as an "addle-minded figurehead beyond his prime," Sam had made a unilateral decision to retire again with no other plan than to be at ease. This decision forced Miriam into retirement too. She feared that Sam was physically decompensating and would, in accordance with the retirement myth, become depressed or die of boredom. Their children shared this concern and became highly critical of her petulant attitude, wanting her to be more solicitous concerning his needs. At the same time, they tried to support her efforts to revitalize their father.

Miriam's efforts had always been successful before, but now Sam adamantly refused to reenter community life or to develop new interests. He seemed not to mind being out of the social loop, and was becoming increasingly withdrawn in response to his wife's pleading attempt to reactivate him. She, in turn, being an outgoing person of action, was becoming increasing agitated by her own feelings of helplessness, loneliness, and deprivation. These feelings were complicated by a certain contractual injunction she believed existed against her voicing any disapproval of Sam's actions. Her marriage role had been to protect, adore, and fix.

Miriam did not know how to contain her resentment at Sam's withdrawal from the public and social life to which she was accustomed. Suddenly, her life had changed, and with it their relationship. Reflecting the intensity of their bonding, Miriam pleaded with Sam to understand her dilemma: "By pulling yourself out of the picture, you're pulling me out too. As strong as I am, my identity is defined by yours." Sam responded angrily: "I'm not holding you back. I've always been more of a feminist than you have. Go find your own identity." Feeling isolated from the world she'd known, and lonely, she turned to her adult children for solace. This offended him because he had always been the shoulder she had leaned on.

It seemed to me that both Sam and Miriam were suffering from the insult of disloyalty: she for his breach of loyalty in not consulting her, he for her turning to others for comfort and companionship. Each change constituted a break in the marital contract, leading to role confusion and an uncomfortable restructuring of their partnership. Miriam wanted Sam to find a comfortable solution to his aging, and Sam wanted Miriam to find an identity, which included people and interests other than those that had previously defined her.

Seemingly a minor infraction (as well it might be for a younger couple), such a breach of loyalty threatens the ties that bind an older couple. Repairs for such a breach are emotionally costly and time-consuming. In their own style, Sam and Miriam kept these feelings to themselves only to find them increasingly difficult to contain.

Tracing the Evolution of a Marital Contract

The dilemma Sam and Miriam were experiencing reflected values formed in their childhoods. Exploring their genograms from a three-generational perspective, the therapist discovered a heart-rending story of immigrant families trying to survive poverty during the depression era. Sam had been abandoned by his father when he was 8 years old. The family were observant Jews who kept the Sabbath (Saturday). His father was a shopkeeper. His mother told his father that since the family was close to starving, he would have to compromise his religious practices by working on Saturday, a busy day for a shopkeeper.

She told him that if he refused, he would have to leave. Rather than compromise his religious principles, he left. Sam became head of the family at age 8 and continued so throughout his life, sharing early meager earnings and later bountiful ones with his mother and sisters, thus honoring the maternal legacy of familial support and participation regardless of the sacrifices required.

Miriam never questioned the extent of Sam's support of his family. She came from an enmeshed family from the same neighborhood, whose father, hardly more than a boy, had run away from his home in Russia to avoid serving in the army. Once in the United States, with hard work and persistence, he was able to fulfill his promise to rescue the rest of his family. Miriam's legacy of loyalty and action remains a driving force in her attitudes and behaviors. It motivates her desire to protect Sam from the unpleasantries of life.

The First Renegotiation

The first renegotiation of the marital contract this young couple was required to make had important ramifications for their marriage, for it firmly established Miriam as the troubleshooter and problem solver and explains the depth of the sense of disloyalty and abandonment she felt when Sam made his unilateral decision to retire. Her story revealed that Sam had received his draft notice shortly after their first child was born. The idea of her becoming a single parent whose husband would be away and probably in extreme danger was not to Miriam's liking. She set about thinking creatively. Her solution was to aggravate an already existing eczema by rubbing undiluted bleach into the palms of her hands until they bled through open sores. She then presented her "eczema" to the draft board, convincing the board that she could not care for her infant, wash diapers, make formula, cuddle the child, and the like without the assistance of her husband. Sam's status was changed to 4F. He was not proud of this resolution but it left him free to build his business and to be with his family.

Sam, like his father, would never have compromised his principles, but Miriam, like Sam's mother, put preservation of family above all else. Her success at circumventing the draft, a proviso that would dominate their partnership and would become part of their history, gave her a role with which she was quite comfortable. In Miriam's words, "He chose the target and I shot the arrows." Through the 54 years of their marriage, that contract saw them through many hard times. It was modified often to comply with changing interpersonal needs and normative life crises, but the core concept remained intact. However, it was just this proviso that now got in their way of negotiating the present crisis. If Sam continues to refuse to make the bullets, Miriam has none to fire, forcing her into unwanted and unsolicited retirement, and they had no alternate scripts to build on.

Their entire structure seemed about to topple. Division of labor had been assigned on pragmatic needs and according to mutually defined roles. His role was to provide financial stability and status in the public sector, hers was to be the hearthmaker and the troubleshooter, being careful to make suggestions but never demands or ultimatums as his mother had done.

Their interaction as a couple was firmly rooted in the principles of communication, cooperation, and compromise, as well as in individuation and connectedness, nurturance of the other's self-image, and affectionate expression toward family, friends, and community. When Sam negated those principles, Miriam felt betrayed. Betrayal at any time is extremely damaging to marital trust, but it is particularly devastating for the older couple because time, resources, and options for repair are limited.

Walking through the past with this couple, revisiting their childhoods, their courtship, and their young to midadulthood lives, was in itself a powerful intervention. The therapist, by guiding, witnessing, and asking for clarification and agreement, helped the couple make those connections with the past that trigger feelings of hurt, anger, and confusion in the present.

Employment has great meaning in our Puritan work ethic culture, particularly for those immigrant couples who were dedicated to making their lives productive, to acquiring community respect and status, and to creating opportunities for their children. The myth of retirement, that it augurs the end of life, lies heavily on Miriam. Doing nothing, however, in her mind, leads to boredom, depression, illness, and death. For Sam, however, doing nothing offers the innocence and joys of the childhood he never had. In putting their stories together, it became clear to me that the distress they were experiencing was a result of their inability to change their roles and alter their expectations and desires in order to accommodate to the life stage in which they now found themselves. The dilemma of change was overwhelming them, threatening both their relationship and their health. I knew that she would never push him off the pedestal she had put him on, nor would she allow the structure to topple due to inattentiveness, but I also saw that she needed help in taking him off, just as he needed help in stepping down from the pedestal that kept them locked into rigid patterns of the past, preventing change from happening.

Giving them some feedback, I said, "Sam, Miriam is worried for a number of reasons. You are no longer interested in socializing, or in going out with her, or even being involved with the family, much less the community. That frightens her because being 'out of the picture' connotes many unpleasant realities. But she is in a bind because if she forces you back into the picture, she will have toppled that 'lord and master' pedestal she's put you on. Preserving your position seems to be more important to her than winning on the issue of getting you connected again. For all of your married life, you have taken care of each other according to the terms of your contract. Through fulfillment of your needs, hers were satisfied. But Miriam was unaware of your letting go of your need to work, and of your desire to abdicate your position on the pedestal."

I asked Miriam, "Would you be willing to take the risk of seeing what would happen if you took him off that pedestal?" She said that she would, but that she did not know how to go about it. I mused that those who worship at the feet of their idol must put aside their own needs. If she were to help him get off the pedestal, she would have to elevate her own position, identify her own needs and desires, thereby giving him the opportunity of addressing them. "Do you think you can do that?" "Well," she said, "I can't stand the boredom of staying home doing nothing. If I'm to build a new life for myself, I need to be able to get around. I don't drive and he's no longer interested taking me places, so I would like a driver."

Sam nodded compliance. "No problem," he said, "I don't need to be in the driver's seat."

"Miriam, what would you do if you were in the driver's seat, if you could get around without him?" I asked.

"Develop interests of my own—which may or may not include him."

"Sam, how does that sit with you?" I asked.

"It's OK. If she needs to do that, she should do that. I'll be OK. I'm perfectly content to be a house-husband."

I noted that their positions were undergoing a change. Sam seemed willing to put aside his own needs in order to validate hers. Curious, I wondered aloud if that was his way of separating from his traditional role of hunter-husband. He shrugged.

I asked Miriam, "What do you feel your greatest loss would be if your desire to 'get around' were fulfilled? In an instant she replied, "His company."

"Sam, would that be a loss for you too—her company?"

"Of course."

I inquired what he might want to do about staying connected to each other even in the process of pursuing separate interests. He thought that her ideas of going out to dinner together, going to the theater, socializing with friends—all those happenings that Miriam was grieving the loss of might be the solution. When I wondered if that would do, she said, "No, it's too easy to just say that. In the long run, I know I would end up having to push him to keep up with that intent." "Well," I said, "You may have to give him a little push to get him off that pedestal. Your role as troubleshooter may not be over yet."

Somewhat sheepishly, Sam owned up to wanting a little push now and again. "When I do go out, I find I usually enjoy it. Sometimes, I'm disappointed when she gives up."

This new information gave impetus to renegotiating, once again, the terms of their marital contract and gave Miriam fresh ideas for getting her needs met without depriving him of his. She suggested that he take on the job of arranging their social and recreational activities, releasing her to pursue some personal interests. Mischievously, she added, "And allow me to decide whether or not to accept your invitations." Even though Sam seemed amenable to that plan, I suggested they put a time boundary round this change to ensure its success: perhaps they could take turns, a week or a month at a time, in which each would control the agenda, allowing for a fresh perspective and equal input to their communal lives.

This renegotiation exposed a more potent issue for the couple. The shadow of death lurked behind them, increasing their awareness of the paucity of their emotional resources to survive without each other. Developing such resources requires individuation, which for this couple can only come from a willingness to become more flexible in their role structure. They agreed that an important piece needing to be addressed was Miriam's concern about taking control of the economic portion of their lives should anything happen to Sam. Sam, who gave her an allowance but doled out extras at his whim, had always handled finances. She'd resented this but kept silent. Even now when illness and death had become more of a reality, she was extremely reticent in bringing up the matter and was surprised at his reaction when she did. He admitted that he too had been concerned about her future in the event of his illness or death, but he had misread her reluctance to discuss the issue as an inability or unwillingness to take control of their financial matters. As a result, he had put his affairs in the hands of strangers.

Their discussion of the unpleasant possibilities attendant to their stage in life permitted them to plan for a future when one of them would be single, a construct they were totally unfamiliar with, and obviously dreaded. Nevertheless, they agreed to initiate a program whereby he would familiarize her with all his financial holdings and introduce her to the lawyers, brokers, accountants, and other professionals who could help her manage their estate.

By agreeing in essence to his taking over some of her former role functioning in exchange for relinquishing some of his control, they were able to renegotiate their marital contract and make a shift in their roles. Keeping the balance if not the roles of the original marital contract increased his interest and involvement in the newly defined partnership. But I made a final suggestion: every time Miriam "pushed" him off the pedestal, regardless of the result, he was to say, "Thank you for your help." She in turn was to say, "You're welcome." My intent was that they experience the pushing as a helpful aid, not the demand or ultimatum so historically toxic to this couple, so that the changes would constitute neither a betrayal of the marital contract nor a betrayal of their legacies. My suggestion was received with amusement, with Sam saying, "Oh, I get it. The new roles need buttering up."

CONNECTING THE PAST WITH THE PRESENT

The expectations couples have of each other as they approach their later years are deeply rooted in the legacy of their past, and are passed on from generation to generation through metaphors, rituals, and stories in order to instruct them in the time-proven methods of surviving life's travails. Although values and expectations change over time as a result of the dilemmas and compromises of life, aging has a way of encouraging a leap back to the predictability and safety of the more innocent times of youth. By making those connections between the past and the present, the therapist can help the older couple to understand their need and their love for each other so that they can appreciate the logic of their interdependence. The basic tool for accomplishing this is the genogram. Reminiscence and storytelling, dates, ages, members, nodal events—all enhance the factual information. The careful selection of events, conscious or not, and the drama of the telling—not to mention a bit of fantasy—combine to weave a tapestry of human connections made tender, alive, and legitimate through the witnessing by an empathic but objective observer, the therapist. In addition to uncovering past injunctions, which may be honored or challenged depending of their usefulness to the couple, new resources may be discovered.

Telling stories from the past enabled me to help another couple change their stance from hostility toward each other to an appreciation of the many life experiences they had shared through the years. Out of this revisiting, resources emerged that allowed the couple to change their circumstances so that they could let go of ineffectual rituals and attachments while staying connected to each other in new and different ways.

Milton and Rose, both 86, have been married for 60 years and are childless. They'd met and worked, until retirement, for the same company but on different shifts. He worked days and she worked nights. As a result, they had few mutual friends, and their interactions with each other were routinized around their work schedules. Since they also had no close relatives, they lived virtually alone and dependent on each other.

They were referred to me by Rose's cardiologist because Milton had become so verbally abusive to her in the last few years that both the doctor and the home attendant were concerned that he might do her bodily harm. Rose was more handicapped by the aging process than Milton. Plagued by the threat of impending heart failure, she was forced to restrict her activities. Crippling arthritis prevented her from accompanying Milton on his forays into the outside world as had previously been her practice. Frantic to maintain a connection with Milton, she questioned him relentlessly for detailed information about his excursions. He responded irritably, becoming increasingly abusive both verbally and physically, thinking that she wanted to restrict his outside activities and curtail his cherished freedom.

The only respite from their arguing was when the home attendant intervened or when Milton went on his frequent and prolonged walks around the neighborhood. Rose whispered loud enough for him to hear that she was worried that he might have early onset Alzheimer disease because of what she perceived as "wandering." Her diagnosis seemed not to be the case: his memory was outstanding and his awareness was acute. These forays into the Lower East Side neighborhood had become an important part of his life. He enjoyed these adventures in which he would quiz the cops on the beat as to the whereabouts of obscure street locations in the neighborhood he knew so well. He would regale tourists with stories of the famous and infamous characters that had lived there and would voluntarily assist local shopkeepers in peddling their wares on the street. He was charming and adored in the community, but he was a hellion with Rose.

Almost everyone working with elderly persons has been witness to outbursts of temper directed by the hardier partner toward the frailer partner—almost as if the intention is to shake by such action the frailer one back into a desired strength or sensibility, perhaps in a desperate attempt to hold on to or bring back previous marital patterns. In addition, older couples may find they have fewer opportunities to socialize outside of the marriage, leaving the gates open for loneliness and depression. Milton's temperamental outbursts were his way of trying to revive the complimentarity the couple had once enjoyed and fight off his feelings of abandonment. This way of angrily expressing that need is experienced by the spouse as rejection and is responded to either by pursuit, as Rose did, or by withdrawal. In any case, this type of aggressive behavior is most often greeted by families and professionals with disgust, disbelief, denial, or rage and leads to interventions that separate the couple oblivious to or perhaps disregarding the need and love they have for each other.

Setting Up a Safety Protocol

Wanting to respect their need for each other, I set up a safety protocol to be supervised by Martha, the home attendant, who lived with them full time and was loved and respected by both. Drawing on Milton's basic ethical and religious values, I was able to get him to promise not to hit Rose and not to threaten to hit her. A devout Jew, he admitted to being deeply ashamed of his violent behavior and offered to talk to his rabbi about it. I agreed that was a good idea, but suggested that he might want to talk to Rose now, in the session, about his feelings of remorse. Tenderly he told her how sorry he was to lose his temper with her to the point where he said and did things that frightened her. He was not proud of that behavior but, he petulantly reminded her, that her nagging triggered memories of his unpleasant childhood in which he had been oversupervised and under constant surveillance by an anxious mother. He needed her to stop being intrusive.

I expressed my concern that if Rose stopped inquiring about his activities, the communication patterns they'd always prized would be broken. Milton exploded, getting out of his chair, threatening to leave. "There is no communication! She does nothing, she sees no one, she has nothing to say. She's like a parasite. She only wants to suck my energy dry and I can't take it anymore."

Rose responded as if she had been hit, as indeed she had been verbally, and began to weep. Citing her crippling arthritis as a major factor in keeping her a recluse, she offered a litany of complaints about the decreasing quality of her life. A subdued Milton sat down and offered his own litany of complaints, citing the emotional, economic, and administrative contributions he had made to the relationship over the many years of their marriage. A tender moment occurred between them as Rose validated his past caring. He both begged and commanded that she promise to stop nagging him or cornering him about his whereabouts. In exchange, he would try to be more attentive.

I asked Martha, the attendant, if the interaction we had just experienced was typical. She said, "No, usually, Rose does not cry. Usually she stands up to him, and the hurt and anger is only resolved by his either threatening her or by his walking out. Sometimes, I have to physically intervene and then he will go to his room. It's very hard."

I wanted to help Rose find a different way, less toxic for Milton, of expressing her anxiety about his health and safety. I suggested that they set aside a time during the day, perhaps before they sat down for dinner, when they could tell each other about their day. However, taking into account that they had few friends left, and Rose's inability to get out, and Milton's impatience, I worried about what she could contribute to the conversation. Remembering that one of Rose's complaints was the vast numbers of cartons and boxes in the apartment in which Milton haphazardly kept his books and photos and memorabilia, I wondered if they might not enjoy setting time aside to sort through them, reminiscing in the process about their lives together. History of all kinds interested Milton, so he agreed to this plan.

Having gotten the couple to calm down with each other, I needed some leverage from caring others to negotiate some permanent

changes in their lives together. A visit to the past uncovered just the resource I was looking for. In exploring Milton's and Rose's genograms,
a story about a nephew came to the surface. This nephew was their only
living relative. Their reluctance to mention him earlier reflected the
pain of the couples' disconnection to their families of origin and revealed their strong desire for independence. This nephew, now a psychiatrist, lived in Arizona with his wife and grown children. He had
been cast out of his family while still a young man in college because he
married out of his religion against his parents' wishes. In spite of their
own strong religious tenets and their awareness that they too would be
ostracized, Milton and Rose welcomed the young couple into their family. Even though this was Rose's nephew, Milton willingly and gener-
ously contributed to his support, enabling him to finish medical school
and establish his career. Their connection continued to be close, with
Rose enjoying his company and Milton delighting in his intellect.

Their nephew had often urged them, in vain, to relocate to Arizona to be near him. As their vulnerability increased with aging, he encouraged them to consider a senior residence with nursing facilities,
which he was affiliated with in Arizona. He had, in fact, set up dates for
admission interviews on three different occasions, which the couple
backed out of at the last minute. I asked them if they would like to reconsider moving to the nursing home in Arizona. Milton felt that the
nephew had given up on them but Rose disagreed. My phone call confirmed Rose's reading. The nephew was eager to cooperate, though
wary that they would once again renege on the arrangements. Indeed,
Milton was still holding out: he had too many books to transport, the
quarters would be cramped, he wouldn't like the food, and he hated
old people—aging was a condition he viewed as contagious. In exploring his ageism, his real concerns came to the surface. Nursing homes
spelled, in his mind, death. He was himself afraid of dying, but he was
even more terrified that Rose would die first. He could not conceive of
living without her, especially in a strange community.

Anticipatory Mourning

Taking time to thoroughly explore the subject of death with aging couples is essential, for it exposes beliefs and rituals, both cultural and spiritual, that will guide the therapist in helping the couple prepare for the
event. Anticipatory mourning can be helpful as a mutual and tender
process of staying connected while letting go. Like many spouses in
long-term relationships, Milton seemed only to be able to let go with

aggression, pushing Rose away, devaluing her as a desirable object in his life in a futile attempt to prepare for a future without her. Rose pathetically responded in the only way she knew: pursuit.

Through the reminiscing process, we were able to evaluate their lifetime successes and regrets, come to terms with dreams never to be realized, and appreciate the rich tapestry they had woven together. Milton became more tender, more connected, and Rose responded by giving him more space. Recognizing their importance to each other but still fearful of surviving the other, they agreed to reopen the dialogue with their nephew about the nursing home. Milton voiced his three remaining fears: being stifled by the regulations of the home, being repelled by the presence of so many old and sick people, and being victimized by anti-Semites. The overriding concern Rose had was one we all shared: without the safety net of Martha, would Milton be able to contain his aggressive behavior toward Rose when alone within the confines of their own small but private suite of rooms? Perhaps he too felt concern. Apprehensive as Rose was about Milton's behavior without Martha's supervision to modify it, living without him was beyond her comprehension.

Using the Resources of Larger Systems

The only way to resolve this dilemma was to consult with every part of the system. I have found that nursing home staff is usually willing to collaborate in the solving of problems; it gives them valuable information from many sources, making their planning and their delivery of service easier and more effective. Milton and Rose agreed to my plan to consult with whatever resources we could find. Working collaboratively with the nephew and the nursing home staff, with me acting as a go-between, checking out possibilities at every turn with Milton and Rose, we were able to arrive at solutions agreeable to all. Rose would have a room by herself in the nursing home where her physical needs could be properly attended. Milton would live separately in one of the cottages set aside for the well elderly. The couple would have their meals and recreational activities together, and they could visit each other as desired, thus ensuring them the opportunity to be together safely and to be apart.

We also networked the Jewish community in Arizona to set up a connection with the rabbi there and with local Jewish organizations so that Milton could anticipate lively conversations, have an audience for his wealth of stories, and participate in cultural activities of meaning for him. Because of their close proximity, this was something Rose might share with him if she chose. Certainly the stimulation by contact with his nephew was a plus, but it was his idea to bequeath his extensive library to his new synagogue in Arizona, certainly a mitzvah that made his commitment to move to Arizona both possible and sweet. This bequest is a sterling example of "letting go and staying connected" in new and fulfilling ways.

COPING WITH ACUTE ILLNESS:
THE DILEMMA OF AUTONOMY VERSUS SAFETY

Normative changes can eventually be integrated into a couple's lifestyle, can sometimes even enhance it. But when acute illness comes into a relationship, the unbalancing of roles and rituals can be so severe as to invite aggressive action by the spouse. Because dependency is anathema for many older people, reflecting as it does the attitudes of our self-oriented culture, autonomy has become a concept of great importance. Older people tend to hang on ferociously to their autonomy because it maintains their sense of identity and allows them to make choices about whom they want to be with and how they want to manage their affairs. This needs to be appreciated when working with older couples because if that autonomy is challenged or threatened, they will often stubbornly hold on to it even at the expense of their own safety. Many older people have retreated into themselves, making themselves unavailable to outside influence or protection just for the sake of maintaining their sense of autonomy.

However, older people become frail and forgetful, and decisions need to be made regarding their safety. These decisions often require input from family and larger systems, such as medical, financial and spiritual helpers. This can be tricky, however, when family members and medical professionals, all trying to protect the ill person, disagree on the means of providing safety and the amount of autonomy to be afforded the patient. Older people's frailty and forgetfulness does not necessarily diminish their desire and need for autonomy. Therefore, ways of balancing safety issues with autonomous decision making often require major but sensitive interventions.

Such a situation came to my attention while consulting on the geriatric psychiatric unit of a major inner-city hospital. Marilyn Frankfurt, a colleague from Ackerman Institute, and I were asked to train the interdisciplinary team of this unit in family systems. We used a combination of training modalities, but the primary clinical training was effected through consultative interviews with the family behind the mirror. Our goal was to glean from the interview the basic dynamics of the system and to interpret for the staff how that dynamic was influencing the interaction not only within the family but also between the family and the larger system, the hospital.

This particular family was special to this team because the husband had been chief of their unit before retirement and was still highly regarded as a mentor. He had also been hospitalized recently on this same unit for evaluation of his confused and disoriented behavior. The current patient, however, is his wife, who is hospitalized for depression. The team's attachment to the couple threatened to interfere with their ability to maintain the neutral distance that would normally allow them to make an accurate assessment and appropriate interventions.

Roger and Grace Carr are a proud, dignified couple in their mid-80s. He is a retired physician, she a retired *schoolteacher*. After 60 years of marriage they still refer to each other in public as "Dr. Carr" and "Mrs. Carr," reflecting the status and the dignity in which they hold their relationship. It also reflected the impermeability of the boundaries they maintained to separate their private and public lives. Their marital contract is traditional and clear, roles being precisely defined on gender lines. The contract had been negotiated many times to accommodate their many life changes, but their dependence on each other never wavered, nor did their devotion.

They had adjusted well to retirement and to the increased frailty that accompanies aging, but when secrecy around illness disrupted their routine, the very foundation of their relationship shook. When Dr. Carr was diagnosed with early Alzheimer disease during a hospitalization, everyone was devastated. So fond and solicitous was the hospital staff of their favorite mentor that they did not inform him directly of his diagnosis, expecting that his wife would. So dignified and honored was this man that even his wife could not see her way clear to telling him either, fearing that he would feel overwhelmed by the very disease he had spent so many years trying to treat.

Complying with medical advice, Mrs. Carr engaged a male home attendant to watch over him but no one told Dr. Carr why this stranger was living in his house, following him everywhere, "spying on him." The elderly, often more protected from reality than younger cohorts, try to make sense out of seemingly illogical events, sometimes constructing explanations based on paranoia and fed by the vibes of secrecy. Dr. Carr resented "being followed." Angered by this intrusion into the family, he could not understand why his wife did not comply with his desire to get rid of the attendant.

This negligence symbolized for Dr. Carr that his wife no longer cared about fulfilling his wishes or that she desired to have the intruder around for her own purposes. Either way, he felt betrayed. Actually, she too resented the aide's presence in her household but was unable to find her voice in the powerful environment of the medical profession.

Their daughter further confused him by attempting to take over some of her mother's responsibilities in the home, and supported the health aide in some domestic conflicts. She thought that she was relieving her parents from some unnecessary stress, but she was in fact increasing their stress since neither parent wanted that kind of help. The power of the secret poisoned the air, and tensions mounted with no outlet for releasing them. Feeling that her role as caregiver and manager of her home was being usurped, thwarted in fulfilling her role as protector, thrown by the unbalancing of their carefully constructed hierarchy, and unable to openly consult with her husband to whom she had traditionally gone to for advice, Mrs. Carr gave into a depression requiring hospitalization. Certainly, this was a plea for help since she not only knew all of the members on the gero-psych team, she knew of their affection for her husband. She felt that since they were the originators of the secret, they were the appropriate dispellers of the secret.

This was an extremely delicate situation for all of us, but it created a particular therapeutic dilemma for me. As the consultant, I obviously was not the person to reveal to Dr. Carr his diagnosis, yet I found myself in the untenable position of knowing it, having been told by the team prior to the interview, but unable to share it, making me a coconspirator. I had not known that it was a secret until Dr. Carr told me during the session that he was distressed because he did not know what his diagnosis was. Reminding myself that the goal of the team, and the reason for the consultation, was to prepare the couple for Mrs. Carr's reentry into the family following her discharge, I decided to expose the secret that there was a secret, and lay the groundwork for an open discussion between the team and the Carrs about Dr. Carr's mental condition. The way that I did this was to weave the information they had given me about their beginnings, their middle years, and later years into the following story that I told to the couple in the presence of their daughter, the home attendant, and the team. This intervention was designed to accomplish two purposes: authenticate the confusion and distress felt by the Carrs, and validate their need and entitlement for autonomy.

"Dr. and Mrs. Carr, you've been married for a very long time. You came together as two young people who understood each other's needs, knew how to make compromises, knew how you could best help each other, how to be there for each other yet keep out of each other's way. You had a couple of children. Then World War II took Dr. Carr away. When he came back, you had to negotiate a new organizational system because you had been a single mother for 4 years. So you had to get tuned in to each other, learning to work once more as a team. Dr. Carr had to begin all over again, starting a new practice, finding an affiliation with this hospital, and you helped him with that. Well, this is another new beginning because Dr. Carr has taken you into a different phase of life and you both are again very vulnerable. You are going into uncharted waters, choppy waters, without a map, without a navigational system."

"Mrs. Carr, you have been confused about the extent of Dr. Carr's condition and distraught about being shackled with the secret of his diagnosis, so much so that you do not know how to help your husband. It has not been your way to withhold information from him and to do so has distressed you mightily. You need time and privacy to work through this phase because the difference now is that you need help from the outside. We will help you both to learn more about Dr. Carr's diagnosis and prognosis, and help you adjust to the changes that you are experiencing."

Turning to the family and the home attendant, and cognizant of the team behind the mirror, I said, "What is most important to Dr. and Mrs. Carr is that they decide how best to utilize outside help so they can continue to be together in a relationship that is still very strong. They know best how to make these changes so that their relationship remains comfortable and familiar. The task you have is to find ways to provide help without intruding into their lives altogether: to listen to and follow their directions, as long as they are able to formulate them; to respect their pace, which may be slower than yours; to honor their dependency on each other for solving in tandem the problems that beset them. There will come a time when more help from you is solicited or required, and certainly I know you will meet that need, but during this transition where Dr. and Mrs. Carr are adjusting to new facts and conditions, it is best to give them the time and space they need to integrate those changes into their lives."

Addressing the couple again, I said, "The team, as you know, is observing this consultation from behind the mirror. I am recommending, now, that they work with you both to open up communication about the diagnosis and why they see the need for a home attendant. Being a physician, you will fill in the gaps and come to your own conclusions, but it is important that you share them with your wife since medicine is not her bailiwick and she depends, as always, on your guidance in such matters. Once the secret is dismantled, you can begin to help each other again."

In a 6-month follow-up, Mrs. Carr reported that the team had been helpful in describing the nature and extent of Dr. Carr's diagnosis and, based on that information, he had accepted the presence of the home attendant, who had in turn become less overbearing. She was aware that the attendant sometimes called their daughter to complain but the daughter did not intervene or even mention it to her parents. Dr. Carr, she said, was holding his own, but she knew that the time was approaching when she would need to lean more heavily on the attendant and her daughter for their help and support. She felt that she could judge when that time would be, and that she could ask and direct them in fulfilling their needs as they arose.

Given the necessary information, time, and appropriate pacing, and the opportunity to work through problems without undue influence by concerned adult children, overzealous professionals, and caregivers, many older couples will find the voice they need to ask for the help they feel is appropriate. It must be remembered that many elders put autonomy before safety and if they are forced to make a choice they will reject any help that threatens their prerogative to make decisions for themselves. This dynamic needs respect and every effort made to preserve it, as it is the juice that nourishes the older cohort, enhancing relationship as well as contributing to healthy longevity.

Options, stressors, and sources of information are more plentiful now for older couples than for any other generation of elders. This abundance in the hands of family members and mental professions may serve to confuse, even paralyze, the decision-making process. In their eagerness to help, they may be unwittingly creating impediments to the couple's successful resolution of their problems by offering solutions rather than useful ideas.

INVOLVING ADULT CHILDREN

The hospital team reported that in the following case they were stymied by two issues: the cyclical reoccurrence of their patient's depression and hospitalization, and the husband's refusal to involve his seven daughters in the matter of discharge planning for their mother. When Pedro faced a forced retirement more than 8 years ago, Helene, his wife became depressed and confused, experiencing delusions and paranoia requiring hospitalization. On her release, Pedro took complete charge of the care of his wife: cooking, cleaning, shopping, bathing, and medicating. His new job as house-husband invited her increased dependency on him, which they all found satisfying, including the daughters.

Each time Helene seemed to retreat from her depression, Pedro would falter in his caretaking, and Helene would lapse into another episode of depression of such proportions as to require another hospitalization. On her release, Pedro would resume his caretaking. Recently, however, Pedro began to show signs of being unable to rise to the occasion. He complained of tiring not only of his caretaking job but also of life itself. Believing that his destiny was such that he would not outlive his father, who died at 74, an age Pedro was fast approaching, he began to talk of taking "one last trip" to Puerto Rico to say goodbye to family and friends. If Helene were stronger he would take her with him, but as long as she was ill he felt that he could not leave her since only he knew how to take proper care of her. Helene misinterpreted this "last trip" as Pedro's intent to go there to die. His daughters, also believing that he was readying himself for death, were not offering to take over the care of their ill mother so that he could return to his native country without her. This kept Pedro stuck in a role guaranteed to keep him alive and functioning here in the States.

We believed it was important at this point to understand the daughters' viewpoint and we asked the couple's permission to involve them. They gave it. Everyone came to the next session. During our discussion, the daughters revealed that even before Pedro had expressed a desire to return to Puerto Rico they did not offer to help him with taking care of their mother because of the family belief that their father benefited emotionally and physically from performing this task. We wondered what they thought would happen if their father could no longer take care of their mother. What options and resources might they draw on? They unanimously agreed: "There's to be no nursing home for our mother; we'd take over the job." We asked what they thought might happen if their mother reached a healthier place in her mental status and no longer required Pedro's care. They speculated that without the job of caretaking, their father would get terribly depressed, his health would deteriorate, and he would die. When we asked where they got that idea, they confided, "That's what happens to our men when they have nothing to do. They get sick or they get into trouble. They need responsibility; they need respect. An idle man gets has no respect for himself." Did they think their mother believed that too? They did.

Many women mindful of a structured hierarchy aimed at preserving the integrity of the family and its members enter into marriage contracts in which showing helplessness secures the honored and powerful position of the patriarch. For women like Helene, schooled in complimentarily, it is a way of respectfully boosting their husband's competency. If they should perceive the impending consequence of their husband's retirement to be anxiety, depression, or even death, they may accelerate their helplessness by exhibiting signs of somatic and emotional deterioration. Pedro's daughters knew well how to honor that legacy.

By identifying this dominant belief underlying the very foundation of the marital contract we were able to understand the daughters' reluctance to override their mother's intent. The logic of this policy, which seemingly flies in the face of culturally approved intergenerational caretaking, lies in the belief that looking after Helene is Pedro's job and his salvation—that without it he would become depressed and die.

In exploring Helene's family background, we discovered that she too came from a small village in Puerto Rico not far from Pedro's. She had many relatives and friends there still, among which she counted Pedro's siblings and cousins. She acknowledged that she missed them, not having seen them since she'd left home. She had not been eager to leave but Pedro thought that life would be better in the United States for a young couple just starting out. She silently complied believing that once they had set aside some money, they would return to Puerto Rico. Years passed and so did her dream. Now that Pedro had expressed his desire to return to his birthplace, presumably to die, she panicked, feeling that her dream of going home had become a nightmare. Desperately she hung on to him by virtue of her ill health and dependency.

Having helped the couple understand the source of their apprehension, we encouraged them to entertain the idea that Helene might be of equal if not more help to Pedro by accompanying him to Puerto Rico, where they would be among relatives and friends. Did she think she was strong enough to do that? She asked Pedro if he wanted her to go with him. He said he did if she was strong enough. She thought maybe she was. The daughters supported this change of plans, seeing it would be beneficial to both their parents. The comfort and security of knowing their daughters approved eased the couple's anxiety.

When we followed up a half-year later, their eldest daughter informed us that Helene's depression had lifted, Pedro had not fallen into one, and that they were together in Puerto Rico visiting their family and friends. Rather than bidding farewell to them, Helene and Pedro were considering making a permanent home there. All of the daughters were involved in providing emotional support to both parents, taking care to maintain a respectful distance from their relationship. The eldest daughter, currently separated from her husband, had moved into their apartment, keeping the home fires burning so that they could return if they so desired. The daughters, who had previously supported their parent's reliance on each other by keeping themselves off stage, revised their stance by actively supporting their parents in ways that the couple found useful, allowing everyone to find innovative ways of letting go while staying connected.

SUMMARY

The later life cycle is a period for review and evaluation, regeneration and experimentation, visualization and empowerment. It is a stage in life when couples must learn to resonate with each other in old and new ways. Older couples also need to resonate with a world they hardly recognize, with values they may not treasure, and with younger generations of loved ones who may themselves be struggling. The cost of failure is isolation, loneliness, and often depression. And there is little time or energy for reparation. Nonetheless, it is an exciting era for those older couples who can open themselves to new perspectives, accept aging as a process, move from known connections to unknown ones, and embrace the opportunity for making changes in a period of abundant resources. Living in this new later life cycle stage is a challenge. Couples who can successfully let go of familiar but empty shells, the baggage that accumulates over time, and still stay connected to life, love, and legacy will lead the way for older couples in the future. What they discover will offer opportunities for enriching the content and texture of late-life coupling, making the transition into this later stage meaningful and rich.

Index